FUNDAMENTALS OF GERIATRIC MEDICINE

Fundamentals of Geriatric Medicine

Editors

Ronald D. T. Cape, M.D.
Professor
Department of Medicine
Section of Geriatric Medicine
University of Western Ontario
London, Ontario, Canada

Rodney M. Coe, Ph.D.
Professor
Department of Community Medicine
St. Louis University School of Medicine
and
Geriatric Research, Education and
Clinical Center
Veterans Administration Medical Center
St. Louis, Missouri

Isadore Rossman, Ph.D., M.D.
Medical Director
Home Care and Extended
Services Department
and Albert Einstein College of Medicine
Bronx, New York

Associate Editors

Richard W. Besdine, M.D.
Alvin J. Levenson, M.D.
Claire W. Maklan, M.P.H.
Jordan D. Tobin, M.D.

Raven Press ■ New York

Raven Press, 1140 Avenue of the Americas, New York, New York 10036

Made in the United States of America

Library of Congress Cataloging in Publication Data
Main entry under title:

Fundamentals of geriatric medicine.

Includes index.
1. Geriatrics. I. Cape, Ronald, 1921–   . II. Coe,
Rodney M. III. Rossman, Isadore J., 1913–   . [DNLM:
1. Geriatrics. WT 100 F981]
RC952.F86   1982   618.97   81-48595
ISBN 0-89004-877-0

Preface

The large and increasing number of Americans over age 65—and especially over 75 and even 85—means that nearly all physicians now have a substantial number of older patients. This assessment is true for almost every specialty and type of practice, and must be faced by both physicians whose education has included adequate attention to geriatrics and by those whose education in geriatrics was minimal or nonexistent. Recent advances in knowledge relevant to geriatric medicine have been extensive. In addition to improved understanding of the underlying biological processes, new tools have become available for diagnosis and management, and major new concepts in care-giving have been developed. There is growing interest and commitment to giving geriatrics appropriate attention in medical education at all levels.

As developed by the Gerontological Society of America, this book is an ideal introduction to geriatric medicine for medical students in their third-year clerkship in internal medicine, in fourth-year subinternships in family medicine and internal medicine, and for residents in these areas, who must treat an ever-increasing number of elderly patients. Every medical student and practitioner in geriatrics and family medicine will find this text to be a valuable contribution to his or her practice.

The text is designed to 1) increase physicians' awareness of the special problems of illness and disease in the elderly; 2) improve understanding of normal anatomical and physiological changes; 3) improve physicians' capacity for effective assessment and treatment of the elderly patient; 4) improve understanding of effective methods for preventing illness and disability in the elderly; and 5) enable the reader to assess his or her comprehension of the multiple factors affecting the health and well-being of the elderly.

As a self-instructional text, this volume presents information in a series of lessons on selected topics. Each concisely written section states educational objectives, includes an introductory overview, and provides multiple-choice examination questions. Also included is a set of six Patient Management Problems (PMPs)—simulated case histories that invite the reader to apply the information reviewed in the text. Each PMP briefly describes a patient's problem, then poses a series of decision-making questions regarding history-taking, physical examination, laboratory tests, and environment. The reader is asked to choose appropriate tests, procedures, or therapies, and then receives a detailed critique of his or her choices.

Fulfilling a previously neglected need in current medical education, *Fundamentals of Geriatric Medicine* offers a practical, effective way for both medical students and practicing physicians to equip themselves with the facts they need to better serve the growing geriatric population.

The Editors

Acknowledgments

This work was produced under a contract between the Health Resources Administration Division of Medicine, U.S. Department of Health and Human Services (HRA 232-79-0089), and The Gerontological Society of America, Washington, D.C.

The work of the steering committee was significantly enhanced by the project director, Claire Maklan, assisted by Anne Middleswarth from the staff of The Gerontological Society of America. Not only did they perform all of the administrative functions for the project, but they also made important substantive editorial contributions.

The cooperation of the authors who prepared the chapters and patient management problems is especially appreciated. They are named in the list of Contributors. I wish also to express our thanks to Victor Vaughan, M.D. and Barbara Muir from the National Board of Medical Examiners who served as consultants to the project.

In the process of evaluating the contributions of the specific authors selected to prepare the lessons and patient management problems, the steering committee was aided by many helpful reviewers. While it is not possible to acknowledge them all individually, I do wish to thank them collectively as representatives of the Clinical Medicine Section of The Gerontological Society of America, eight Veterans Administration Centers, the Ontario Association of Medical Directors of Homes for the Aged, and the medical schools of the University of Western Ontario and George Washington University.

Special thanks are due officers of the Clinical Medicine Section of the GSA, who supported this project from its conceptualization to completion: Drs. Eugene Towbin, Gilbert Rosenberg, Jordan D. Tobin, John A. MacDonell, and Uriel Barzel. Rosemary Yancik, Ph.D., Associate Director for Projects Development for the GSA from 1977–79, developed the idea of producing a self-instructional text for physicians and was responsible for the proposal that eventually made it feasible.

Contents

Management

Controversies in Geriatric Medicine

Falling, not due to accidents, in a 79-year-old woman
Persistent fever in a 72-year-old physician
Complications of hip fracture in a 79-year-old widow
Congestive heart failure in a 74-year-old woman
Forgetfulness and withdrawal in a 75-year-old widower
Agitation in an 82-year-old nursing home patient

Associate Editors

Richard W. Besdine, M.D.
Harvard Medical School
Hebrew Rehabilitation Center for Aged
Boston, Massachusetts

Ronald D. T. Cape, M.D.
Department of Medicine
Section of Geriatric Medicine
University of Western Ontario
London, Ontario, Canada

Rodney M. Coe, Ph.D.
Department of Community Medicine
St. Louis University School of Medicine
St. Louis, Missouri

Alvin J. Levenson, M.D.
Section on Geriatric Psychiatry
University of Texas Medical School at
  Houston

Baylor College of Medicine
Houston, Texas

Claire W. Maklan, M.P.H.
The Gerontological Society of America
Washington, D.C.

Isadore Rossman, Ph.D., M.D.
Home Care and Extended Services
  Department
Montefiore Hospital and Medical Center
Albert Einstein College of Medicine
Bronx, New York

Jordan D. Tobin, M.D.
Metabolism Section and Human
  Performance Section
Gerontology Research Center
National Institute on Aging
Baltimore, Maryland

Contributors

Owen W. Beard, M.D.
Department of Medicine
University of Arkansas School of
Medicine
Division of Geriatrics
Veterans Administration Medical Center
Little Rock, Arkansas

David W. Bentley, M.D.
Department of Medicine
University of Rochester School of
Medicine & Dentistry
Infectious Diseases Unit
Monroe Community Hospital
Rochester, New York

Frederick N. Brand, M.D.,
M.P.H.
Section on Preventive Medicine and
Epidemiology
Boston University School of Medicine
Boston, Massachusetts

Stanley J. Brody, J.D., M.S.W.
Department of Physical Medicine and
Rehabilitation, and the
Rehabilitation Research and Training
Center in Aging
University of Pennsylvania
Philadelphia, Pennsylvania

S. George Carruthers, M.D.
Department of Medicine and
Pharmacology
University of Western Ontario
University Hospital
London, Ontario, Canada

Joan I. Casey, M.D.
Division of Infectious Diseases
Montefiore Hospital and Medical Center
Department of Medicine
Albert Einstein College of Medicine
Bronx, New York

Faith B. Davis, M.D.
Department of Medicine
State University of New York at Buffalo,
School of Medicine
Erie County Medical Center
Buffalo, New York

Paul J. Davis, M.D.
Department of Medicine
Endocrinology Division
State University of New York at Buffalo
School of Medicine; and
Veterans Administration Medical Center
Buffalo, New York

William S. Fields, M.D.
Department of Neurology
University of Texas Medical School
Houston, Texas

Barbara A. Gilchrest, M.D.
Department of Dermatology
Harvard Medical School
Boston, Massachusetts

James C. Grotta, M.D.
Department of Neurology
University of Texas Health Science
Center
Houston, Texas

Leonard Hayflick, Ph.D.
Center for Gerontological Studies
University of Florida
Gainesville, Florida

Philip J. Henschke, M.D.
Department of Geriatric Medicine and
Rehabilitation
Repatriation General Hospital
Daw Park, South Australia
Geriatric Assessment Unit
Flinders Medical Centre
Bedford Park, South Australia

David E. Johnson, M.D.
St. Mary's General Hospital
Lewiston, Maine

William B. Kannel, M.D., M.P.H.
Department of Medicine
Section on Preventive Medicine and
Epidemiology
Boston University School of Medicine
Boston, Massachusetts

Edith R. Kepes, M.D.
Pain Treatment Center
Montefiore Hospital and Medical Center;
and Department of Anesthesiology
Albert Einstein College of Medicine
Bronx, New York

Ian R. Lawson, M.D.
Department of Community Medicine and
Health Care
University of Connecticut Health Center
Farmington, Connecticut

Bernard S. Linn, M.D.
Department of Surgery
University of Miami School of Medicine
Veterans Administration Medical Center
Miami, Florida

Daniel L. McGee, Ph.D.
National Heart, Lung, and Blood
Institute
Bethesda, Maryland
Honolulu Heart Program
Honolulu, Hawaii

James T. Moore, M.D.
Department of Psychiatry and Community
and Family Medicine
Duke University School of Medicine
Duke University Center for the Study of
Aging and Human Development
Durham, North Carolina

Howard L. Moscovitz, M.D.
Department of Cardiology
Mount Sinai Medical Center
New York, New York

W. Bradford Patterson, M.D.
Sidney Farber Cancer Institute
Harvard Medical School
Boston, Massachusetts

Charles W. Pollak, M.D.
Sleep-Wake Disorders Center
Montefiore Hospital and Medical Center
Department of Neurology

Albert Einstein College of Medicine
Bronx, New York

Manuel Rodstein, M.D.
The Jewish Home and Hospital for Aged
Department of Clinical Medicine
Mount Sinai School of Medicine
New York, New York

John W. Rowe, M.D.
Division on Aging
Department of Medicine
Harvard Medical School
Boston, Massachusetts

Kenneth J. Ryan, M.D.
Department of Obstetrics and Gynecology
Harvard Medical School
Brigham and Women's Hospital
Boston, Massachusetts

Leonard P. Seimon, M.D.
Department of Orthopedic Surgery
Albert Einstein College of Medicine
Pediatric and Spinal Orthopedic Services
Montefiore Hospital and Medical Center
Bronx, New York

Nathan W. Shock, Ph.D.
Gerontology Research Center
National Institute on Aging
Baltimore, Maryland

Franz U. Steinberg, M.D.
Department of Rehabilitation Medicine
Jewish Hospital of St. Louis
Department of Clinical Medicine
Washington University School of
Medicine
St. Louis, Missouri

Alan D. Whanger, M.D.
Department of Psychiatry
Duke Geriatric Psychiatry Service
Duke University Medical Center
Durham, North Carolina

Frederick L. Willington, M.D.
Department of Medicine
University of Western Ontario
London, Ontario, Canada
University Hospital of Wales
Cardiff, Wales, United Kingdom

Fundamentals of Clinical Geriatrics

Fundamentals of Geriatric Medicine, edited by
Ronald D. T. Cape, Rodney M. Coe, and Isadore
Rossman, Raven Press, New York © 1983.

1

Comprehensive Care of the Elderly

Rodney M. Coe

There are at least three important reasons why physicians must become informed about gerontology and geriatrics: (a) the population of elderly persons is increasing in absolute numbers and proportionately; (b) there is a strong association between age and morbidity and disability from chronic diseases; and (c) the health care system, as it is presently organized, has not been able to meet all of the needs of the elderly. These conditions suggest (a) a continued increase in demand for health-related services by the elderly who have relatively greater health needs but fewer resources to meet those needs and (b) an expanded role for physicians in providing comprehensive care for older patients.

POPULATION INCREASES

The elderly have increased steadily in number and in proportion to the total population of the United States. In 1900 approximately 4% of the U.S. population of 76 million persons were age 65 and over. By 1950 the proportion had increased to 8% (12.4 million). In 1980 the elderly population is estimated to be 24 million, or about 11% of the total population. By 2020 the proportion is projected to be about 16% of the total population (7).

The rapid increase in the very old (those age 75 and over) is of key importance. Between 1950 and 1975 the percentage growth of persons 75 and over was 119% compared with a 65% increase for those 65 to 74 years of age. The significance of the very old group (which includes many of the "frail elderly") lies in its disproportionately high prevalence of disabilities and requirements for health services.

Other characteristics of the elderly are also important for geriatric practice because they are linked to the disabling aspects of limitations imposed by diseases of senescence and therefore to potentials for treatment effectiveness. Recent population statistics (6) reveal, for example, that

1. The number of elderly women exceeds that of elderly men (life expectancy at birth in 1978 was 7 to 8 years more for females than for males and 4 to 5 years more at age 65).
2. The majority of elderly females who were married are widowed, whereas most elderly men are still married. Men thus may have an advantage over women if therapy at home requires some assistance or supervision.
3. Ninety-five percent of all older persons live in the community. Most of them live independently in their own homes or apartments. About one in six older persons lives in a household with relatives other than their spouse.
4. About one-fourth of all elderly have incomes at or below the designated poverty limit.
5. Many urban elderly live in older parts of cities with restricted access to medical care, stores, churches, clubs, transportation, and other needed facilities.

AGE AND MORBIDITY

The dramatic increase in average length of life because of better sanitation, improved nutrition, and technological advances (e.g., immunization and antibiotics) is associated with an increased prevalence of chronic diseases and disabilities. Prevalence rates for heart disease, cancer, hypertension, diabetes, and arthritis all show marked age-related increases. Disabilities associated with these chronic conditions also are more common among the elderly. For example, the percentages of persons with limitations, by age, are shown in Table 1.

The significance of these data, of course, is that they represent information typically used as a measure of health care need. With the preponderance of chronic conditions among the elderly, the conclusion is that this age group has more health care needs than other age groups. At the same time, the elderly generally have fewer resources—economic, social, and psychological as well as physiological—to meet these needs, many of which are health-related but not strictly defined as medical so as to be provided for under health insurance programs.

TABLE 1. *Persons with activity limitations*

Age	Any limitation (%)	Major limitation (%)
All ages	14.3	10.8
Males, 65 +	48.3	43.7
Females, 65 +	43.4	36.4

From ref. 4.

ORGANIZATION OF HEALTH SERVICES FOR THE ELDERLY

Many observers have noted that the success of public health measures and medical technology in controlling many infectious diseases has not yet been duplicated for chronic diseases (2). By almost any conventional yardstick of health or illness (life expectancy at age 65, bed disability days, morbidity rates), there has been less improvement for the elderly than for other age groups. There are many reasons for this "failure of success" beyond the limitations of medical technology. One is that health services in the United States are organized and financed to deal primarily with acute illness, hence the heavy emphasis on inpatient care, episodic treatment, and specialized facilities. Care of persons with chronic conditions does involve acute care, but mostly it requires services that emphasize out-of-hospital care, continuous monitoring, and coordination of medical with support services. Thus the multifaceted demands of care for the chronically ill require a multidisciplinary approach. This can be achieved by coordination of the specialized skills of many health professionals and services of community agencies, which suggests that the therapeutic role of the physician must be expanded to include coordination of these services.

Another factor is the attitude of health care providers toward aging as a process and toward the care of the elderly. To some extent, providers share prevailing societal values, which may include negative stereotypes of elderly persons. It is important that health professionals be aware of their own attitudes and the influence they may have on providing care for elderly patients.

ROLE OF THE PHYSICIAN IN CARE OF THE ELDERLY

This kind of critique suggests the need for a more coordinated system to provide comprehensive care for the elderly. Indeed, one definition of comprehensive care involves supplementing biomedical knowledge and skills with psychosocial knowledge and skills to provide a more holistic approach to service (1). However, a definition of comprehensive care should extend beyond direct medical services; it should include services in the community and social support systems as well as the means for financing such care.

Such an "ideal type" system, to the extent that it could be developed, still leaves some unanswered questions. In what ways do the needs of the elderly, which differ from those of other age groups, impose special requirements on a comprehensive system? Many of the characteristics often associated with the concept of elderly (e.g., chronicity of illness, frailty, long-stay institutionalization) are not exclusively the province of the elderly, and many if not all conditions of the elderly can be treated. However, diseases in the elderly often do present differently and require special consideration of risks of treatment and substitution of maximizing functional independence for cure as a therapeutic goal.

A second question relates to the role of the physician in a comprehensive care program. The physician interacts not only with the patient but also with the patient's family, medical colleagues, allied health professionals, institutional managers, and many others who could be part of the care program for any given patient. Should only specialists in geriatrics direct the activities of a health care team? Should physicians specialize in geriatrics at all? There is some controversy in the United States about the need for geriatrics as a board-certified specialty. The Institute of Medicine of the National Academy of Sciences (3) recommended against board certification but suggested that the skills and knowledge of all physicians who care for elderly patients should be increased. Others, however, take the view that the specialist model found in some European medical care systems is adaptable and appropriate in the United States (5). Regardless of the degree of specialization, every clinician who provides care for elderly patients encounters some situations in which the age of the patient modifies the "traditional" approach to patient care. For example, a physician may be tempted not to be a therapeutic activist with a patient just because he is very old. Geriatric care certainly requires more collaboration between physician and other members of the health care team than would be necessary for a young patient, and care more often should be given in such settings as the patient's home or a long-term care institution rather than in the acute care hospital.

The community's care system often fails to provide integrated, comprehensive services for the elderly. A community's health care system includes not only health professionals who provide direct care and the settings in which they work (e.g., doctors' offices, clinics, hospitals, nursing homes) but also a host of supporting personnel and agencies that serve administrative, financial, planning, and supply functions. There are many areas of duplication as well as gaps in services at federal, state, and local levels. The lack of coordination of services prevents effective use on behalf of the elderly. The physician has the most important role in the system and is central to making the system work more effectively.

SUMMARY

This overview identifies some trends which indicate the importance of gerontology and geriatrics for physicians and other health personnel. As this and succeeding chapters in this section point out: (a) the number and proportion of elderly are still rising rapidly, increasing the demand for health-related services; (b) there are some specific characteristics of the elderly and their diseases which require special consideration in treatment; (c) physicians must acquire a better understanding of the nature of health problems of the elderly, who often require a different approach; and (d) most communities have a wide range of services available to serve the elderly, but often they are uncoordinated, expensive, and ineffective. There is much that can be done to increase the capacity to deliver comprehensive care to the elderly.

When caring for elderly patients, the physician should:
1. Know the factors which contribute to the increased importance of gerontology and geriatrics to modern medical practitioners.
2. Know the specific characteristics of older persons that can influence decisions about diagnosis and therapy.

3. Understand the significance of personal and societal factors that influence physicians' attitudes toward aging as a process and older people as patients.
4. Be familiar with the purpose, availability, and capability of services in the community to provide comprehensive care to the elderly.

REFERENCES

1. Engel, G. L. The need for a new medical model: A challenge for biomedicine. *Science*, 196:129–136, 1977.
2. Gruenberg, E. W. The failure of success. *Milbank Mem. Fund. Q.*, 55:3–24, 1977.
3. Institute of Medicine. *Aging and Medical Education.* National Academy of Sciences, Washington, DC, 1978.
4. National Center for Health Statistics. *Persons with Activity Limitations.* Series 10, No. 80, 1978.
5. Portnoi, V. A. What is a geriatrician? *JAMA*, 243:123–235, 1980.
6. Sternlieb, G., and Hughes, J. W. *Current Population Trends in the United States.* Transaction Books, 1978.
7. U.S. Bureau of the Census. *Current Population Reports.* Series P-25, 1978.

Fundamentals of Geriatric Medicine, edited by
Ronald D.T. Cape, Rodney M. Coe, and Isadore
Rossman, Raven Press, New York © 1983.

2

The Geriatric Patient

Ronald D. T. Cape

Most physicians have a mental picture of those elderly people whom they describe as "geriatric patients." The picture is of a rather frail, perhaps partially paralyzed, partially immobilized, mildly confused old person who is finding it difficult to remain independent in the community. Often these patients are brought to the physician's notice by relatives or neighbors; a few are brought by public health nurses or even, on occasion, by the police. There is a general air of hopelessness about these individuals, and until recent years the physician's first reaction was to look for a nursing home or other institution in which they may comfortably end their days. Such situations do arise, but in truth these persons constitute a very small minority of elderly patients.

DEFINITION

"Geriatric" means the medical care of elderly people, being derived from the Greek words *geron* (old man) and *iatros* (medical care). Geriatric medicine is the medical care of all old people and is practiced by a wide range of physicians involved in primary care and many of the subspecialties. There has, however, been an unwillingness to accept geriatrics as a specialty oriented to a specific age group. The reason for this is not difficult to find. Because geriatrics is concerned with people who are aged or aging, its relevance is to the stage of life when aging changes become obvious and begin to influence health. It is well known that aging occurs at rates which vary from person to person. The pace of aging is dictated by genetic makeup and, to a lesser degree, environmental factors. For these reasons, there are people who are already aged and failing in their sixties and others who show little evidence of the decremental processes of biosenescence even in their eighties. Hence it is difficult to identify a specific age at which people become "geriatric patients." Age 65, for years the age of retirement, has come to be accepted and regarded as the entry point to the latter part of life. From the clinical standpoint, however, this is almost certainly too soon. The majority of individuals who come under the care of physicians in geriatric medicine are over the age of 75.

This is confirmed by a number of studies, most of which have been carried out in Great Britain where geriatric medicine developed to a much greater extent than elsewhere during the two decades following the Second World War. The results of a study comparing the clinical situations in two groups of patients aged 65 and over who were admitted to a Glasgow hospital are shown in Table 1 (2). Approximately half of these patients were admitted directly to a geriatric unit, and half came in through the emergency department to be admitted to general medical wards. Although all patients were technically old (i.e., over 65), it is obvious from the figures that those admitted to the geriatric unit were significantly older—the majority having reached the age of 75— than those admitted to the general medical wards. In North America the same age pattern is seen, with more than 70% of old people in institutions being 75 or over. Table 1 also illustrates another feature of geriatric medicine: the recurring frequency of certain major clinical problems.

CHRONIC ILLNESS

The geriatric patient conjures up a picture of chronic and continuing disease and disabilities. It should be emphasized, however, that chronic disease and age do not always go hand in hand. Recent work demonstrates the fallaciousness of the idea that geriatric cases are invariably "bed-blockers." A study from Winnipeg has shown that patients who occupy beds in acute hospitals for more than 1 month—the "long-stay" cases—are by no means exclusively elderly people. Shapiro (3) found that more than half of the patients remaining for more than a month in hospital were people under the age of 65, and this has been confirmed by experience at a large teaching hospital in London, Ontario. It is important, therefore, to distinguish between those unfortunate sufferers from chronic disabilities and the elderly. The latter have multiple disease problems which may, in some cases only, lead to continuing complex disabilities that result in loss of independence; in others, the prospect of achieving a satisfactory return to independence is good. It must be stressed, therefore, that chronicity and geriatric medicine are in no sense synonymous.

TABLE 1. *Presenting symptoms and age of geriatric and medical patients*

Age/symptom	Geriatric patients		Medical patients	
	No.	%	No.	%
Age 65–74	67	26	166	66
Age 75 and over	188	74	84	34
Stroke	38	15	36	14
Immobility	176	69	33	13
Falls	120	47	39	16
Incontinence	129	51	19	8
Mental abnormality	125	49	13	5

Adapted from ref. 2.

Elderly patients suffer from a number of chronic disease states, notably atherosclerotic vascular disease, chronic obstructive pulmonary disease, maturity-onset diabetes, and chronic arthritis. The first and most common of these, atherosclerosis, usually presents as a series of acute episodes of myocardial infarction, gangrene from peripheral vascular disease, or a stroke. Although some less fortunate individuals do become chronically disabled from these conditions, the majority continue to maintain independent living apart from occasional acute episodes. It should be stressed that even the group with continuing disability can be greatly assisted by thoughtful management. Chronicity does not mean that treatment cannot be offered to reduce the problem and help maintain independence.

GOALS OF MANAGEMENT

The importance of goals cannot be overemphasized. For patients in their forties, it is paramount to achieve a quick cure and a return to work and family roles. For patients in their late seventies, the most important aspect of any illness may be whether it is going to cost them their independence. This is the key issue and is often of even greater importance than the question of whether the illness is life-threatening. To make this point clear, one can envisage an illness in an elderly person for whom the outcome is, broadly speaking, likely to be one of three events. The first is that the illness proves terminal, and the individual dies within 2 to 3 weeks; the second is that the illness responds to treatment and appropriate rehabilitation, and the patient regains full independence; the third is that as a result of the illness there is a significant loss of functional ability, so the individual becomes dependent on the support of others. More than 20 years devoted almost exclusively to the medical care of the very old lead me to believe that such patients fear the third possibility most. The philosophy of managing disease in the elderly should be to avoid the third situation as much as possible. This can be done by having the patient continue rehabilitation programs—at home if necessary with Day Hospital and Home Care support—in order to encourage and maintain independence, whether complete or partial. This philosophy is a commonsense approach which the great majority of people will understand, particularly those in their latter years.

THE ELEMENT OF RISK

Another aspect of care of the elderly is concerned with the inevitable risks everyone faces in life. Not unnaturally, most families of very old people are concerned for their safety and take precautions to make the environment in which they live as safe as possible. In spite of these efforts, however, there are a significant number of subjects who sustain falls from time to time who are thus exposed to the danger of having to lie on the floor for some hours before they are found. Steps can be taken to organize call systems, but even with these the risk remains. The question frequently arises about an old person's ability to live alone in an apartment (e.g., if he or she has sustained one or two falling episodes). In some cases the appropriate decision is to have the individual in question admitted to a nursing home or similar institution. On the other hand, if when evaluating the cause of the falls a reasonable way to prevent them is available, there is no reason why old people should not continue to live in their own homes, accepting the danger of a further fall. Such risks are part of living. To try to avoid them altogether and to attempt to "wrap old people in cotton" is quite wrong. The effect of such an approach is often to reduce the individual's desire for living.

INDEPENDENCE, NOT CURE?

One example of a situation which may arise in an octogenarian is the discovery of an asymptomatic abdominal aortic aneurysm, a condition not uncommon at this age. Comparing the risk of surgical mortality with that of rupture while continuing to lead an active life is difficult. There may be compelling reasons to arrange for the removal of the aneurysm; however, faced with an active, independent person who reports for a checkup at the age of 82 and is found to have an aneurysm, what is one to do? Should one suggest removal of the aneurysm? The facts are: (a) The individual has a potentially lethal condition because rupture of the aneurysm will almost certainly cause sudden death. (b) The mortality from this type of surgery in a healthy octogenarian is significant, perhaps as high as 10%. (c) The surgery may be associated with a period of catabolic negative nitrogen balance and loss of tissue, with resultant deterioration in the physical capacity of the individual.

The questions that have to be asked are: Will this 82-year-old enjoy the last months or years of a long life more effectively with no operation or will surgery enable the individual to live longer and remain vigorous without any significant adverse effects? There is no universally correct answer to these questions, but, on the whole, discretion is probably the better part of valor. Certainly the issues should be explained to the patient in these terms and in a way which can be understood. The patient can then have some relevant input into the final decision that is reached.

A second example relates to the management of hypertension. Evidence is steadily accumulating that adequate control of high blood pressure reduces the incidence of stroke, and, on the average, increases the life expectancy of the individual. This is well documented for patients under the age of 75. Two facts should be carefully considered in this situation. The first is the increasing amount of carotid artery disease, and the second is the increased danger of postural hypotension in elderly people. The former situation means that by lowering systolic blood pressure in some predisposed individuals it is possible to slow blood flow through the narrowed internal carotid artery to a point which results in cerebral infarction. The second danger lies in life becoming a series of episodes of dizziness whenever the individual stands up, possibly associated with occasional falls, as a result of severe postural hypotension. This occurs in 10 to 20% of elderly people who are having *no* anti-hypertensive treatment and almost certainly to a greater extent in persons being treated with such medications. The dilemma is whether one should aim for increasing longevity at the possible risk of causing a stroke on the one hand or making life so uncomfortable that it is scarcely worth living on the other, or whether one should accept the risk of offering no therapy at all. Again the decision of the physician should be made in consultation with the patient and the patient's relatives. (The controversy regarding treatment of hypertension is further discussed in Chapter 23.)

These two examples underline the fact that the physician should always treat the patient, not the disease. This is a principle which applies at all ages. Nonetheless, it is probably of paramount importance when managing the geriatric patient. This individual may have multiple problems, many of which have appropriate remedies or medications that might modify or improve them. The therapeutic enthusiasm of the physician, however, should be tempered by a realization of the possible adverse effects of the drugs on the one hand and the need to maintain the independence and clarity of mind of the patient on the other. The goal is to aim for independence and health rather than to expend efforts on maximizing the chance of longevity. Experience suggests that the majority of elderly people, if offered the choice, would prefer a shorter period of independent life to a longer period of invalid existence when they are dependent on others for their care.

EXPECTATIONS OF OLD AGE

Often elderly patients explain to their doctors in almost apologetic terms that their symptoms are probably due simply to their age. What can one expect at age 75 or 80? Such ideas are encouraged by many well-meaning relatives and friends, who tell old persons that they should not do this or that; it is too much for them! Often these members of the old person's immediate circle offer assistance when it is unneeded. Therefore in many ways, some of which are subtle and some obvious, it is conveyed to the very elderly that good health is a thing of the past: They are bound to be weak and feeble and can expect only to become worse before ultimately dying.

Current demographic projections dramatize how important it is that we dispel the myth of helplessness in old age. During the last quarter of this century in the developed nations, the percentage of octogenarians in the total population will be as high as 10 to 12%. Longevity will have a direct bearing on the health and clinical care of the elderly. So long as individuals—both patients and physicians—accept aches and pains, dizziness, weakness, shortness of breath, tiredness, and other symptoms as part and parcel of advanced age, much disease will go undetected and untreated.

Elderly patients require a physician who is truly interested in them as people and who encourages them to report new and disturbing symptoms as soon as they appear. Such well educated physicians know from experience the situations that repay careful study, and they can offer sensible reassurance and advice about those conditions which are better left alone.

REHABILITATION

The geriatric patient, like modern patients of any age, expects an almost magic potion or pill to relieve symptoms and restore strength. One of the most basic facts about weakness and strength of muscle is that the only way in which strength can be increased is by using the muscle. The athlete accustomed to training to build up muscle strength as well as cardiac and respiratory reserve is well aware of this fact. It is not easy, however, to convince some old people that the only way to retrieve some physical strength and ability is by getting out of bed and using muscles for short, acceptable periods, gradually building them up over a period of time. The efficacy of rehabilitation programs for elderly people has been proved time and time again in both Britain and North America. This aspect of care is one which the physician should bring into play no matter how trivial or short-lived an illness may be.

The critical part of an illness for geriatric patients is the final stage, i.e., the restoration of mind and body to their pre-illness state. There is an interesting contrast in the way in which human beings react to illness and recover from it at different ages in their life cycle. Children who appear at death's door one minute, may, in a remarkably short space of time, throw off the effects of a severe infection and recover all their normal boisterous muscular activity and good health. The mature individual struck down by a myocardial infarction or pneumonia often recovers remarkably fast when rehabilitation is stimulated by the need to return to work and family responsibilities. For the elderly geriatric patient, however, the future may hold little that seems exciting or important. The effort of the rehabilitation process, which inevitably demands considerable persistence by the patient, holds little appeal. Careful thought and persuasion must go into achieving the objective.

PERSPECTIVE ON HEALTH FOR THE GERIATRIC PATIENT

Few studies have examined the health of random samples of old people living in their own homes. There is one study, however, conducted in three counties of southwest Ontario (1), that provides estimates of the proportion of people at different ages who have lost some or all of their independence (Fig. 1). Based on an analysis of simple activities (e.g., walking, showering, going up or down stairs, and dressing), this study found that the great majority of elderly people do retain completely independent life styles to the end. Between the ages of 65 and 75, the incidence of significant disability rose slowly from 5 to 10%. Only beyond the age of 80 did this increasing loss of independence reach 20 to 30% of the population at risk.

The significance of this simple study is to draw attention to the false nature of the idea that old age must be a time of debility and lost health. Most old people lay greater store on health than on any other one aspect of life, and it is therefore important that this message is broadcast far and wide and is well understood and recognized. It will encourage the elderly to have higher expectations for their own health than they otherwise might. If physicians recognize this, they can help many elderly people understand that disabilities they expect need never occur.

LOSS OF RESERVES

To sum up the clinical nature of the geriatric patient in a few words, one can say that he or she is an individual whose relatively enormous reserves of function

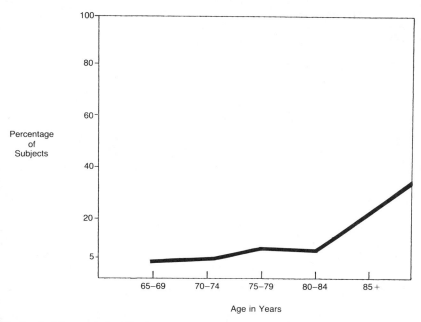

FIG. 1. Incidence of disability in 385 subjects living in their own homes. (Adapted from ref. 1.)

which everyone has during development and early maturity have largely been lost. For this reason, any illness or injury that befalls the geriatric patient has much more profound effects and consumes much more time in the recovery process. In spite of the reduced reserve, most systems continue to function quite adequately, if at an appreciably slower pace. There is very seldom any need to forbid old people to undertake specific activities, provided these do not demand unusual strength or agility. The only required qualification to that statement is that older people should be warned that many activities require much more time to accomplish; they should be encouraged to accept this and not attempt to hurry.

Although morbidity and mortality steadily increase with age, many old people can enjoy a full and active life. The proportion that do so falls slowly from about 95% at age 65 to perhaps 85% at age 80 and to 70% or less at age 90. This means that, for the majority, old age can be a time to look forward to, a time when unfulfilled ambitions may be achieved, and a time when a slower pace of life may allow the individual to enjoy and cherish each moment to the fullest extent.

REFERENCES

1. Cape, R. D. T., and Henschke, P. Perspective on health in old age. *J. Am. Geriatr. Soc.*, 28:295–299, 1980.
2. Isaacs, B. *Studies of Illness and Death in the Elderly in Glasgow*, Vol. 17, p. 13. Scottish Health Services Studies, Edinburgh, 1971.
3. Shapiro, E. The reality and the myth of "geriatric bed-blocking." *Essence*, 3:179–184, 1980.

Fundamentals of Geriatric Medicine, edited by
Ronald D.T. Cape, Rodney M. Coe, and Isadore
Rossman, Raven Press, New York © 1983.

3

Physician as Geriatrician

Isadore Rossman

The very nature of disease processes in aging organisms makes a geriatric practice more difficult, slower-paced, and more subject to disappointment than any other. The physician who requires frequent or dazzling therapeutic triumphs to maintain his self-esteem and mood had best avoid geriatrics. It is especially important also to recognize that the interaction between physician and patient is subject to more complexity in geriatrics than elsewhere in medicine. Troublesome value judgments arise more frequently. Conscious and unconscious personal and societal orientations interpose themselves more often into daily practice. Unless these are examined down to their roots and mastered, the geriatrician may flounder in the same ambivalence exhibited by many others in the medical care system. Some of these difficulties are bound to continue in an era of unprecedented basic questioning of almost all role relationships. One has only to contrast the simple ethical behavior decreed by the categorical imperatives of the eighteenth century, such as its well-defined intrafamilial roles, with the complex oedipally tainted ambivalence of the twentieth century family to see one measure of the change. It seems to be true *a priori* that when once formalized or rigid family relationships become tenuous so too will many institutionalized relationships, including the doctor-patient one.

A substantial modification has occurred since the original administration of the Hippocratic Oath which adjured the physician "into whatsoever house you shall enter it shall be for the good of the sick to the utmost of your power...." The Oath was meant to lay definitive guidelines for medical graduates embarking on the new career. Now the utmost of the doctor's powers extends to keeping the excessively old, and even the brain-dead alive, and it is clear that there is no longer an unswerving path to follow. Once the cultural anthropologists revealed how attitudes were shaped by society, the categorical imperatives disappeared. This left a void which has not been filled.

Changes in the culturally defined age for application of our high technology point up some of the difficulties in this area. The highly arbitrary age of 65 was initially a time for entry into a governmentally sponsored pension system, then into its health insurance system. Concurrently, there were many in the health care system who proposed age 65 as a cutoff for such new expensive technology as renal dialysis and coronary bypass surgery. In at least one example of considerable notoriety, a British hospital considered 65 as a cutoff age for cardiopulmonary resuscitation. Although these delimitations have collapsed under the weight of their own illogicality and arbitrariness, a prejudicial age factor, "ageism," the more dangerous when it is unconscious, persists.

A basic question is whether there is an age past which the geriatrician can become less of an activist when treating his patient and, if so, what that age should be. Has the average 80-year-old or 90-year-old "lived long enough" so as to dilute the physician's energy for one or another diagnostic work-up? If chronological criteria are tossed out, what others are reasonable and worthy of consideration? It must be conceded that a major degree of frailty can make it difficult if not impossible for the patient to cooperate in diagnostic procedures, and this often vitiates attempted even-handedness in the treatment approach. Perhaps of greater consequence is impairment of cognitive functioning. In the presence of a severe organic brain syndrome, cataract surgery will improve only the quality of the stimulus falling on the retina, not a vacuous cortical response. There doubtless would be general agreement that to use renal dialysis for someone with dementia would be a *reductio ad absurdum*. However, organic brain syndrome is a spectrum which emerges without sharp distinction from the common mental impairments of the aging process. Thus those who furtively tell their colleagues they would not give antibiotics to a demented patient for pneumonia are faced with defining where on the continuous spectrum the departure from antibiotic therapy is applicable. Even then the withholders may be confronted by families demanding that all measures be utilized.

It is perhaps evident from the above that there are no clear-cut boundaries that separate an elderly group that should be treated with benign neglect. Rigid criteria for withholding care may muddle a clinical situation as often as resolve it. It seems equally true that application to any group of patients of a double standard in which full measures and half measures can hopefully coexist is extraordinarily difficult. Over a very wide range, a simple solution to the dilemma is to hold that the middle-aged, the old, and the very old should, within reason, be treated equally. Only under such a banner of equality can both geriatrician and patient be liberated. Further, strict adherence to this principle will prevent the return of the always old/always new geriatric chamber of horrors that in one century is the alms house and in the next can be the nursing home and the state mental hospital.

Although doctrinal equality may resolve troubling aspects of the diagnostic role, it may not suffice for the geriatrician's therapeutic role. This patient population is, in fact, characterized by greater frailty and lessened adaptability, which at once creates difficulties. These characteristics affect all aspects of practice whether it is drug administration or the question of hospitalization. Whereas middle-aged patients brought into hospitals may react with depression, some older patients react with confusion, which is much more difficult to handle. This potential for confusion is omnipresent in geriatric practice.

An everyday example may suffice: It is a common disservice—rather than good service—to a homebound, febrile, slightly confused, older patient to order him to the hospital. In contrast, on a routine house call one can (a) determine that the patient does not have pneumonia; (b) collect a urine sample, which when centrifuged in the office can validate or exclude urinary tract infection; and (c) draw blood for culture and counts which may indeed support the diagnosis of a viral infection. Carrying a patient through such an illness at home is an important contribution to both the patient and his Medicare society, and here the geriatrician's role has an expanded dimensionality not always appreciated in hospital confines. Frailty and homebound status mandate a continued role for the house call in geriatric practice despite its virtual banishment from the other specialty areas. The geriatric house call is not simple; there are always questions of housing and its safety, the quotidian question of the distance from bathroom to bed, issues of availability of supportive services, and identification of the capacity of the spouse or other caring persons.

A sophisticated level of care in the home can be delivered to the elderly in organized home care programs. Using the team approach, comprehensive and co-ordinated services at a high level can be delivered to the elderly. The basic team consists of doctor, nurse, and social worker, and many programs also utilize physical therapists, occupational therapists, meals-on-wheels services, and visits from volunteers. However variable in development and distribution, home care programs have a demonstrable application to the elderly and are widely believed to be the major alternative to the soaring institutionalization rate of the geriatric population. The key person in such a program is the geriatrician, who makes the major decisions regarding the feasibility of home care and its continuation in changing circumstances, and who writes the basic therapeutic orders. Home care often conforms to the patient's or family's wishes; for geriatricians familiar with the home care potential, it is often tragic to witness a forced institutionalization. The house call and home care add an important dimension to the patient–practitioner relationship and give first-hand insight into the home as an environment for geriatric care. The physician who does not make house calls deprives patients of a valuable service and may deprive himself of a valuable data base.

Even with a major thrust into the area of home care, the realities of geriatric practice mandate the utilization of institutions, e.g., the nursing home. Roughly 5% of the population over 65 are in such institutions, perhaps half with significant organic brain syndromes. Major diagnostic categories also include cerebrovascular disease, cardiac and pulmonary disease, and peripheral vascular disease including amputation. Often the major impairments are frailty and dependence. Not only is the total number of beds devoted to such geriatric patients formidable (it greatly exceeds the number of acute hospital beds), but perhaps one in five of the patients the geriatrician serves will, at one time or another, spend time in such an institution. The levels of nursing and medical care afforded the nursing home population vary from good to bad. Unfortunately, as with the home, this environment is often not sufficiently familiar to the geriatrician. Diagnostic facilities are seldom good, and the level of surveillance is often inadequate, so that the nursing home population is a constant source of surprise to the unwary: Missed carcinomas keep surfacing, congestive heart failure results from missed myocardial infarcts, and pneumonia turns out to be pulmonary embolus. The care of nursing home residents demands patience, good diagnostic skills, and expertise in geriatrics. Thus the geriatrician has a vital role not only in the office and hospital but also in the home and institution.

MEDICAL CARE

The intelligent clinician quickly learns the necessary adaptations for working with older patients. It may be an elementary courtesy to speak in a loud voice. It may be the better part of discretion when prescribing several medications to write out their names and identify their purposes, e.g., "heart pill," "sleeping pill," "water pill." Compliance problems may be no worse in the elderly than with other age groups, but they may have different origins. Thus forgetting to take a medication may not be due to denial of illness or rejection of treatment but more often to a basic memory impairment. Many an elderly patient coming across his diuretic pills after breakfast, for example, is unsure whether it is time to take one or he has already done so. "Should I or did I? That is the question," remarked one of my older patients. Relating the taking of pills to meals, brushing of teeth, or other daily routines may reduce noncompliance. The problem is sufficiently weighty that the experienced geriatrician from time to time insists that patients come in with all their medicines to check on possibilities of confusion, omission, and double-dipping. Advance loading of memory-aid devices (e.g., boxes with compartments labeled for day and time) may prove useful to both patient and geriatrician. In older persons, sensitivity to medications and adverse effects of drugs are part of the expected rather than the unexpected, and these enter into differential diagnoses in many interesting ways. As nowhere else in medicine, in geriatrics it is clear that our drugs are not specifically targeted.

Of the diseases that are highly age-related and which cause considerable disability during old age, those in Table 1 are perhaps the most prominent. Causes of morbidity and mortality have a good deal of confluence, although there are important exceptions. Symptomatic osteoarthritis is virtually universal in a geriatric population, but rarely is it a mortal illness. Major causes of death overwhelmingly fall into the two large categories of cardiovascular and neoplastic diseases, with infections often playing the terminal role. Thus the battlelines are more clearly drawn in geriatric medicine than elsewhere. Although life-threatening illnesses seem remarkably small in number, their differential diagnoses remains complicated and often presents the clinician with a difficult task. For example, a small drop in the hematocrit from one annual examination to another may be the only signal to the existence of cancer. Intermittent mild episodes of nocturnal angina may be the first warnings of atherosclerotic heart disease and congestive heart failure. Osteoporosis progresses silently until revealed by the first major fracture. Diabetes can be hard on the organism and difficult to diagnose. A wide variety of useful drugs may mimic or worsen an organic brain syndrome.

TABLE 1. *Leading causes of death in the elderly, U.S., 1977*

Cause of death	No. of deaths	Rate per 100,000
Age: 65–74 years		
Heart disease	182,354	1,250
Cancer	115,587	792
Stroke	37,896	260
Diabetes mellitus	9,611	66
Accidents	9,006	62
Pneumonia	8,335	57
Cirrhosis of liver	6,208	43
TOTAL OF ALL CAUSES	445,595	3,054
Age: 75 years and over		
Heart disease	366,141	4,106
Stroke	116,753	1,309
Cancer	116,675	1,308
Pneumonia	30,487	342
Arteriosclerosis	23,683	266
Accidents	15,175	170
Diabetes mellitus	13,993	157
Emphysema	6,190	69
TOTAL OF ALL CAUSES	797,318	8,941

From ref. 2.

It soon becomes clear to the geriatrician that his role is not only to treat illness but, importantly, to preserve structure and function as long as possible and to anticipate omnipresent threats. The problem and difficulties in preventive geriatric medicine are well illustrated by the patient with osteoporosis. Some degree of osteopenia is universal during old age and is likely to be clinically most marked in light-boned Caucasian females of Northern European extraction. There are hundreds of thousands of serious bone fractures each year ascribable to osteoporosis. Although a negative calcium balance may be only a secondary contributor to this multifactorial disease, there is evidence that it plays an important role. Dietary analysis reveals that many middle-aged women have insufficient calcium intakes, certainly one remediable factor. In osteoporosis, as in many areas of geriatrics, an iatrogenic contribution is also to be reckoned with: For example, furosemide is often prescribed for chronic administration in older women, even though it is a potent calcium excretor. Hydrochlorthiazide, on the other hand, does not affect calcium stores and, everything else being equal, is the preferred diuretic. One cannot always comfortably assume that vitamin D intake is adequate in a geriatric population. Further, the evidence of declining renal conversion of vitamin D to its active form with aging may be an important therapeutic lead to the osteoporosis problem. The use of fluorides, estrogens, and other steroids is still under active investigation and is discussed in the standard textbooks on geriatric medicine. It is clear that the geriatrician has an important role to play, if not in prevention at least in slowing down the rate at which osteoporosis progresses.

Results of epidemiological studies strengthen the geriatrician's role in the primary prevention of cardiovascular disease. Risk factors identified in the Framingham study which are modifiable or preventable include hypertension, elevated serum cholesterol, cigarette smoking, glucose intolerance, and left ventricular hypertrophy (1).

The impact of systolic hypertension alone is currently under study, but the results will not be known for some 5 to 6 years. However, informed opinion is increasingly swinging toward treatment of elevated systolic pressures alone, and it currently seems as reasonable to treat this as to treat significant diastolic hypertension in the geriatric age group. As the link between hypertension and stroke is unequivocal, the geriatrician must recognize how rewarding the somewhat tedious routine of treating hypertension is.

In geriatrics an ounce of prevention is worth more than a pound of cure, for it may lead to a significant prolongation of the life span. Pediatricians who have never seen diphtheria, pertussis, or tetanus unhesitatingly give DPT immunizations. This should be an example to geriatricians who have seen much mortality from influenza and pneumonia but have not been as compulsive about immunizing against these two important diseases. There is evidence that such immunization is rewarding and should be embraced as a routine measure. The frailty and diminished capacity of patients to cope are an unending source of worry to the geriatrician. A few unexpected deaths from pneumonia or influenza may emphasize the applicability of preventive medicine.

There are many other everyday opportunities to practice prudent medicine. Antithrombotic measures should be employed in some postoperative situations, especially after hip surgery, and in all other instances where immobilization makes pulmonary embolus an imminent threat. Even in the absence of a statistical demonstration, I routinely prescribe aspirin for elderly patients prior to their going on long airplane trips. The recent return to the use of antibiotics preoperatively and prophylactically surely is most applicable to the geriatric population. Even though the incidence of cancer of the lung declines in smokers past 75, it seems unlikely that geriatric smokers will escape the life-shortening impact of cigarette smoke. They can be harangued as successfully as much younger patients. Granted that in geriatric medicine there are vast areas of ignorance, it seems likely *a priori* that some of the facts established for younger organisms should hold for elderly ones. Thus excessive obesity, hypercholesterolemia, hyperglycemia, high saturated fat diets, patterns of immobility, and excessive alcohol intake (in contrast to one cocktail per day) are illustrations of conditions or habits on which the geriatrician may have to take a stand. As geriatric medicine becomes stronger, guidelines will become sharper; until then rational opinions and prudent judgments continue to be applicable in many everyday clinical situations.

REFERENCES

1. Kannel, W. B. Some lessons in cardiovascular epidemiology from Framingham. *Am. J. Cardiol.*, 37:269, 1976.

2. *Vital Statistics of the United States, Vol. 2: Mortality, 1977.* Mortality Statistics Branch, Division of Vital Statistics *(to be published).*

SUGGESTED READING

Austrian, R. Prevention of pneumococcal infection by immunization with capsular polysaccharides of streptococcus pneumoniae: polyvalent vaccines. *J. Infect. Dis.*, 136:538–542, 1977.

Kannel, W. B. Some lessons in cardiovascular epidemiology from Framingham. *Am. J. Cardiol.*, 37:269, 1976.

Moser, K. M. Pulmonary embolism. *Am. Rev. Resp. Dis.*, 115:829, 1977.

Rossman, I. Environments of geriatric care. In: *Clinical Geriatrics*, 2nd ed., edited by I. Rossman. Lippincott, Philadelphia, 1979.

Rossman, I. Mortality and morbidity overview. In: *Clinical Geriatrics*, 2nd ed., edited by I. Rossman. Lippincott, Philadelphia, 1979.

Rossman, I., Rodstein, M., and Bornstein, A. Undiagnosed diseases in an aging population. *Arch. Intern. Med.*, 33:366, 1974.

Fundamentals of Geriatric Medicine, edited by
Ronald D. T. Cape, Rodney M. Coe, and Isadore
Rossman, Raven Press, New York © 1983.

4

Formal Long-Term Support System for the Elderly

Stanley J. Brody

Evaluation of any system is keyed to identifying the goals of that system and measuring the relevance of its service components and their organizational relationships to those goals. An assessment of the formal health support system for the elderly must determine if the services, whether in the home, community, or institutions, are responsive to the needs of the target population.

Chronic care is the major health need of today's elderly. Chronic diseases are now the leading cause of death, and chronic disabilities are the principal modifiers of well-being. Acute diseases have long been superceded as the major cause of death in the United States, and researchers have recognized this change. During the last 20 years their efforts to assess the health status of the American population have made a corresponding shift. Instead of mortality measurements, which are more applicable to a very young population characterized by acute infectious disease, attention has focused on the measurement of functional disability in a population typified by chronic illness and aging.

The health care system, however, has lagged in responding to the new disease pattern. Medicare was designed as an acute care medical program. During the 15 years since its enactment, it has become even more so. As a result, much of the acute care delivered in short-term general hospitals and in private offices is in response to chronic illness.

The net result of the reduced importance of infectious disease as a cause of death has been a population shift. Although life span has not been much altered, life expectancy has. Life expectancy at birth in 1900 was 49.2 years; in 1976 it had increased to 72.8 years. For those reaching 75 years of age, life expectancy is now 10.1 years, 3 years more than it was for this age group at the turn of the century. Consequently both the number and proportion of the elderly in our population have increased dramatically.

The new phenomenon we will experience during the next two decades is the "graying" of the gray. During the first seven years of the 1970s, whereas the total population 65 and over rose by 18%, the number over 85 grew by a full 50%. This aging of the aged will continue and will produce a population shift having substantial implications for the health care system.

Health, as commonly understood, represents the ability to adapt. Medical care makes a major contribution to that capacity, but with the limitations of current knowledge and skill it cannot cure those diseases which are termed "chronic." Chronic illnesses lead to long-term physical and mental disabilities and further limit the individual's adaptability, thus increasing vulnerability to disability. The effects of chronic disease are exacerbated by adverse psychological, socioeconomic, and environmental factors. Limitation of activities and loss of functional effectiveness take both physical and mental tolls.

Once a chronic disease has been medically stabilized, the main role of the health system is to help those with residual disability to function at their highest possible capacity. Mobility and activity levels are the best available indicators of their need for assistance. About 80% of older people are mobile; of the 20% who suffer significant limitation in mobility, 1 in 10 is bedfast, another 1 in 4 housebound (9). More than half (57%) of all elderly persons are free of functional limitations. Of those who are limited, about 39% are unable to carry out their major activity, 49% are limited in the amount or kind of major activity, and 12% are limited but not in their major activity (15). Estimates vary, but approximately 30% of all elderly require some form of assistance.

In response to these varied health needs, public policy has been largely irrelevant. The major public resources, Medicare and Medicaid, have focused an acute care medical response. In 1977 about $20 billion was spent through Medicare on acute hospital ($15 billion) and physician ($4.2 billion) care for the elderly. Expenditures under this program for other than acute care were less than $1 billion. For those elderly who are medically indigent, Medicaid provides the capacity to buy coverage for physician services and skilled nursing home care under Part A of Medicare. A federal-state matching program administered at the state level, Medicaid provides benefits that vary widely from state to state. Nationally, skilled nursing home care represents the greatest portion ($7 billion) of Medicaid spending. Other benefits (e.g., home health services and prescription drugs) are a very small percentage of these two major programs (8).

Paralleling and overlapping Medicare and Medicaid is the health program of the Veterans Administration (VA). During the next 20 years, as many as 60% of all males over 65 will be veterans. By definition, the VA considers all veterans over 65 disabled and, under that rubric, offers a full range of medical and health benefits. Thus although the VA accounted for only 4% of the total per capita health care outlay for the elderly in 1977, it is reasonable to anticipate that this proportion will increase significantly as more individuals become eligible.

The fourth major public source of funds, primarily derived from state expenditures, is the psychiatric hospital system. Following the emphasis on "deinstitutionalization" during the 1960s, there was a wholesale transfer of the elderly into what is euphemistically called "the community." In reality these placements were made in skilled nursing homes and boarding homes; many of the latter have been described as substandard nursing care facilities (16). It may be anticipated that the state psychiatric hospital system will not increase in population.

Other minor contributors to the medical care system are the CHAMPUS program of the Department of Defense, Workmen's Compensation, and Medical Vocational Rehabilitation. Only the latter program shows any indication of an increase in expenditure on behalf of the elderly, and very little at that.

Supplementing the medical care system are the health/social services for the vulnerable and impaired aged. These are financed primarily by four funding streams, although as many as a dozen public programs make modest contributions. Although it might be argued that transportation, information and referral, multipurpose senior centers, home-delivered and congregate meals, and protective services are all part of the health support system for the elderly and chronically disabled, consideration here is restricted to home health services.

The problem of identifying the home health service component within the health system is compounded by the peculiar description of some aspects as medically oriented and others as socially focused. The net result of this phenomenon is a clear division into two multifaceted systems of support. Medicare and Medicaid provide funding only for home health services which are directly relevant to a medical condition. This includes home nursing and occupational, physical, audio, or speech therapy. Medicare currently offers 100 units of these services and only when they are needed immediately subsequent to a hospital stay. Medicaid, too, provides home health services but limited to as many units as the particular state will fund. The medical component of home nursing services is perceived as the provision of intermittent personal care. The social component is focused on personal maintenance or homemaker services. These are administered by the states under the Social Services Title XX of the Social Security Act or through Title III of the Older Americans Act. These programs are funded by the federal government under a close-ended appropriation, whereas Medicare and Medicaid are open-ended federal appropriations. Furthermore, the Social Services, Older Americans Act, and Medicaid programs are all subject to limitations of state funding. The VA provides both home health care and homemaker services, either directly or through personal grants, but these too are limited by close-ended federal appropriations.

It has been estimated that as few as 6% of those in need are receiving either home health or homemaker services in any quantity from the formal health care system (10). Most health/social services are provided by informal sources, especially families and friends (2).

In summary, virtually all personal medical care has a substantial base of public support, whereas the health/social services are severely restricted in terms of public funding. In another context, this has been termed "the thirty-to-one paradox" (4).

COMMUNITY HEALTH SERVICES

Dividing health services into two subsystems of medical and social services is a problem that exists in virtually all developed societies. Its net result is that health

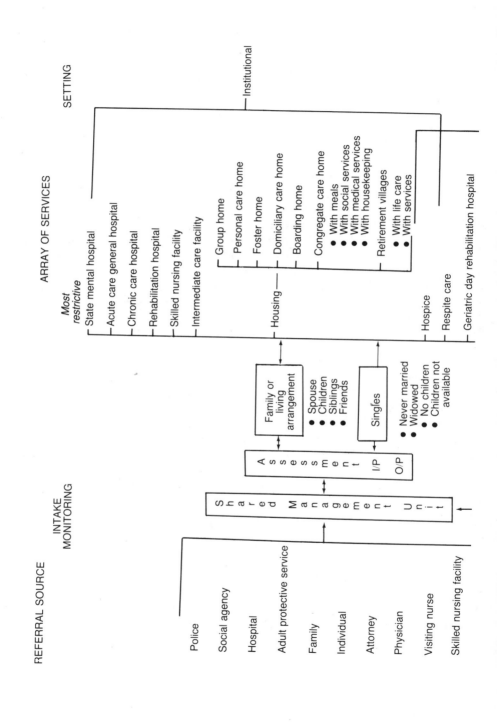

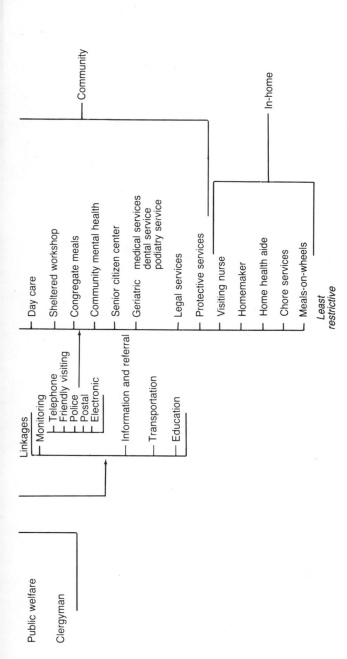

FIG. 1. Long-term support system: a paradigm. I/P, O/P = inpatient, outpatient. The classification of from most to least restrictive is a general view of services and may vary within each service. (From ref. 3.)

services for the aged are multiple, parallel, overlapping, noncontinuous, and, at best, confusing to the consumer. Rarely do they meet the collective criteria of availability, accessibility, affordability, adequacy, and accountability or offer continuity of care in a systematic way.

Planning for services is in similar disarray. Parallel systems of services have their own planning mechanisms. As a result, the various planning efforts overlap, contradict, and are unrelated to one another. Congress had given the Health Systems Agency (HSA) the role of planning for the long-term support system. When carrying out this responsibility, the HSA found itself limited by national funding policies which are focused on the medical response and which include the skilled nursing facility as the only significantly funded option to acute hospital care. Paralleling the HSAs are the socially oriented Area Agencies on Aging charged with planning, allocating, and coordinating services to the aged. Other special disease-focused planning units (e.g., community mental health agencies) also have congressionally authorized planning roles. Separate from all the other planning efforts is the VA, which, it has been pointed out, will be concerned during the next 20 years with health care of almost two-thirds of the elderly males in this country.

ROLE OF THE PHYSICIAN

The physician is assigned the single most important role within this complex health care system. S/he is called on to certify need for five of the most quantitatively significant services. Aside from the physician's own one-on-one direct services, s/he must decide on the appropriateness of admission to a hospital (acute, chronic, or rehabilitative), to a state psychiatric institution, and to the skilled nursing facility before the public dollar will be expended. Furthermore, the physician is required to certify and recertify the need for home health care. Beyond these formal roles, s/he participates with the patient and family on multiple decisions as to treatment, support, and care of the elderly, and advises on the use of the formal support system.

UTILIZATION OF HEALTH SERVICE

The utilization of this system by the elderly may be derivative of Roemer's law: that services follow funding. Twenty percent of all aged are admitted to the acute-care hospital at least once a year. One-fourth of that group will be admitted more than once during the year, for a total of 10 million admissions. As their average length of stay is longer than for persons under 65, the aged will account for 39% of all patient days. In the same vein, almost one-fourth of the aged use hospital outpatient departments at least once a year, for a total of 10 million visits. They use physicians' services half again more often than those under 65 years of age (5).

Most (89%) of the residents of skilled nursing facilities (SNF) are elderly, and as many as one-fourth of the aged will enter nursing homes at some time in their lives. As the likelihood of an SNF stay for a given individual increases with his or her age, the general aging of our population will eventuate in even higher utilization of these facilities unless there is a major change in the formal health system. The net result is that the aged, who comprise 11% of the population, use up almost 30% of our nation's health care resources.

It is suggested that the confusion and inappropriateness of response by the formal health system lie in the inability to define or recognize the health care needs of the aged. None of the proposals for national health insurance receiving executive or congressional consideration (as of this writing) are health-oriented. Rather, they are medically oriented programs, virtually extensions (insofar as benefits are concerned) of Medicare or Medicaid. Even the so-called Catastrophic Health Insurance Bill is limited to acute hospital care—this in the face of the government's own research pointing out that the catastrophic expenses for the aged are for skilled nursing home care (1).

More than a quarter-century of gerontological research has led to agreement on two main understandings: (a) The conditions of the elderly that require support are chronic, dictating the need for continuous, sustained services; those services are medical and medically related and health/social supports; and (b) the principal providers for the dependent elderly are family members. However, family resources are being strained, so that the family requires assistance to sustain its support. As a corollary, elderly persons without family resources require an alternative form of assistance.

The established facts supporting the second of these propositions have been summarized:

1. Intergenerational ties are strong and viable. Most older people (84%) live close to at least one adult child and see their children frequently (12).
2. Family members, not professionals, give the bulk of care to the impaired elderly: 80% of medically related care and personal care (14) and 90% of home help services (7), to say nothing of emotional support, response in crises, and the like.
3. In general, widowed older people look to daughters rather than sons for assistance, and those daughters respond (11,13). In fact, the word "alternative" is a euphemism for adult daughter.
4. Families do not "dump" their elderly. In the main, institutionalization of an impaired older person is the last resort for families, used when all other efforts fail. Families continue their concern and involvement after placement has occurred.

Recognition of the substantial contribution made by individuals providing informal support to the care of their elderly relatives lends weight to the view that the service system should return some form of support to the family to encourage and maintain them in their effort to retain the impaired elderly relative in the community.

The initiation, augmentation, and control of the quality of service in the home, community, or institutions is a community affair. Each locality has its own special resources, often with unique service agencies taking special leadership responsibilities. Furthermore, each community has its own value system which intimately relates to service acceptability. The most developed local organizational base in recent years is that of the catchment area. The community mental health system and the Area Agencies on Aging each have approximately 600 locations across the country. In most communities there is a variety of planning organizations in housing, mental health, vocational rehabilitation, and transportation. Professional Standard Review Organizations (PSROs) increasingly are taking responsibility for the quality of local medical services.

All of these local efforts must be rationalized into a long-term support system aimed at providing a full spectrum of services for the disabled which will ensure assessment and continuity of care (Fig. 1). Many of these services are already in place. For example, virtually every community is served by an acute-care general hospital. Most have access to skilled nursing home beds. Visiting nurse services are often available. Any one of these or other services can be built on, depending on the motivation, resources, and self-perception of the particular agency. Thus a rehabilitation unit in a general hospital may become the center for assessment not only for inpatients but for the community population as well. A community mental health unit could broaden its focus to include physical as well as psychosocial evaluation. Skilled nursing homes, particularly those with a voluntary auspice, are exploring ways of expanding their community role by providing functional and resource assessment along with other services. Currently, there are about 20 federally funded long-term care demonstration programs, all requiring medical school participation. Another group of local projects concerned with the organization and mobilization of services is being initiated by the federal government as channeling demonstrations.

The role of the federal government has been confusing, ranging between the provider of direct services to that of the funder of block grants with few restrictions. If we are committed to a community-oriented long-term health system, the federal role must be refocused, giving the local group maximum control over all public medical and health/social service funds. Thus the national responsibility would be for provision of funds, perhaps with state or local matching, and for the enunciating of the goals of the long-term health system together with establishment of generally applicable standards and methods of evaluation. The political problems are very substantial. Sooner or later the issue of many systems (i.e., for the poor, the aged, the disabled, veterans, etc.) versus a universal system must be confronted. Dr. J. Grimley Evans describes the goal of the British Health and Social Services system for the elderly as that of enabling "old people suffering from physical or mental disability to live where they would wish to live if they were not disabled. . . . The aim of assessment, treatment, and rehabilitation services is to improve their functioning to a maximum consistent level, and if this is still inadequate we must reduce the demands of the environment" (6). This is a long distance from the current climate of the American health care system, which is oriented to acute scientific medical care and to curative, rather than supportive, goals. To a large degree, these goals are reflective of the values of our society. The task of redirecting these values from the quantity to the quality of life is a major one. It is, however, the *sine qua non* to the achievement of a sound national system of long-term support and care.

REFERENCES

1. Birnbaum, H. *A National Profile of Catastrophic Illness.* DHEW Publication No. (PHS) 78-3201. Department of Health, Education, and Welfare, National Center for Health Services Research, Washington, DC, 1978.
2. Brody, E. M. The Informal Support System of the Functional Dependent Elderly. Paper prepared for Conference on the Role of the Nursing Home in the Continuum of Care of the Functionally Dependent, American College of Physicians, Washington, DC, June 13–16, 1980.
3. Brody, S. J. *Planning for the Long-Term Support/Care System: The Array of Services to be Considered.* Health Services Council, Philadelphia, 1979.
4. Brody, S. J. The thirty-to-one paradox: health needs and medical solutions. *National J.*, 11:1869–1873, 1979.
5. Brody, S. J. Health care for the aged: the graying of America. *Hospitals*, May 16, 1980.
6. Evans, J. G. Care of the Aging in Great Britain: An Overview. Paper presented at the Anglo-American Conference on New Patterns of Medical and Social Supports for the Aging, Fordham University, New York, May 12–13, 1980. Royal Society of Medicine, London *(in press)*.
7. General Accounting Office. *Home Health—The Need for a National Policy to Better Provide for the Elderly.* Report to the Congress by the Comptroller General of the United States. U.S. General Accounting Office, Washington, DC, December 30, 1977.
8. Gibson, R. M., and Fisher, C. R. National health expenditures, fiscal year 1977. *Social Security Bull.*, 41:11, 1978.
9. National Center for Health Statistics. *Current Estimates from the Health Interview Survey: United States, 1976*, Series 10, No. 96. National Center for Health Statistics, Rockville, MD, 1977.
10. Reif, L. Expansion and merger of home health care agencies. *Home Health Care Q.*, 1:No. 3, 1980.
11. Shanas, E. Family help patterns and social class in three countries. *J. Marriage Family*, 29:257–266, 1967.
12. Shanas, E. Older people and their families: the new pioneers. *J. Marriage Family*, 42:9–15, 1980.
13. Troll, L. E. The family of later life: a decade review. *J. Marriage Family*, 33:263–290, 1971.
14. U.S. Department of Health, Education, and Welfare, Public Health Service. *Home Care for Persons 55 and Over, United States: July 1966–June 1968.* Vital and Health Statistics, Series 10, No. 73. Government Printing Office, Washington, DC, 1972.
15. U.S. Department of Health, Education, and Welfare, Public Health Service, Office of the Assistant Secretary for Health. *Health United States, 1978*, Table 56. DHEW Publication No. (PHS) 78-1232. Government Printing Office, Washington, DC, 1978.
16. U.S. Senate, Special Committee on Aging. *Nursing Home Care in the United States: Failure in Public Policy*, Supporting Paper No. 7: The role of nursing homes in caring for discharged mental patients (and the birth of a for-profit boarding home industry). Government Printing Office, Washington, DC, 1976.

SUGGESTED READING

Brody, E. M. *Long-Term Care of Older People.* Human Sciences Press, New York, 1977.

Brody, S. J. Comprehensive health care for the elderly: an analysis (the continuum of medical, health and social services for the aging). *Gerontologist*, 13:412–418, 1973.

Brody, S. J., and Masciocchi, C. Data for long-term care planning by health systems agencies. *Am. J. Public Health*, November 1980, pp. 1194–1198.

Scanlon, W., Difederico, E., and Stassen, M. *Long-Term Care*. The Urban Institute, Washington, DC, 1979.
Veterans Administration. *The Aging Veteran: Present and Future Medical Needs*. Government Printing Office, Washington, DC, 1977.

The Biology of
Aging

Fundamentals of Geriatric Medicine, edited by
Ronald D. T. Cape, Rodney M. Coe, and Isadore
Rossman, Raven Press, New York © 1983.

5

Overview

Ronald D. T. Cape

Physiology and anatomy have traditionally been taught to medical students in terms of the ideal 70-kg man. It is only during the twentieth century and particularly during the past 20 to 30 years that medical science has begun to appreciate that this hypothetical adult is largely a myth. Throughout our lives we are constantly changing. The genetic impulse which gives us our initial developmental thrust almost certainly influences the pace of aging and length of life. Growth and development achieves its peak as we reach maturity in our early twenties. Biologically speaking, that is the point at which all of our bodily functions have the maximum potential, the greatest reserve of function, and optimum capacity. Thereafter, the detrimental effect of biosenescence takes over. During the first 20 to 30 years beyond the point of optimum maturity, deterioration in biological systems is slow and gradual; beyond that period it speeds up.

During youth and maturity there is a range of function among individuals which slowly widens during senescence. As a result, there are individuals at age 90 who constitute a biologically elite group, still functioning fully and independently, whereas others of the same age function poorly.

For this reason it is important to include in this text details of some of the main physiological changes which accompany aging. These modify and alter the behavior of disease and thus have relevance to clinical medicine. As function tends to be reduced with aging, morbidity increases. From 60 years onward there is an intermingling of aging and morbidity which results in the complexity of clinical presentations and the frequency of multiple pathological changes found in the old. To unravel these, the physician's knowledge of aging must include the aspects most relevant to medicine, several of which are covered in the succeeding six chapters.

LEAN BODY MASS

The general shape and configuration of the human frame depends to a large extent on its muscular covering. Muscles, composed of nonmitotic cells, achieve their optimum size and strength when the individual reaches full maturity, in the middle twenties. Thereafter there is a decline in the musculature, which is accelerated after age 50. Sedentary patterns contribute to this, though the more robustly physical the life style the bulkier the muscles remain. Eventually, for everyone, there is considerable atrophy, which may be due not only to primary degeneration of muscle cells but also to some loss of anterior horn cells responsible for motor units. Wasting of muscles is often concealed by an increasing quantity of adipose tissue, which not only compensates for the loss of bulk but may create new bulges in unwanted places!

Lean body mass is made up chiefly of muscles, liver, brain, and kidneys, its total weight diminishing by 20 to 30% between the ages of 30 and 80 years. Novak (4) studied 215 men and 305 women volunteers between the ages of 18 and 85, determining total body potassium by counting naturally occurring radioactive ^{40}K in the whole body counter. Total body potassium has been found to be reduced with age in men from 56 to 43 mmol kg^{-1} and in women from 46 to 38 mmol kg^{-1}. Fat increased with age from 18 to 36% in men; fat-free mass diminished from 82 to 64% and cellular mass from 65 to 36% (Fig. 1). Similar but less striking changes occurred in women, the process commencing in both sexes at about the age of 45. The same type of loss occurs in the organs which combine with muscle to constitute lean body mass. Only the lungs appear to be spared, with liver, brain, kidneys, spleen, and pancreas all showing a significant loss over the life span.

The reduction in lean body mass results in a progressive decrease in total body protein. The total albumin pool is reduced in the elderly by about 20%, the serum concentration decreasing slowly from the fifth decade. Albumin levels in the serum depend on a homeostatic mechanism that operates in the liver; osmotic pressure variations in the plasma cause the liver to produce more or less albumin as required. One reason for the reduced albumin pool may be that this mechanism becomes less effective with increasing age.

There is a similar picture in the skeleton. Garn (3) reported that bone loss has been quantified in both men and women in a number of ways. Based on innumerable absorptiometric assessments and radiographs, he found that, over the years from maturity through the ninth decade, there is a 12% loss of tissue bone in the male and a 25% loss in the female. This bone loss begins at the end of the fourth decade, and from the fifth decade onward there is a steady, slow loss of bone substance from both men and women. Unfortunately, women, with a smaller initial bone mass, lose a higher proportion than their male counterparts.

Changes in lean body mass have obvious relevance to clinical pharmacology and are discussed in another section. The tendency to osteopenia plays a major role in the occurrence of fractures, particularly spinal compression fractures and limb fractures.

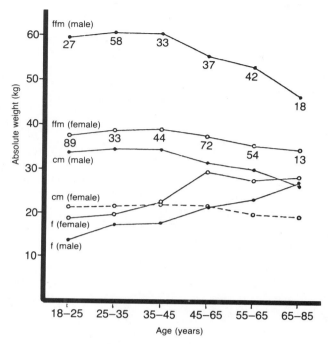

FIG. 1. Fat (f), fat-free mass (ffm), and cell mass (cm) of males and females at various ages. Mean values are given, and the number of subjects in each age group is noted. (From ref. 2, with permission.)

AGING OF BRAIN

There are 15,000 to 20,000 million nerve cells in the human body, each with 10,000 dendritic processes linking it to other nerve cells. These are responsible for five main attributes of the central nervous system:

1. The extreme sensitivity of receptors in skin, eye, ear, and tongue.
2. The versatility of the motor system with its thousands of units ranging from the small muscles of the hand, concerned with delicate, skillful movements, to the large muscles of strength in proximal segments of limbs.
3. The complexity of sensorimotor links with input from many parts of the brain.
4. The reliability of the autonomic system which controls most visceral functions in a largely involuntary manner.
5. The capacity of memory and cognitive function.

As we age we lose cerebral cells from areas of the brain, and there is a slow development of certain pathological changes which are seen in abundance in senile dementia of the Alzheimer type. Senile plaques, neurofibrillary tangles, and granulovacuolar degeneration represent, however, only part of the aging changes. Pigment accumulates in neuronal and glial cells. This represents inert material of no further value to the cell, fatty in nature and possibly derived from lysosomes. It has been suggested that it may be an end-product of an effete enzyme system. It is unlikely to improve cell function and probably indicates the reverse. There are quite striking changes in the gross chemistry of the brain between youth and old age. Water content falls from 92% at birth to 76% at age 90; total lipids increase from 3.5% at birth to 10.5% at age 30, and thereafter decline to 7.5% during old age. At maturity 140 g of the brain's dry weight is protein. This is reduced to 100 g by the ninth decade. A significant reduction in muscarinic receptor binding sites in the frontal lobes of 23 brains which exhibited slight or no senile plaque formation and no neurofibrillary degeneration has been described.

Associated with these histological and chemical changes are alterations in electrical patterns, exhibited by the functioning brain on electroencephalography. Visually evoked responses demonstrate slowing and reduced amplitude among the old, compared with the young or middle-aged (1).

MEASUREMENT OF CEREBRAL FUNCTION

With most visceral organs and systems, there are methods by which function may be assessed. With the brain, securely enclosed in its bone case and inaccessible to our attempts to learn its secrets, the situation is more difficult. We do know that the elderly individual who continues physical activities that require strength and suppleness in his or her muscles must have a brain in which the motor units are in good condition. Similarly, we can judge that the elderly musician who continues to play or conduct with vigor into his or her eighties must have a brain which is continuing to function well. How can we assess humbler mortals without such revealing habits?

There are two types of measure that can be used. The first is an assessment of intelligence and cognitive functions, and the second is an assessment of the individual's ability to perform activities of daily living (ADL) in a competent manner. Some physicians regard attempts at defining and marking intelligence to be an activity of dubious utility. Psychologists have developed these tests with skill and care, however, and they provide a great deal of valuable information helpful to the clinician. An argument in favor of the authenticity of psychological testing as a measure of brain function is the fact that young people with above-average intelligence (IQ > 100) are physically healthier and live longer than those with less intelligence. On the basis of cross-sectional and longitudinal testing of groups of subjects of varying ages, it appears that cognitive function, as measured by a variety of intelligence tests, is maintained reasonably well until the sixth decade, after which it begins to fail, as do physiological functions. Those individuals who begin with above-average intelligence are likely to retain intellectual powers longer and more effectively.

The second method of assessing cerebral function is to note the individual's skill at ADL. Normally we think of these skills in relation to progress in a rehabilitation program or need for various types of assistance. If one widens the concept to include all of the physical and mental activities people engage in each day, it is possible to document the more obvious differences between the way we do things as we grow older. Between ages 30 and 40 we may find we cannot continue to play in violent competitive sports, e.g., hockey or football. We may blame this on cardio-respiratory problems, but equally if not more important is eye-hand-foot coordination and speed, achieved by our brains.

It is reasonable to hypothesize that both psychometric tests and ADL assessments point to a reduction in cerebral competence in the elderly. The question should now be asked: "Does this fact have any implications for clinical medicine?"

The authors of this volume, and particularly this section have borne in mind the clinician's need for information relevant to patient care. It is thought that the chapters in this section provide the scientific base on which later sections dealing with diagnosis, management, and controversies are constructed.

REFERENCES

1. Beck, E.G., Dustman, R. E., and Schenkenberg, T. Life span changes in the electrical activity of the human brain as reflected in the cerebral evoked response. In: *Neurobiology of Aging,* edited by J. M. Ordy and K. R. Brizzee, pp. 175–192. Plenum Press, New York, 1975.
2. Cape, R. D. T. *Aging: Its Complex Management*, p. 20. Harper and Row, Hagerstown, MD, 1978.
3. Garn, S. M. Bone loss and ageing. In: *Nutrition of the Aged*, edited by W. W. Hawkins, pp. 73–90. Proceedings of a symposium. The Nutrition Society of Canada, 1978.
4. Novak, L. P. Aging total body potassium, fat-free mass, and cell mass in males and females between ages 18 and 85 years. *J. Gerontol.*, 27:438–443, 1972.

SUGGESTED READING

Botwinick, J. Intellectual abilities. In: *Handbook of Psychology of Aging*, edited by J. E. Birren and W. K. Schaie, pp. 580–605. Van Nostrand Reinhold, New York, 1977.

Bromley, D. B. *The Psychology of Human Ageing*. Penguin Books, London, 1974.

Cape, R. D. T. *Aging: Its Complex Management*. Harper & Row, New York, 1978.

Kane, R. A., and Kane, R. L. *Assessing the Elderly: A Practical Guide to Measurement*. Lexington Books, Lexington, MA, 1981.

Rossman, I. Anatomic and body composition changes with age. In: *Handbook of the Biology of Aging*, edited by C. E. Finch and L. Hayflick, pp. 189–221. Van Nostrand Reinhold, New York, 1977.

Fundamentals of Geriatric Medicine, edited by
Ronald D.T. Cape, Rodney M. Coe, and Isadore
Rossman, Raven Press, New York © 1983.

6

Theories of Aging

Leonard Hayflick

There is probably no other area of biological inquiry that is as susceptible to so many theories as is the science of gerontology. This is true not only because of a lack of sufficient fundamental data but also because manifestations of biological changes with time affect almost all biological systems from the molecular level to that of the whole organism. It is therefore easy to construct a theory of aging based on a biological decrement that may be observed to occur in time in any system at the level of the molecule, cell, tissue, organ, or whole animal. The significant question will always be: Is the change observed a direct cause of aging, or is it the result of changes that occurred at a more fundamental level?

As modern notions of biological development are rooted in signals originating from information-containing molecules, it seems reasonable to attribute postdevelopmental changes to a similar system of signals occurring at the molecular level. This is one compelling reason why changes in the genetic signal in cells are thought to play the leading role in producing manifestations of aging. Furthermore, the life spans of animals, presumably genetically determined, are remarkably constant for each species. Among mammalian species, life spans may differ by a factor of 30 or more; yet within each species life spans are played out with notable uniformity.

Selective processes do not seem to have played an important role in species longevity. Few, if any, selective mechanisms appear to favor long-lived members of a species. This is so because, beyond the age of sexual maturation and the rearing of progeny, longevous members of a species have little survival value for which to be selected. In fact, as soon as feral animals reach ages slightly beyond sexual maturity, their declining functional capacities make them easier prey for predators and disease. We can conclude, therefore, that aging in its extreme manifestations is a phenomenon confined only to humans and the animals that humans choose to protect.

Although the evidence is not altogether convincing, species' life spans may be indirectly determined by the genetically based developmental changes that lead to sexual maturity. Developmental processes may have a built-in overcompensation momentum which ensures that an animal will reach sexual maturity. The overcompensation then permits the animal to survive beyond sexual maturation, but with ever-increasing decrements in physiological function.

These decrements lead to an increased vulnerability to disease processes. Diseases of old age therefore must be distinguished from normal age changes. The latter are the ultimate causes of death because they lead to a diminished capacity to cope with disease and environmental insults.

If age changes are caused by fundamental changes in information-containing molecules that result, in chain-reaction fashion, in physiological decrements at higher organizational levels (i.e., cell, tissue, organ, whole animal), then the most tenable theories of aging are those based on molecular events that occur in the genetic apparatus. Nevertheless, several nongenetically based phenomena may induce age changes, and these are considered also.

GENETIC THEORIES OF AGING

Error Theory

In 1963 Orgel (9) proposed a model for biological aging that was based on a decrease in the fidelity of protein synthesis. Protein synthesis involves two steps in which discrimination between related molecules occurs. A unique amino acid must be selected by each activating enzyme, and this must be attached to the appropriate tRNA. A codon of messenger RNA must then pair with the anticodon of an appropriate tRNA. These processes are probably prone to a small degree of error. The fidelity of protein synthesis could also be decreased by errors in RNA synthesis. A repetition of events such as these, in which errors in proteins occur, could result in convergence to a stable value of errors or it would diverge. If the former were the case, aging would not occur. In the latter case, the error frequently would eventually become great enough to impair cell function. Although Orgel originally maintained the latter possibility, he has now abandoned this position because it is possible that a protein-synthesizing system containing a small number of errors might be capable of synthesizing a new protein-synthesizing system containing fewer errors. It is more plausible that this is the case in view of evidence for the existence of enzymes capable of scavenging error-containing proteins.

It has also been conjectured that it may not be possible to distinguish between contributions to cellular aging caused by errors in protein synthesis from those due to an accumulation of somatic mutations. Inaccurate protein synthesis may be indistinguishable from inaccurate DNA synthesis, and in that sense they may be coupled phenomena. The accuracy of both processes may be completely dependent on the fidelity of the other. Orgel now subscribes to this more general notion in which positive feedback occurs where "the greater the number of errors that have accumulated in the macromolecular constituents of the cell, the faster the accumulation of further errors" (8). It is also envisioned that extracellular and intracellular mechanisms of aging are coupled, as inaccurate protein synthesis must affect extracellular events.

In spite of this proposal, which enjoyed some popularity when it was first suggested, a preponderance of experimental evidence does not now support the error theory. The contrary evidence reveals that: (a) aging is not accelerated when misspecified amino acids are purposely introduced, and (b) misspecified molecules do not accumulate to a significant level in aged cells.

Redundant Message Theory

Although the redundant message theory is closely allied to the error theory, it is sufficiently unique to bear separate consideration. Medvedev is the chief proponent of this notion, which has considerable merit as a fundamental theory of species longevity and perhaps individual aging. He proposes that the selective repetition of some definite genes, cistrons, operons, and other linear structures on the DNA molecule, the bulk of which are repressed, behave as redundant messages to be called into action when active genome messages become faulty (7). He argues that the total genome of mammals is composed of not less than 10^5 structural genes or cistrons, but that in each cell only about 0.2 to 0.4% of this number are expressed during biological development and maturity. If 1/500 of all genes are active and 499/500 specifically repressed, and if mutagenic factors act equally on the repressed and active cistrons, the mutation rate of repressed genes must yield more mutations than those occurring in active genes. Medvedev asserts that different species' life spans may be a function of the degree of repeated sequences. Long-lived species should then have more redundant messages than do short-lived species. As errors accumulate in functioning genes, reserve sequences containing the same information take over until the redundancy in the system is exhausted, resulting in biological age changes. The differences in species' life spans, then, are thought to be manifestations of the degree of gene repetition.

Thus the phenomenon of linear repetition of some genes can have not only evolutionary but also gerontological implications when there is a protective role of gene repetition against random molecular accidents. Conceptually, this has merit not only as an explanation for the wide differences found in the life span of species but also for the less variable life span of individual members within a species. A repeated nucleotide sequence simply has a greater chance of preserving intact the final gene product during evolution or during a long life span than does any unique sequence. It follows therefore that if errors accumulate in unique genes, age changes may result from this kind of event. Certainly not all unique genes would be expected to have equal value for cell function or maintenance of cell life. The really vital unique sequences are likely to be restricted to some universally important genes of general metabolism. They may represent the essential group of genes whose failure ultimately results in manifestations of biological aging. Medvedev prefers the view that the derepression of unique genes during postembryonal or adult stages in development are the real initiators of age changes. This suggests a manifestation of the deterioration with time of nonrepeated nucleotide sequences.

The theory that aging is due to the accumulation of gene mutations and chromosome anomalies has many advocates, yet the failure of this theory to explain the quantitative aspects of normal and radiation-induced aging has been repeatedly observed.

Transcription Theory

The transcription theory, championed by von Hahn (11), suggests that the control of cellular aging is functional at the level of the transcription of genetic information from DNA into the intermediary messenger RNA. The thesis maintains that: (a) with increasing age, deleterious changes occur in the metabolism of differentiated postmitotic cells; (b) the alterations are the result of primary events that occur within the nuclear chromatin; (c) there exists in the nuclear chromatin complex a control mechanism responsible for the appearance and sequence of the primary aging events; and (d) this control mechanism involves the regulation of transcription, although other regulated events may occur.

Von Hahn notes that there are several *a priori* assumptions involved in this hypothesis, the most important being that there is a universal physiological aging process deleterious to the cell that is due to intrinsic causes and which progressively acts with increasing chronological age. These are the essential criteria characterizing biological aging that have been proposed by Strehler (10) and appear to be generally valid.

The central event of aging, at whatever level of biological complexity, seems to be the progressive diminution in adaptation to stress and in the capacity of the system to maintain the homeostatic equilibrium characteristic of the adult animal at the end of growth and full development.

Von Hahn suggests that two types of primary events can interfere with transcription. One is genetically controlled and based on a genetic program; the other is random, involving stochastic processes similar to those discussed in the error hypothesis.

Von Hahn offers data suggesting that there is an age-related increase in the stability of the DNA double helix which is dependent on the presence and degree of binding of certain proteins. In old nucleoprotein a particular protein fraction is bound to DNA in such a way as to increase the energy required for the separation of the two strands of the helix. As strand separation is an essential step in transcription, blocking the process will block transcription, leading to a loss of genetic information within the cell.

As attractive as this hypothesis might seem, it suffers from a lack of sufficiently compelling experimental data. This should not imply that the hypothesis is wrong but only that it has not attracted enough interest to subject it to extensive experimental analysis.

Programmed Theory

A final proposition offered to explain age changes at the genetic level is based on a continuation of those genetic events that result in the development and maturation of any animal. This notion assumes that the switching on and off of genes during developmental processes also determines age changes. That is, age changes, like developmental changes, are "programmed" into the original pool of genetic information and are "played out" in an orderly sequence just as developmental changes are. The graying of the hair is not generally thought of as a disease associated with the passage of time. It is regarded to be a highly predictable event that occurs later in life after the genetic expression of a plethora of other programmed developmental events that occur in orderly sequences.

This one example is typical of the thousands of normal age changes that are not regarded as evidence of pathology but as expressions of normal postmaturation decrements in physiological function over time. Aging might therefore be attributable to an underlying series of orderly programmed genetic events that shut down or slow down essential physiological phenomena after postreproductive age is reached. The programming may be the result of specific gene determinants that, like the end of a tape recording, simply trigger a sequence of events that ultimately shuts down the machine. The sequence of events may include the incorporation of "errors" in a cell's metabolic machinery that are less readily repaired or whose frequency of occurrence simply overwhelms any existing repair processes.

We may call the span of time during which functional decrements ultimately express themselves in death of the organism as the "mean time to failure." This concept is applicable to the deterioration of mechanical as well as biological systems and can be illustrated by considering the mean time to failure of, for example, automobiles. The mean time to failure of the average machine may be 5 to 6 years, which often varies as a function of the competence of the repair processes. Barring total replacement of all vital elements, deterioration is inevitable. Similarly, failure of cell function may occur at predictable times that are dependent on the fidelity of the synthesizing machinery and the degree of perfection of cellular repair systems. As biological systems do not appear to function perfectly and indefinitely, we are led to the conclusion that the ultimate death of a cell or loss of function is genetically programmed and has a mean time to failure. The mean time to failure may vary among individual cells, tissues, or organs. It is proposed that the genetic apparatus simply runs out of accurate programmed information that might result in different mean times to failure for all of the dependent biological systems. The existence of different species' life spans may be the reflection of more perfect repair systems in those animals that have greater longevity.

Finally, one must consider two metazoan cell lineages that seem to have escaped from the inevitability of aging or death. These are the germ cells (precursors of egg and sperm cells) and continuously reproducing cancer cell populations. It may be possible to explain the immortality of cancer cell populations by suggesting that in order to maintain immortality genetic information is exchanged between these cells in the same way that the genetic cards are reshuffled when egg and sperm fuse. Thus some process of rearrangement or genetic information may serve to reprogram or reset a more perfect biological clock.

Although genetically based theories of aging seem to be the most tenable, they probably do not act alone. Superimposed on one or more genetic mechanisms may be nongenetic processes of aging that may also contribute to functional decline in some essential organ or organ system.

NONGENETIC THEORIES OF AGING

Immunological Theory

Immunological theories, championed by Walford (12), Burnet (1), and Makinodan (6), argue that alterations in the immune system contribute to decrements associated with old age. With increasing age, the immune system is thought to become less efficient, with a reduced capacity to deal with infection (Chapter 21) and/or a greater likelihood of immunocompetent cells reacting against the body's own constituents. The breakdown of immune tolerance would then lead to the formation of antibodies against one's own cells. The autoimmune diseases are an example of this kind of event. Although this hypothesis has much to recommend it, it may not be universally applicable as age changes occur in nonvertebrates that lack an immune system. Also, known alterations in the immune system with age may be caused by more fundamental changes in the genetic apparatus of its constituent cells. These facts would remove this theory from a nongenetic phenomenon to one of the more generalized genetic theories described above.

Connective Tissue Theory

Many age-related changes are known to occur in the collagen, elastin, or ground substance surrounding cells in most tissues. Kohn (5) argues that most of the age changes found in vertebrates can be attributed to changes in these extracellular substances. As these substances are widespread and are involved in the transport and exchange of materials among cells, changes in their physics and chemistry can produce profound effects on physiological function. Many changes are known to occur in the ground substance, with particular attention being paid to collagen because it comprises 25% of total body protein. Collagen changes with age in several ways that seem to be independent of environmental influences. More molecular cross-linking occurs, and this could give rise to age-associated changes in the skin. More important is the likelihood that these cross-linkages affect the flow of nutrients and waste products from cells. These, in turn, are thought to produce age changes. Nevertheless, there is no convincing evidence that these changes represent the ultimate cause of aging. Their presumptive detrimental effects, however, may be superimposed on more fundamental causes.

Free-Radical Theory

Free radicals are chemicals whose outer orbit contains an unpaired electron and, as such, are highly reactive entities. They are produced as short-lived chemicals during normal metabolic reactions. It is hypothesized that they contribute to age changes by combining with essential molecules. Harman (3) is the chief exponent of this concept, for which some convincing experimental evidence exists. Free radical damage to proteins or DNA could produce profound effects and lead to cross-linking in some of these important molecules. They are also known to induce peroxidation of fatty acids and thereby affect vital membrane functions. Lysosomes, for example, might become leaky and release damaging hydrolytic enzymes.

Substances which inhibit free-radical activity are called antioxidants. When fed to experimental animals, these substances increase longevity. It is not known whether free-radical production is the fundamental cause of age changes or is simply an ancillary phenomenon that can perturb age-related changes induced by other, more basic causes.

Other Organ Theories

Several other nongenetic theories of aging have been proposed which depend on functional decline in some organ or organ system. All suffer from the same criticisms: (a) They may simply be the result of more fundamental causes; or (b) the organ system in question may not be universally present in all aging animals. Good examples of this kind are theories based on known neuroendocrinological changes that occur with age (2). There is little question that changes do occur in this system, but the likelihood that it represents the fundamental cause of age changes is in serious doubt.

CONCLUSION

Most gerontologists agree that there is probably no single cause of aging. A phenomenon which probably comes closest to a unifying theory relates to those concepts based on a passive (random) or an active process of genetic programming (4). The latter would operate in precisely the same fashion as do those active genetic processes that lead to biological development and maturation. Age changes might be viewed as being caused by the same fundamental processes that produced the mature animal. Superimposed on genetically based causes could be one or more of the nongenetic mechanisms that together result in increased vulnerability.

When caring for elderly patients, the physician should be familiar with the principal current theories of aging, but understand that no current theory of aging is regarded universally as being adequate.

ACKNOWLEDGEMENTS

Supported in part by grant AG 00850 from the National Advisory Council on Aging, NIH, Bethesda, MD, and the Glenn Foundation for Medical Research, Manhasset, NY.

REFERENCES

1. Burnet, F. M. An immunological approach to aging. *Lancet*, 2:358–360, 1970.
2. Finch, C. E. Neuroendocrine and autonomic aspects of aging. In: *Handbook of the Biology of Aging*, edited by C. E. Finch and L. Hayflick. Van Nostrand Reinhold, New York, 1977.

3. Harman, D. Free-radical theory of aging: effect of amount and degree of dietary fat on mortality rate. *J. Gerontol.*, 26:451–456, 1971.
4. Hayflick, L. Current theories of biological aging. *Fed. Proc.*, 34:9–13, 1975.
5. Kohn, R. R. *Principles of Mammalian Aging*. Prentice Hall, Englewood Cliffs, NJ, 1971.
6. Makinodan, T. Immunity and aging. In: *Handbook of the Biology of Aging*, edited by C. E. Finch and L. Hayflick. Van Nostrand Reinhold, New York, 1977.
7. Medvedev, Zh. A. Repetition of molecular-genetic information as a possible factor in evolutionary changes in life span. *Exp. Gerontol.*, 7:227–238, 1972.
8. Orgel, L. E. Ageing of clones of mammalian cells. *Nature*, 243:441–445, 1963.
9. Orgel, L. E. The maintenance of the accuracy of protein synthesis and its relevance to ageing. *Proc. Natl. Acad. Sci. USA*, 49:517–521, 1963.
10. Strehler, B. L. *Time, Cells and Aging*, 2nd ed. Academic Press, New York, 1977.
11. Von Hahn, H. P. The regulation of protein synthesis in the aging cell. *Exp. Gerontol.*, 5:323–334, 1970.
12. Walford, R. L. *The Immunologic Theory of Aging*. Williams & Wilkins, Baltimore, 1969.

SUGGESTED READING

Comfort, A. *The Biology of Senescence*, 3rd ed. Elsevier North Holland, New York, 1979.

Finch, C. E., and Hayflick, L. *Handbook of the Biology of Aging*. Van Nostrand Reinhold, New York, 1977.

Hayflick, L. The cell biology of human aging. *Sci. Am.*, 242:58–66, 1980.

Kohn, R. R. *Principles of Mammalian Aging*. Prentice Hall, Englewood Cliffs, New Jersey, 1971.

Rockstein, M. *Theoretical Aspects of Aging*. Academic Press, New York, 1974.

Strehler, B. L. *Time, Cells and Aging*, 2nd ed. Academic Press, New York, 1977.

Walford, R. L. *The Immunologic Theory of Aging*. Williams & Wilkins, Baltimore, 1969.

Fundamentals of Geriatric Medicine, edited by
Ronald D. T. Cape, Rodney M. Coe, and Isadore
Rossman, Raven Press, New York © 1983.

7

Aging of Regulatory Mechanisms

Nathan W. Shock

Aging represents the irreversible progressive changes that take place in the performance of a cell, tissue, organ, or total individual animal with the passage of time. As the probability of an individual's death increases with age, most of the changes associated with aging are apt to represent decrements in performance.

Numerous studies have described changes with age in the performance of specific organ systems. The pattern of age changes differs across organ systems, but the general tendency is for performance to decrease gradually over the entire age span after the attainment of maturity. On the other hand, the rate of change varies markedly across different types of performance. Complex performances requiring the integrated activities of different organ systems and the ability of an individual to adapt to displacing stimuli show greater decrements with advancing age than do performances which can be accomplished by a single organ system. It is apparent, therefore, that aging in an individual is primarily related to the effectiveness of a number of the body's regulatory mechanisms. These mechanisms depend heavily on communication among cells, tissues, and organs mediated by the nervous and endocrine systems.

In adapting to the stresses involved in daily living, the individual must first be able to detect the presence of a displacement, its direction, and its magnitude. The sensing mechanism must then be able to activate the appropriate organ or groups of cells to counteract the stress, either by generating or releasing some substance (e.g., a hormone or enzyme) or by stimulating other cells or organs to action. Thus the major result of aging may be the breakdown of regulatory mechanisms, primarily those involving the endocrine, neurological, and immune systems.

No doubt the ultimate biological mechanisms of aging lie at the cellular level, with special reference to cells involved in regulatory processes. Nevertheless, much can be learned about aging from studying the effects of age on performances of varying degrees of complexity. Studies to define the status of regulatory processes in an individual may lead to predictions about the rate at which he or she is aging, and thus predictions about survival. In short, aging must be viewed as a complex multidimensional process that cannot be identified with any single organ system. The ability to survive, which depends on the integrated responses of many organ systems, is the key to aging.

Studies on the effects of age on the performance of a number of organ systems in humans show the following:

a. There are wide individual differences in the rate of aging.
b. Different organ systems age at different rates.
c. Different organ systems, even in the same individual, may age at different rates.
d. With increasing age, the range of variance among different subjects of the same chronological age increases in many measurements.
e. Age changes are greater in complex performances (which require integrated activity among different organ systems) than in simple performances.
f. Aging has the greatest effect on the time required to achieve adaptive responses—the aged require more time than do the young.

Specific experimental data can be cited to illustrate these generalizations about aging and to indicate some of the consequences.

VARIANCE IN PERFORMANCE AMONG INDIVIDUALS

The effect of age on renal plasma flow as determined by the clearance of Diodrast in a group of 96 normal males is shown in Fig. 1. On the average, renal blood flow falls significantly with advancing age. It can be seen that the kidney function

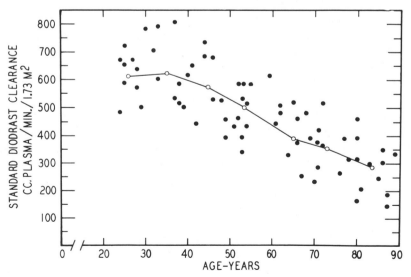

FIG. 1. Change in standard Diodrast clearance or effective renal plasma flow with age. Results shown are average values. (From ref. 1.)

of some individuals 80 to 90 years of age was as good as the average for 60-year-olds. Furthermore, the range of variability was greater among the 80-year-old subjects than among the 30-year-olds. Similar patterns of age changes are found in many other physiological parameters, e.g., pulmonary functions (vital capacity, maximum breathing capacity), cardiac output, creatinine clearance, maximum work output, and maximum oxygen uptake during exercise.

Statistical analysis of these observations led to the derivation of linear regression curves which indicate the average decrement in specific functions with age. The variation between subjects is so large that it is impossible to decide whether the age decrement is linear over the entire age span from 20 to 90 or the rate of decline increases during the later years.

However, when longitudinal observations are made by measuring the same subject at frequent intervals (1 to 2 years) over a period of 15 to 20 years, it is possible to show that, at least in the case of renal function, the rate of decline increases with advancing age. That is, the decrement in function between age 75 and 80 years is greater than the decrement between 65 and 70 years.

These data show that chronological age alone is a poor predictor of performance for most physiological characteristics. Thus although it is important to take age into account when setting norms for physiological performance (i.e., blood pressure, basal metabolism, lung functions, kidney functions, glucose tolerance), the range of "normal" values may be great.

The use of percentile ranking of an individual among other subjects of the same age has proved a useful device to avoid the problems of defining a "normal range." This method simply indicates the rank order of an individual within a group of persons the same age. A nomogram constructed from data on creatinine clearance tests conducted on normal males, aged 20 to 80, is shown in Fig. 2. A straight line drawn between the creatinine clearance measured on a given subject and his age intersects the percentile scale to give his percentile rank. As normative data accumulate for more and more tests, rank orders for individual subjects can be determined for many types of performance.

AGE REGRESSIONS FOR DIFFERENT PERFORMANCES

Figure 3 compares the average values for a number of physiological functions over the age span 30 to 85 years. For each function, values at ages over 35 years are expressed as the percentage of the mean value for male subjects aged 25 to 35 years. The average decrements over the age span 30 to 85 years ranged from 15% for the speed of conduction of the nerve impulse in the ulnar nerve to a 60% decrement in maximum breathing capacity (maximum amount of air that the subject could voluntarily breathe in and out of his lungs in 15 sec).

Examination of such plots for various tests indicate that age trends are quite different and that age decrements are least for functions that depend on a single organ system, such as that for nerve conduction velocity, which on the average falls by only 15% between the ages of 30 and 90 years; the age trends are greatest

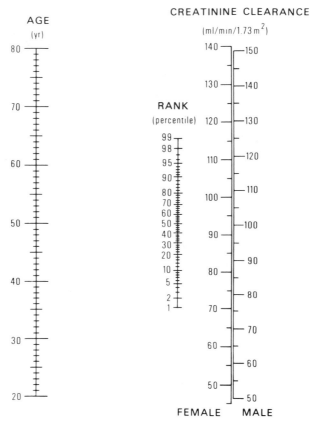

FIG. 2. Nomogram for determining the age-adjusted percentile rank in true creatinine clearance for males aged 20 to 80 years. (From ref. 3.)

for performances such as maximum work output, which requires the integration of many organ systems (cardiovascular, pulmonary, muscular, endocrine, and nervous systems).

Performances which require the coordination of organ systems show much greater decrements with age. Maximum breathing capacity, showing a decrement of 60% between the ages of 30 and 80, is an example of a performance that requires close coordination between the nervous and muscular systems in order to achieve maximum performance.

The process of turning a crank with the arms requires close coordination between periodic contractions of certain muscle groups associated with relaxation of opposing muscles. Figure 4 compares the age change in the strength of specific muscle groups and the maximum power generated by the same muscle groups when involved in turning an ergometer to achieve maximum work output. It is apparent that the coordinated performance (i.e., cranking) shows a greater age decrement than does the static strength of the same muscles.

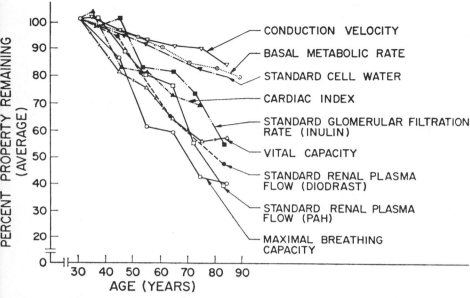

FIG. 3. Average age differences in physiological functions among normal male subjects aged 30 to 90 years. (From ref. 4.)

Other evidence for the influence of task complexity on the degree of age decrements in performance can be found by comparing age changes in simple reflex time with more complicated performances which involve choices. For example, simple reflex time to the stimulus of a single scratch to the sole of the foot does not change significantly over the entire age span from 30 to 80 years. This response, which operates primarily through the spinal cord, involves transmission of nerve impulses over short distances through only a few synapses.

In contrast, when the subject must make a choice between responses, response time increases markedly in proportion to the number of alternative responses available to the subject. Choice reactions involve transmission through many synapses and include inputs from the central nervous system as well. There is, in fact, a linear relationship between reaction time and the amount of stimulus information that is provided. For a given increase in stimulus information (i.e., the number of possible responses from which the correct response must be selected), the increase in time required to make the selection is significantly greater for the old than for the young subjects.

AGE CHANGES IN DIFFERENT ORGAN SYSTEMS WITHIN THE SAME SUBJECT

It is only within the past 10 years that the effect of age on the performance of organ systems has been measured in the same normal subjects. Data from the

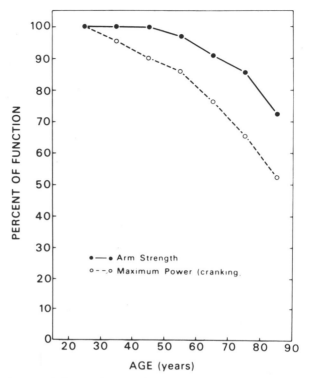

FIG. 4. Age decrements in muscle strength (●——●) compared with maximum power developed in a coordinated movement (cranking) utilizing the same muscle groups (○——○). (From ref. 6.)

Veterans Administration Study of Normal Aging (Boston) and the Baltimore Longitudinal Study of Aging have been analyzed in an attempt to isolate a general aging factor. Factor analyses of the data from both studies have thus far failed to provide evidence for any such factor. In other words, elderly subjects who show a significant reduction in kidney function may or may not show a similar reduction in cardiac performance. A 70-year-old subject may have kidneys that are as good as the average man of 60. Studies of normal subjects as they age emphasize the individual nature of aging. Aging has its primary effects on the cardiovascular system in some subjects, whereas in others the primary effects may be on the muscular system or the kidneys. Thus aging is a complex, multidimensional process which must be evaluated in each individual.

AGING AS A REDUCTION IN ADAPTABILITY: ROLE OF THE NERVOUS SYSTEM

One of the primary characteristics of aging is the gradual impairment of the effectiveness of physiological control mechanisms. Old animals require more time to adjust to physiological displacements induced by environmental factors than do young animals.

The rate of recovery of heart rate, blood pressure, oxygen uptake, and CO_2 elimination following exercise is slower in old subjects than in young, even though the degree of displacement induced by exercise may be less in the old than in the young.

Many regulatory mechanisms operate primarily through the nervous system. The regulation of body temperature, for example, is highly dependent on the activity of the autonomic nervous system, which plays a role in regulating peripheral blood flow.

Aging is associated with a reduction in the ability to maintain body temperature in the face of both increases and decreases in environmental temperature. The regulation of body temperature is a complex process; a primary factor is the regulation of heat loss, which is effected by altering blood flow through the skin. In hot environments cooling is provided by increasing blood flow to the skin, where heat is lost from the body by convection, radiation, and evaporation. In cold environments heat loss is minimized by reducing blood flow to the skin. With increasing age there is a reduction in the ability to maintain body temperature in the face of alterations in environmental temperature. For example, exposure to ambient temperatures of 5° to 15°C for 45 to 120 min produced only insignificant changes in rectal temperature in young subjects, whereas aged subjects showed a fall of 0.5° to 1°C. It is also known that old subjects are much more sensitive to hypothermia than are young ones.

The ability of aged subjects to adjust to increases in environmental temperature is impaired. This is reflected in death rates from heat stroke, which rise sharply after age 60. For example, death rates from heat stroke are reported to increase from 8 per 100,000 deaths for those 70 to 79 years old to 80 per 100,000 deaths for those 90 to 100 years old.

One of the mechanisms involved in the regulation of heart rate in mammals is a lowering of the heart rate when blood pressure rises. This regulatory mechanism operates through the nervous system: The rise in blood pressure is sensed by specific nerve endings in the carotid sinus, which in turn transmit impulses to nerve centers in the central nervous system. These then transmit impulses to the heart to slow its rate. Systolic blood pressure was increased by 50 mm Hg in young and old rats by a continuous intravenous phenylephrine infusion. The rise in blood pressure induced a lowering of the heart rate which was significantly less in the old than in the young animals (Fig. 5). Although the magnitude of the stimulus was the same in the young and old animals, the response was significantly less in the old than in the young.

AGING AS A REDUCTION IN ADAPTABILITY: ROLE OF THE ENDOCRINE SYSTEM

Many physiological processes are regulated by hormones which have specific effects on cellular metabolism. In order to influence cellular processes, hormones

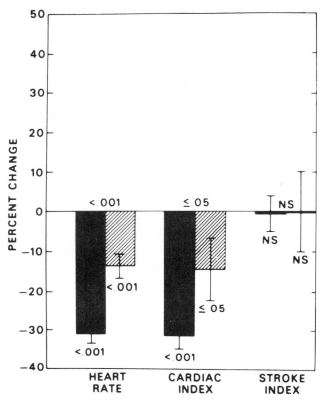

FIG. 5.   Effect of 50 mm Hg increment in systolic blood pressure on heart rate, cardiac index, and stroke index in young (12 months) and old (24 months) unanesthetized rats. The percentage reduction in heart rate and cardiac index was significantly greater (p < 0.001) in the young than the old rats. Young: ■; old: ▨. (From ref. 5.)

must be attached to specific binding sites. Some of these sites are located on cell surfaces (as are binding sites for insulin, epinephrine, and glucagon) or on genetic material located in the nucleus of cells (sites for sex hormones, cortisone, and thyroid hormones). Studies on animals and humans have shown that most target organs which show reduced function during old age respond when exposed to increased levels of the appropriate hormone stimulus. Thus ovaries in postmenopausal women do not secrete estrogens and progesterone in sufficient quantity to maintain the normal menstrual cycle. However, the senescent ovary responds to the administration of estrogenic hormones, and endometrial bleeding can be experimentally re-established in postmenopausal women. From these experiments and others, it is inferred that any reduction of the effectiveness of a physiological process dependent on hormones is a reflection of reduced hormone production rather than a failure in the ability of the target organ to respond, although the degree of responsiveness may be reduced (Chapter 8).

However, more extensive research has shown that some regulatory mechanisms, mediated by the endocrine system, are limited by a reduction in the number of receptors present in cells of old animals. For example, steroid hormone receptor concentrations appear to be reduced in a number of tissues including brain, fat, liver, muscle, and prostate gland in the rat. The receptors present in old tissues, however, show no reduction in their binding capacity. Thus the aging effect seems to depend more on the ability of tissues to maintain normal tissue concentrations of receptors than on the functional capacities of those receptors which are present.

Some metabolic processes are regulated by the formation of specific enzymes. Animal studies have shown that the impairment of these processes with advancing age is primarily due to the reduced rate of enzyme synthesis in senescent animals. Therefore the age effects are a reflection of slower rates of reaction.

The rate at which excess glucose can be removed from the blood falls progressively with advancing age. Measurements of the amount of insulin present in the blood at specific blood glucose levels showed that the reduced rate of glucose removal from the blood in older subjects was due to a reduction in the amount of insulin released into the blood in response to a given blood glucose level. The reduced response of the elderly was due to the lowered sensitivity of the beta cells of the pancreas to a given glucose level in the blood. No age difference in the peripheral utilization of glucose was found.

The cells of the tubular epithelium in the kidney regulate the excretion of water and electrolytes. The level of antidiuretic hormone (ADH) in the circulating blood regulates the amount of water excreted. Normally, when the level of ADH in the blood is increased, the tubular cells of the kidney respond by returning more water from the glomerular filtrate to the blood. Figure 6 shows the response of the kidney in young, middle-aged, and old subjects to an intravenous administration of a standard dose of pitressin (ADH). The low urine/plasma (U/P) ratio for inulin at the beginning of the experiments shows that maximum water diuresis was induced in subjects of all ages at the beginning of the experiment, but the response (inhibition of diuresis with a rise in U/P ratio) was much greater in the young than in the old subjects when a standard dose of pitressin was administered intravenously.

AGING AND REGULATORY MECHANISMS: SITES OF FAILURE

It is my belief that aging is primarily the result of the impairment of control mechanisms rather than impaired performance of any single system.

Any regulatory system must have sensing mechanisms which detect deviation of the critical variable from the normal value and initiate processes to correct the deviation. The effectiveness of the control depends on the sensitivity of the sensing system. Experimental data have been presented to show how aging may reduce the sensitivity of a control mechanism and thus permit deviations in some critical variable. Reduced sensitivity of beta cells of the pancreas to changes in blood glucose concentration which induces the release of insulin into the blood is one example of such an age impairment.

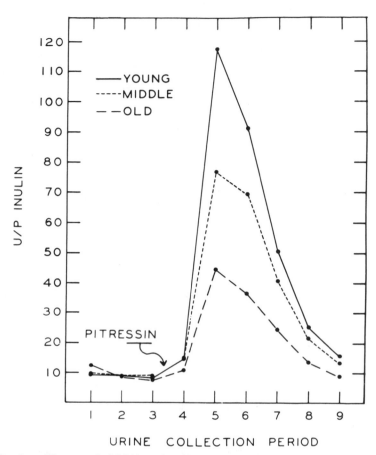

FIG. 6. Age differences in inhibition of water diuresis from intravenous administration of an antidiuretic hormone (pitressin). Mean values of U/P ratio for inulin in each of three age groups are shown for successive 10-min urine collection periods. The response of the old subjects was significantly less than that of the middle-aged or young subjects. (From ref. 2)

However, an effective control mechanism must also have the capability to induce changes that correct deviations. These mechanisms may involve the production of a chemical substance (enzyme, hormone). As aging is often accompanied by the loss of functioning cells, the ability of the old organism to meet these demands may be compromised. For example, the impaired immune response observed in old animals may be a reflection of the reduced rate of cell division. Thus aging may also affect control mechanisms by reducing the capability of the animal to adjust to the stresses of daily living.

SUMMARY

Aging is the overall result of many processes which place limitations on performance and adaptation to environmental stresses. The interrelationships between cells, tissues, and organs are of primary concern in determining the effects of age. Aging in the total animal is more than a simple summation of changes that take place at the cellular, tissue, or organ level. Life in the individual depends on the integrated activity of all of the body's organ systems to meet the varied stresses of daily living. Aging is characterized by a reduction in reserve capacities.

When caring for elderly patients, the physician should:

1. Understand the multivariate nature of aging.
2. Understand how changes in regulatory mechanisms play a central role in determining the alterations of function which occur with aging.
3. Know the wide range of individual differences in the effects of age on physiological performance.
4. Understand how important it is that each elderly patient be evaluated and understood as a unique individual.

REFERENCES

1. Davies, D. F., and Shock, N. W. Age changes in glomerular filtration rate, effective renal plasma flow, and tubular excretory capacity in adult males. *J. Clin. Invest.*, 29:496–507, 1950.
2. Miller, J. H., and Shock, N. W. Age differences in the renal tubular response to antidiuretic hormone. *J. Gerontol.*, 8:446–450, 1953.
3. Rowe, J. W., Andres, R., Tobin, J. D., Norris, A. H., and Shock, N. W. The effect of age on creatinine clearance in men: a cross-sectional and longitudinal study. *J. Gerontol.*, 31:155–163, 1976.
4. Shock, N. W. In: *Proceedings of Seminars*, edited by F. C. Jeffers, pp. 123–140. Center for the Study of Aging and Human Development, Duke University, Durham, NC, 1962.
5. Shock, N. W. In: *Theoretical Aspects of Aging*, edited by M. Rockstein, pp. 119–136. Academic Press, New York, 1974.
6. Shock, N. W., and Norris, A. H. Neuromuscular coordination as a factor in age changes in muscular exercise. In: *Physical Activity and Aging*, edited by D. Brunner and E. Jokl, pp. 92–99. Karger, Basel, 1970.

SUGGESTED READING

Behnke, J. A., Finch, C. E., and Moment, G. B. *The Biology of Aging.* Plenum Press, New York, 1978.

Cander, L., and Moyer, J. H., editors. *Aging of the Lung.* Grune & Stratton, New York, 1964.

Comfort, A. *The Biology of Senescence*, 3rd ed. Elsevier, New York, 1978.

Finch, C. E., and Hayflick, L., editors. *Handbook of the Biology of Aging.* Van Nostrand Reinhold, New York, 1977.

Maletta, G. J., editor. *Survey Report on the Aging Nervous System.* DHEW Publication No. (NIH) 74-296. U.S. Dept. Health, Education and Welfare, Public Health Service, NIH.

Reichel, W., editor. *Clinical Aspects of Aging.* Williams & Wilkins, Baltimore, 1978.

Shock, N. W. Systems integration. In: *Handbook of the Biology of Aging*, edited by C. E. Finch and L. Hayflick, pp. 639–665. Van Nostrand Reinhold, New York, 1977.

Shock, N. W. The process of aging. In: *Health Handbook*, edited by G. K. Chacko. North-Holland, Amsterdam, 1979.

Shock, N. W. Systems physiology and aging. *Fed. Proc.*, 38:161–162, 1979.

Strehler, B. L. *Time, Cells and Aging*, 2nd ed. Academic Press, New York, 1977.

Fundamentals of Geriatric Medicine, edited by
Ronald D.T. Cape, Rodney M. Coe, and Isadore
Rossman, Raven Press, New York © 1983.

8

Age-Related Physiological Changes in the Cardiovascular System

Owen W. Beard

There are a large number of physiological changes in the cardiovascular system with aging. The most significant of these changes in terms of affecting function of the aged cardiovascular system fall into two categories: physiological changes in the vascular system and those in the heart.

PHYSIOLOGICAL CHANGES IN THE VASCULAR SYSTEM

Effect of Aging on Blood Pressure

Systemic blood pressure increases with age. The greater mean systolic pressure during the older decades is offset by a lower heart rate response to exercise, with the result that both the tension time index and the calculated cardiac work do not reflect an age effect on the workload of the heart. The diastolic blood pressure response to exercise is not different in the young and the aged. However, compared to pre-exercise values, aged individuals have a greater increase in their systolic blood pressure levels after exercise than do young adults. In addition, the time required for the systolic blood pressure to return to normal or pre-exercise levels is longer in the aged. The decrease in cardiac output of about 1% per year in mature adults, coupled with the increase in arterial blood pressure, makes it obvious that the total peripheral resistance increases with aging.

Effect of Aging on Baroreceptors

Experimental studies suggest the presence of stretch receptors (baroreceptors) at many sites in the cardiovascular system, including the abdominal vessels, cerebral vessels, descending thoracic aorta, pulmonary vessels, atria, and even the walls of the ventricles. Few of these have been clearly implicated, however, in the control of blood pressure. The two most important reflexes involved in regulating arterial pressure are the baroreceptor reflexes, with the receptors located in the aortic arch and the carotid sinus regions. These two reflexes have been shown to become less sensitive as one ages. This decrease in sensitivity is not the result of an altered blood pressure; rather, because these are stretch reflexes and the aorta and carotid sinus areas are favorite sites for atherosclerotic changes, it seems likely that the reduced sensitivity of these baroreceptor reflexes results from the decreased distensibility of the arterial wall in which the baroreceptors are located.

The best understood arterial stretch receptor is that located in the carotid sinus. At the bifurcation of the common carotid artery into the external and internal carotids, there is a dilatation of the first portion of the internal carotid artery, called the carotid sinus. It has a thinner wall than arteries of the same caliber, being somewhat deficient in smooth muscle and having an unusual amount of elastic tissue. Such an arrangement appears to make the area particularly suitable for monitoring intravascular pressure or stretch by baroreceptors located there. The frequency with which a stretch receptor discharges is dependent on the arterial pressure and the distensibility of the vessel. A drop in arterial pressure leads to a decrease in pressoreceptor impulse frequency, which in turn leads to a decrease in vagus nerve impulses and an increase in the rate of sympathetic nerve impulses, thus leading to an increase in the heart rate. An increase in activity of the sympathetic vasoconstrictor fibers leads to an increase in peripheral resistance. The net effect is to raise blood pressure. If the arterial pressure rises above the "normal set value," the impulse frequency of carotid sinus nerves increases, leading to a reduced sympathetic discharge and an increasing vagal discharge. This leads to slowing of the heart rate and peripheral vasodilatation, which returns the blood pressure to normal.

It is easy to see how the age-related decreased sensitivity of these baroreceptors could interfere with the ability of the aged vascular system to make immediate and precise readjustments to such stresses as changes in body position and activities which involve a valsalva maneuver. When the aged individual stands, with a resultant decrease in return of blood to the heart, the cardiac output decreases and the pressure in the aortic arch and carotid sinus area drops. Because of the decreased sensitivity of these baroreceptor reflexes, there may not be a compensatory increase in blood pressure and an increase in heart rate sufficient to maintain adequate cerebral blood flow. Thus the aged individual is apt to develop symptomatic orthostatic hypotension and may even lose consciousness upon standing.

It should not be surprising that measurable postural falls of blood pressure occur in otherwise healthy old people. The magnitude of the postural drop in systolic pressure is greater in those over 75 years of age, almost one-third of whom demonstrate a decrease in standing systolic pressure of at least 20 mm Hg. Most elderly people can tolerate this drop without any loss of consciousness. However, when an elevation in body temperature or a decrease in blood volume due to bleeding, inadequate fluid intake, or overenthusiastic use of potent diuretics is added to the already compromised vascular system, postural syncope and falls may result. When the decreased systolic standing pressure is accompanied by an inability to increase the cardiac output by increasing the heart rate, syncope is likely to occur. The absence of a rate response may be the result of the decreased sensitivity of the baroreceptor reflexes with age, or it might result from a decreased automaticity of the sinoatrial node.

Effect of Aging on Maintenance of Stable Central Venous Pressure

When a person arises from a supine to a standing position, about 650 to 750 ml of blood leaves the chest and is pooled in the abdomen and legs; the distending pressure on the right atrium then falls to or below the mean intrathoracic pressure. Before this can result in an absence of right atrial filling and failure of the left side of the heart to deliver blood, several compensatory reflexes normally restore the status quo. These adjustments are so effective and prompt in the fit young adult that systemic arterial pressure measured at the level of the upper arm drops only transiently upon standing. As individuals become older, these control mechanisms become less efficient, making the aged subjects more prone to develop symptomatic postural hypotension, especially when getting out of a comfortable chair in a warm room or when rising from a prolonged hot bath.

Maintenance of central venous pressure within a very narrow critical range requires that the venous system compensate for variations in blood volume and changes in its distribution. The transmural pressure in the thoracic portions of the inferior and superior vena cava is of great importance because it represents the filling pressure of the right heart. A positive effective filling pressure must be maintained in those veins regardless of the magnitude of blood volume, the redistribution of blood in dilated capillary beds, the accumulation of blood in distended veins, or the position of the body. Excessive pressure in these veins would raise the pressure gradient in both the venous and lymphatic systems and lead to accumulation of extravascular fluid.

In the erect position the hydrostatic columns of blood produce distension of vessels below the heart and venous collapse above the heart. Unless compensatory adjustments are promptly effective, the central venous pressure may fall below the right atrial level, and the effective filling pressure (intravenous pressure minus extravascular pressure) could drop to zero. A decrease in central venous pressure of only a few centimeters of water could result in a serious impairment of right ventricular filling and hence a decrease in cardiac output. This is prevented by precise and continuous adjustments in the venous reservoir system to maintain the central venous pressure at levels only slightly above that of the right atrium, regardless of the position of the body. The aged individual can still make adjustments, for to do otherwise is not compatible with life. However, the adjustments are neither as precise nor as continuously effective in the aged, thereby making them more vulnerable to conditions which add extra stress to these physiological mechanisms. Conditions such as dehydration or loss of blood volume, varicose veins, and infection may seriously impair the aged individual's ability to maintain the filling pressure necessary for an adequate cardiac output. Disturbances in consciousness and falls may be the result.

PHYSIOLOGICAL CHANGES IN THE HEART WITH AGING

Effect of Aging on Ventricular Compliance

Aging produces an increase in collagenous and amyloid deposits in the heart. Although the relationship may not be proved, these increases in collagen and heavy ventricular amyloid are thought to be factors in the decreased compliance with impairment of ventricular filling that occurs with aging. This decreased ventricular compliance may also be responsible for the increased S4 gallop sounds in the elderly patient. The left and right ventricular filling pressures at rest are normal, or the same, in both young and old individuals. During exercise, however, these filling pressures increase significantly more in the aged. The increased filling pressures during exercise in old age are thought to be necessary adjustments to overcome the decreased ventricular compliance and are therefore an essential step in increasing the stroke volume.

Effect of Aging on Cardiac Output

Cross-sectional studies suggest that cardiac output during exercise in both the sitting and supine positions, or at rest in the supine position, is lower in elderly men than in young men. The decrease in cardiac output at rest and during sub-maximal exercise is the result of a reduction in stroke volume. The cardiac index has been estimated to decrease by 0.8% per year with aging (Chapter 5, Fig. 3). Older subjects cannot develop as great an increase in cardiac output during maximal exertion as young subjects. The left ventricular ejection fraction at peak exercise is lower in older individuals, and the magnitude of change from resting values to exercise values is inversely related to age.

Effect of Aging on Sinus Node Function

There is a decreased automaticity of the sinoatrial node, with a decrease in the maximal heart rate response to stress. There is no significant change with age in the resting heart rate or with the heart rate response to submaximal workloads. There is an increase of fibrotic tissue in the sinoatrial node and in the intranodal tracts with muscle fiber loss. As it is universally accepted that automaticity is a function of these muscle fibers, this may account for the increased frequency with which old age is accompanied by a disturbance in rate and rhythm. Slowing of the sinus node rate allows other areas in the heart to become the site for initiation of arrhythmias. Atrial arrhythmias are common and easily induced in the elderly. This is perhaps related to the fibrosis and dilatation of the atria with damage to atrial muscle which occurs in the aged. The exact role of decreased ventricular compliance in the production of atrial arrhythmias is not known.

Effect of Aging on Valvular Function

The thickening and increased rigidity of the heart valves that occur with age are usually not severe enough to produce hemodynamic consequences unless they are superimposed on an underlying organic heart disease. These changes do present problems in the interpretation of the decreased E-F slope of the anterior mitral leaflet as seen on the echocardiogram of elderly patients. The decreased E-F slope might indicate that the rate of early diastolic filling of the left ventricle was diminished; conversely, the changes in the leaflets themselves might account for the decreased E-F slope.

Effect of Aging on Myocardial Function

The tension period phase and the ejection period are prolonged in the elderly. Diastole is somewhat shortened, and the maximum rate of rise of left ventricular pressure decreases. Extracardiac nervous influences on the heart are weakened with age. The heart synthesizes less norepinephrine, so the catecholamine content per gram of wet heart tissue is less in aged than in young animals. The sensitivity of the cardiovascular system to acetylcholine and catecholamines increases with age, but its reactive capacity diminishes. There are no detailed, *in vitro* studies of the contractile characteristics of human cardiac muscle. However, it is well known that the aged myocardium is not capable of withstanding stress as well as that of young individuals. Thus congestive heart failure is apt to be precipitated by infections, especially of the pulmonary system, as well as by anemia, thyrotoxicosis, fluid overload, and tachyarrhythmias. For this reason, congestive heart failure in elderly individuals is apt to be transitory and often responds satisfactorily to treatment or removal of the stressful condition.

SUMMARY

The normal physiological changes in the cardiovascular system with aging are those which impair the body's ability to make the prompt and sudden adjustments necessary to maintain an adequate cardiac output at all times and under all conditions. Compensatory adjustments can be made up to a point, but they require more time to restore the cardiac output to an adequate level. Thus the aged individual is more vulnerable to the development of transitory episodes of heart failure as well as to syncope or falls which may result from a sudden discrepancy between the cardiac output and that necessary to maintain adequate cerebral flow.

When caring for elderly patients, the physician should:

1. Know the changes in physiological function of the cardiovascular system which usually occur with aging.
2. Know how such changes produce impairment of function or modify the expression of cardiovascular diseases in the aged.
3. Know how orthostatic hypotension may develop and be expressed in the elderly patient.

4. Know how the changes that occur with aging may make the cardiovascular system vulnerable to temporary dysfunction under a variety of stressful circumstances.

SUGGESTED READING

Caird, R. I., Andrews, G. R., and Kennedy, R. D. Effect of posture on blood pressure in the elderly. *Br. Heart J.*, 34:527–530, 1973.

Norris, A. H., Shock, N. W., and Yiengst, M. J. Age changes in heart rate and blood pressure responses to tilting and standardized exercise. *Circulation*, 8:521–526, 1953.

Ostfeld, A. M., and Gibson, D. C. *Epidemiology of Aging*, pp. 137–160. DHEW Publication No. (NIH) 75–711. NIH, Bethesda, MD, 1972.

Port, S., Cobb, F. R., Coleman, R. E., and Jones, R. H. Effect of age on the response of left ventricular ejection fraction to exercise. *N. Engl. J. Med.*, 303:1133–1137, 1980.

Rushmer, R. F. *Cardiovascular Dynamics*, 3rd ed. Saunders, Philadelphia, 1970.

Sebban, C., Job, D., Caen, J. L., et al. Ventricular compliance and aging. *Biomedicine*, 22:56–61, 1973.

Strandell, T. Cardiac output in old age. In: *Cardiology in Old Age*, edited by F. I. Caird, J. L. C. Dall, and R. D. Kennedy, pp. 81–100. Plenum Press, New York, 1976.

Fundamentals of Geriatric Medicine, edited by
Ronald D. T. Cape, Rodney M. Coe, and Isadore
Rossman, Raven Press, New York © 1983.

9

Influence of Age on Renal Function

John W. Rowe

Advancing age is associated with a progressive reduction in renal mass. Studies have shown the normal human kidney to shrink from 250 g at age 40 to 200 g at age 80. A progressive reduction in renal plasma flow (RPF) with advancing age is well established and is contributed to by age-related decreases in cardiac output and reduction in the renal vascular bed. (Also see Chapter 5, Figs. 1–3.)

HISTOLOGICAL CHANGES

The loss of renal mass is primarily cortical, with relative sparing of the renal medulla; it seems to be secondary to very distinctive intrarenal vascular changes that are associated with advancing age (8). Two patterns of changes in arteriolar-glomerular units have been noted with senescence. In one type, hyalinization and collapse of the glomerular tuft is associated with obliteration of the lumen of the preglomerular arteriole and a resultant loss in blood flow. This type of change is seen primarily in the cortical area. The second pattern, seen primarily in the juxtamedullary area, is characterized by the development of anatomical continuity between afferent and efferent arterioles during glomerular sclerosis. The endpoint is thus loss of the glomerulus and shunting of blood flow from afferent to efferent arterioles. This maintains blood flow to the arteriolae rectae verae, the primary vascular supply of the medulla, which are not decreased in number with age.

The functional reflections of these histological changes can be seen in the studies of Hollenberg et al. (5), who, by employing xenon washout techniques, demonstrated that the decline in renal plasma flow with age actually represents a decrease in perfusion per gram of renal tissue and is not just a reflection of diminished renal size. The decreased flow is most profound in the cortex, with relative sparing of flow to inner zones. As juxtamedullary glomeruli have a greater filtration fraction (that fraction of plasma flow filtered at the glomerulus) than cortical glomeruli, this shunting from cortex to medulla may account for the slight but definite increase in filtration fraction with advancing age. These cortical vascular changes probably also account for the patchy cortical defects commonly seen on renal scanning of healthy elderly persons. The intrarenal vascular changes are associated with loss, from age 30 to 80 years, of approximately 30% of the glomeruli. Of the remaining, more than 10% of identifiable glomeruli are sclerosed in 80-year-olds, compared to only 1% in young adults. Electron microscopic studies of the basement membrane of remaining intact glomeruli in aged kidneys have shown a prominent reduplication and focal thickening. These findings are also present in tubular basement membranes in aged kidneys. Studies of the filtration characteristics of intact glomeruli have shown no changes in glomerular pore size with advancing age.

CHANGES IN GLOMERULAR FILTRATION RATE

The major, clinically relevant defect in renal function arising from these histological and physiological changes is a progressive decline after maturity in the glomerular filtration rate (GFR). As creatinine clearance is frequently used as a measure of the presence and severity of impaired GFR, age-adjusted "normative" standards for creatinine clearance are needed. These have recently been established in studies at the Gerontology Research Center of the National Institute on Aging based on 24-hr urinary creatinine clearance values on a large, healthy, community-dwelling male population, age 17 to 96 years (6).

Results in the 548 normal subjects showed that creatinine clearance is stable until the middle of the fourth decade, when a linear decrease of about 6.5 mg/min/1.73 M^2/decade begins. The reduction in creatinine clearance with age is attended by a parallel reduction in daily urinary creatinine excretion, reflecting decreased muscle mass. The net effect is that there is no significant change in serum creatinine with age. Therefore a healthy 80-year-old man will have creatinine clearance of 32 ml/min/1.73 M^2 less than his 30-year-old counterpart but with the same serum creatinine. Thus depression of GFR so severe as to result in elevation of serum creatinine (above 1.5 mg/dl) is rarely due solely to normal aging; it indicates the presence of an additional disease. These considerations affect the dosage of drugs such as digoxin and aminoglycosides, which are primarily excreted by the kidneys (Chapter 16).

FLUID AND ELECTROLYTE BALANCE

The changes in GFR with advancing age influence the elderly person's adaptive mechanisms which are responsible for maintaining constancy of the extracellular fluid. Because of these physiological changes, acute illness in geriatric patients is often complicated by derangements in fluid and electrolyte balance which delay recovery and prolong hospitalization.

These changes in homeostasis are best understood in terms of renal sodium and water excretion after acute alterations in salt and fluid intake. The aged kidney's response to sodium deficiency is blunted. Studies on the renal response to acute reduction in salt intake (100 to 10 mEq sodium diet) have shown that, although aged patients are capable of sodium conservation and reaching salt balance on this markedly restricted intake, their response is sluggish when compared to that of younger adults (2). The half-time for reduction in urinary sodium after salt restriction is 17 hr in the young and 31 hr in old subjects. The cumulative sodium deficit before daily renal losses equal intake is thus greater in the elderly. As old patients are more likely to experience confusion, loss of thirst, and disorientation when acutely ill, this "salt-losing" tendency is aggravated by not having adequate salt intake, leading to further depletion of the extracellular fluid volume as well as impaired cardiac, renal, and mental function. This vicious cycle too often continues after hospitalization when physicians, dreading pulmonary edema, are reluctant to administer substantial amounts of sodium-containing fluids intravenously to the acutely ill volume-depleted geriatric patient. This salt-losing tendency of the senescent kidney is a function of both nephron loss, with increased osmotic load per nephron, and mild osmotic diuresis.

Another important age-related alteration that mimics a specific pathophysiological entity is the change in the renin-aldosterone system (3,9). It is now well established that basal renin, whether estimated by plasma renin concentration or renin activity, is diminished by 30 to 50% in the elderly in the face of normal levels of renin substrate. This basal difference between young and old is magnified by maneuvers designed to augment renin secretion, e.g., salt restriction, diuretic administration, or upright posture.

The lowered renin levels are associated with 30 to 50% reduction in plasma concentrations of aldosterone as well as significant reductions in the secretion and metabolic clearance rates of aldosterone. That aldosterone deficiency of old age is a function of the coexisting renin deficiency and not secondary to intrinsic adrenal changes is suggested by studies showing that plasma aldosterone and cortisol responses after ACTH stimulation are not impaired with advancing age (Chapter 10).

The impact of normal aging on plasma renin must be considered when designating hypertensive patients to specific pathophysiological groups based on renin levels. A hypertensive geriatric patient, or occasionally a normotensive patient with the normal elevation of systolic blood pressure seen with advancing age, may be diagnosed as having "low renin hypertension" when in actuality the renin level is not low but normal for the patient's age. This can lead to confusing or inappropriate conclusions in clinical studies, as the relationship between the normal reduction in renin with aging and the low renin levels seen in some young hypertensive patients is unknown. These alterations in the renin-aldosterone system may contribute to the increased risk of elderly patients developing hyperkalemia in a variety of clinical settings. Through its action on the distal renal tubule, aldosterone increases sodium reabsorption and facilitates renal excretion of potassium. Aldosterone represents one of the major protective mechanisms preventing hyperkalemia during periods of potassium challenge. As glomerular filtration rate, another major determinant of potassium excretion, is also impaired in old patients, these individuals are apt to develop serious elevations of plasma potassium, especially when given potassium salts intravenously. This tendency toward hyperkalemia is further aggravated in any clinical setting associated with acidosis, as the senescent kidney is sluggish in its response to acid loading, resulting in prolonged depression of pH and concomitant potassium elevation. Similarly, diuretics which impair renal potassium excretion (e.g., spironolactone or triamterene) should be administered to the elderly with caution.

Just as old patients are more likely to develop volume depletion when salt-deprived, volume expansion is also a commonly encountered problem. Primarily because of its lower GFR, the senescent kidney is less able to excrete an acutely administered salt load than the younger kidney. Geriatric patients with or without pre-existing myocardial disease are thus at risk of expansion of the extracellular fluid volume when faced with an acute salt load (e.g., inappropriate intravenous fluids, dietary indiscretion) or, as commonly happens, after the administration of sodium-rich radiographic contrast agents such as those employed in intravenous pyelography.

The clinical impact of the aged kidney's inability to properly regulate salt balance when stressed is compounded by similar abnormalities in water metabolism. Old patients are less able to concentrate their urine after water deprivation or the administration of high doses of vasopressin (Chapter 5, Fig. 6), and maximal urine concentration at age 80 is about 70% of that at age 30 (7). The cause of this defect is uncertain, but the defect is most likely due to the age-related reduction in GFR, as well as the relative shunting of blood to the renal medulla with advancing age. This conservation of medullary flow, in the face of a reduction in nephron number and cortical flow, might result in enhanced removal of solute from the medullary interstitium, a "washout" effect that could reduce the efficacy of the countercurrent system. Although this decline in water-conserving capacity is not so severe as to have clinical significance under conditions of free access to water, it becomes important when fluid intake is limited and in the presence of higher than ordinary insensible losses, e.g., with fever. Under such conditions, elevations of the serum sodium concentration to levels which impair mental function are commonly seen in the geriatric age group. Thus both the salt- and water-losing tendencies of the senescent kidney contribute to the common clinical presentation of acutely or sub-acutely ill elderly patients with hypertonic volume depletion.

Perhaps the most serious and least well recognized electrolyte disorder in geriatric patients is their tendency to develop water intoxication. The clinical presentation of hyponatremia is nonspecific, with depression, confusion, lethargy, anorexia, and weakness the most common findings. When hyponatremia is severe (serum sodium concentrations below 110 mEq/L), seizures and stupor may be seen. Most frequently the water intoxication complicates an acute or subacute illness, or is associated with the administration of diuretics or medications known to impair water excretion. However, in our experience it is not unusual for geriatric patients to become hyponatremic in the setting of any stress, whether it is surgery, fever, or acute virile illness. Clinical evaluation of the elderly hyponatremic patient usually reveals a constellation of findings consistent with oversecretion of antidiruetic hormone (ADH) as a cause of the water retention. These include, in addition to the low serum sodium, evidence of good renal function (low blood urea nitrogen), mild extracellular fluid expansion (normal to slightly full neck veins, trace edema), and evidence of inappropriate renal water retention (urine osmolality greater than maximally dilute and, in many cases, more concentrated than serum). In addition, excess ADH secretion, because of the slight extracellular fluid expansion and the subsequent reduction in aldosterone secretion and elevation of GFR, is associated with the presence of modest to large amounts of salt in the urine.

Excess ADH secretion is commonly associated with pneumonia, tuberculosis, stroke, meningitis, subdural hematoma, and a variety of other pulmonary and central nervous system disorders. Although all age groups may develop hyponatremia in these settings, the elderly seem particularly prone to this complication. This may also hold true for drug-induced ADH excess; in one study elderly patients accounted for most cases of hyponatremia developing from use of chlorpropamide. The stress of anesthesia and surgery have also been shown to result in water intoxication with excess ADH secretion, a complication seen most often in elderly patients (1). We have seen, over the past 2 to 3 years, several elderly patients who developed hyponatremia with laboratory concomitants of excess ADH secretion in a variety of clinical settings, including fever, psychological stress, and acute viral illness. While hyponatremic these patients are unable to excrete a water load, but after resolution of the acute illness water metabolism is normal. In many cases the same patient has returned several weeks or months later with another acute illness and, again, hyponatremia.

These clinical data suggesting oversecretion of ADH with advancing age are supported by anatomical studies showing an increased size of the supraoptic and paraventricular nuclei (hypothalamic sites of ADH production) in the elderly. In order to clarify the impact of normal aging on ADH secretion, Helderman and co-workers (4) studied the response of healthy young and old subjects to infusions of hypertonic saline (as a stimulus for ADH release) and ethanol (as a test of pharmacological inhibition of ADH).

In the hypertonic saline studies, the ADH levels in the young subjects were 2.5 times the basal concentration in response to an increase in plasma osmolality from 290 to 306 mOsm/kg. In the old subjects, on the other hand, the circulating ADH level increased 4.5-fold in response to the same osmolar challenge. During ethanol infusion, which is known to inhibit ADH secretion, the plasma ADH level steadily declined throughout the 1-hr infusion in the young group. In the older subjects, after an initial decrease there was no pharmacological inhibition and the ADH secretion began to increase, returning to basal values by the end of the infusion. These data provide physiological support for the concept that the clinically observed excess in ADH secretion in the elderly represents a result of normal aging and underlines the importance of a high degree of suspicion for hyponatremia in geriatric patients, particularly in view of the slow, insidious nature of the development of water intoxication and its nonspecific clinical presentation. Physicians caring for the elderly should be cautious when prescribing medications known to increase

ADH secretion, as well as in the administration of hypotonic fluids in the setting of recent surgery or any acute illness.

SUMMARY

As the body ages, so too does the renal tissue. Its weight is reduced by 50 g between ages 40 and 80, and renal plasma flow is decreased, as is the GFR. The creatinine clearance is reduced with age, but there is no change in serum creatinine. Hence if the serum creatinine is elevated in an elderly person, it usually signals the presence of some pathological process.

The GFR alterations seen in old people are often responsible for the derangements in fluid and electrolyte balance seen in acutely ill patients. Sodium deficits are common, and this salt-losing tendency may result in impaired cardiac, renal, and mental function. The renin–aldosterone system also suffers, which is important to hypertensive patients.

"Water intoxication" is a danger to elderly patients due to their electrolyte imbalance. Although not well known among physicians, it is perhaps the most serious of these complications.

When caring for elderly patients, the physician should:

1. Be aware of the influence of age on "normal" laboratory measures of kidney function.
2. Be familiar with the physiological basis of increased risk of fluid and electrolyte problems in the elderly.
3. Be familiar with fluid and electrolyte complications of acute illness in the elderly.

REFERENCES

1. Deutsch, S., Goldberg, M., and Dripps, R. D. Postoperative hyponatremia with the inappropriate release of antidiuretic hormone. *Anesthesiology*, 27:250–256, 1966.
2. Epstein, M., and Hollenberg, N. K. Age as a determinant of renal sodium conservation in normal men. *J. Lab. Clin. Med.*, 87:411–417, 1976.
3. Flood, C., Gherondache, C., Pincus, G., et al. The metabolism and secretion of aldosterone in elderly subjects. *J. Clin. Invest.*, 46:960–966, 1976.
4. Helderman, J. H., Vestal, R. E., Rowe, J. W., et al. The response of arginine vasopressin to intravenous ethanol and hypertonic saline in man: the impact of aging. *J. Gerontol.*, 33:39–47, 1978.
5. Hollenberg, N. K., Adams, D. F., Solomon, N. S., et al. Senescence and the renal vasculature in normal man. *Circ. Res.*, 34:309–316, 1974.
6. Rowe, J. W., Andres, R., Tobin, J. D., et al. The effect of age on creatinine clearance in men: cross-sectional and longitudinal study. *J. Gerontol.*, 31:155–163, 1976.
7. Rowe, J. W., Shock, N. W., and DeFronzo, R. A. The influence of age on the renal response to water deprivation in man. *Nephron*, 17:270–278, 1976.
8. Takazakura, E., Wasabu, N., Handa, A., et al. Intrarenal vascular changes with age and disease. *Kidney Int.*, 2:224–230, 1972.
9. Weidmann, P., DeMyttenaeu-Bursztein, S., Maxwell, M. H., et al. Effect of aging on plasma renin and aldosterone in normal man. *Kidney Int.*, 8:325–333, 1975.

Fundamentals of Geriatric Medicine, edited by
Ronald D.T. Cape, Rodney M. Coe, and Isadore
Rossman, Raven Press, New York © 1983.

10

Age-Related Change in Endocrine Function

Paul J. Davis and Faith B. Davis

Several changes in endocrine function are observed in the course of normal aging:

1. Primary alterations in hormone secretory rates may occur. Progressive loss of secretory cell mass is involved in loss of estrogen secretion in women; this change is unique to the ovary, rather than a model of aging for the endocrine system, and its mechanism is unknown.
2. Rates of hormone degradation by nonendocrine tissues may decline with age. Through widely known negative feedback loops, these changes in hormone metabolism lead secondarily to proportionate decreases in hormone secretory rates. As a result, levels of these hormones in blood (e.g., cortisol and thyroxine) are unchanged with age.
3. Alterations in end-organ sensitivity to hormones may develop. Examples of such end-organs are the pituitary gland—whose response to thyrotropin-releasing hormone (TRH) administration in men falls with age—and the distal renal tubule, which becomes less responsive to antidiuretic hormone (ADH) (Chapter 7).
4. Recent evidence suggests that tissue insulin responsiveness declines with normal aging. This finding may contribute to changes in carbohydrate tolerance which are typical of aging but do not imply the presence of diabetes mellitus.
5. Sensors which modulate endocrine feedback loops may change during the course of aging. Perhaps the glucose sensor for insulin secretion in the β-cell is less sensitive with increased age, and certainly the responsiveness of the renin-angiotensin-aldosterone axis to assumption of the upright posture and volume depletion is depressed in normal elderly subjects (Chapter 7).

This chapter emphasizes changes in endocrine physiology and points out that the expression and epidemiology of endocrine *diseases* may change with age. Adrenocortical diseases, for example, are uncommon in the elderly, whereas as many as 20% of hyperthyroid patients are over 60 years of age. The absence of goiter in older thyrotoxic patients is common, as is single-system (e.g., heart or gastrointestinal tract) expression of thyroid disease.

PITUITARY-THYROID AXIS

When subjects with nonthyroidal illness are meticulously excluded from study, it is clear that there are no age-specific changes in serum concentrations of thyroxine (T_4), triiodothyronine (T_3), or thyrotropin (TSH) in adult man (25). Serum levels of reverse T_3, free T_4, and free T_3 are also unaltered by age. In the context of these observations, it is not surprising that the basal metabolic rate (BMR), expressed as a function of lean body mass (see *Overview* to this section), is unchanged over the life span (33). Earlier evidence that serum levels of thyroid hormone decline with age depended on the inclusion of data from "euthyroid sick" subjects in whom changes in hormone metabolism could be expected independent of the factor of age. There is, however, an age- and sex-specific change in pituitary gland responsiveness to the administration of TRH, so that normal elderly men can have depressed secretion of pituitary TSH after TRH injection (29). The physiological significance of this change is unknown. Failure to appreciate this age-dependent change in TRH response can lead clinically to an erroneous conclusion in a healthy man that hypopituitarism or excess thyroid hormone action is present. The response of the thyroid gland itself to TSH is intact in terms of the ability of the gland to secrete thyroid hormone.

Although levels of circulating thyroid hormone are stable thoughout healthy adult life, it is known that normal aging has a substantial effect on thyroid hormone metabolism and secretion. The half-life ($t_{1/2}$) of T_4 increases over the normal life span (16). Because serum T_4 levels are constant, a decrease in hormone secretory rate must accompany the change in peripheral (i.e., extrathyroidal) degradation of T_4. The alteration in secretory rate is presumably accomplished via reduced basal levels of endogenous TSH. One would predict that thyroid hormone replacement dosage in elderly patients with thyroidal hypothyroidism is lower than that needed in younger subjects. Recent preliminary evidence in fact indicates that replacement dosage of thyroid hormone—expressed on the basis of dose per kilogram body weight per day—in elderly hypothyroid subjects is 30% lower than that required in younger patients (7).

Decreased iodide trapping by the thyroid gland is also a concomitant of normal aging (11), perhaps as a function of the downward adjustment of secretion described above or due to age-dependent change in renal iodide excretion. The clinical correlate is an age-related decline in thyroidal radioiodide accumulation rate.

No satisfactory data are available to clarify the issue of advancing age and tissue ("end-organ") sensitivity to thyroid hormone in man. A clinical bias exists that "sensitivity" of certain organs (heart, gastrointestinal tract) may be altered differentially with age and account for "monosystemic" hyperthyroidism (8). Expression of certain manifestations of hyperthyroidism may reflect changes in end-organ sensitivity to catecholamines, e.g., control by thyroid hormone of the ratio of cell α- and β-adrenergic receptors, as shown in animal models (21). These animal studies have not, however, focused specifically on a possible aging effect.

There is no clinical evidence to support the possibility raised in animal studies that the pituitary-thyroid axis materially influences the aging process. Nor is there evidence that a pervasive change in hypothalamic function occurs during aging and results in an altered hormone feedback loop.

PARATHYROID GLAND AND CALCIUM METABOLISM

Little is known about the effect of normal aging on serum total calcium concentration. Wiske et al. reported that serum ionized calcium content falls slightly with age (36), as does serum phosphate [in the face of an age-dependent decrease in glomerular filtration rate (GFR)]. A putative corollary of the change in serum ionized calcium content is an increase in circulating levels of intact and carboxy-terminal (C-terminal) immunoreactive parathyroid hormone (iPTH). A fall in GFR would result in increased iPTH levels. A preliminary report from another laboratory, however, indicates that serum iPTH levels are constant over the adult life span.

More relevant is the contention that the action of PTH may be potentiated in elderly women as a function of estrogen lack (12); it has been proposed that estrogen deficiency also predisposes women to hyperparathyroidism (23). Thus even if iPTH levels were constant with age, a change in end-organ (bone) sensitivity to this hormone could lead to bone demineralization. The possibility that osteoporosis is mediated by PTH is not widely accepted, however.

Evidence of both decreased and normal dietary calcium absorption in elderly normal subjects has been reported (14,30). It has been suggested that the amount of dietary calcium required to maintain positive calcium balance increases with age, reaching levels not consumed by most elderly persons. Intestinal calcium absorption is directly influenced by levels of vitamin D metabolites. Decreases in 25-hydroxylation of vitamin D (31), and renal 1-hydroxylation (13) of this substance have been reported in older subjects. These biochemical steps are important in the activation of vitamin D; impairment of hydroxylation leads to decreased mineralization of osteoid (osteomalacia). In the United States osteomalacia is not currently acknowledged to be a frequent finding in elderly subjects. It should also be pointed out that some observations dealing with vitamin D metabolism have been drawn from geriatric hospital populations, and it may not be possible to distinguish the effects of age and of debilitation and lack of exposure to sunlight on circulating levels of vitamin D and its metabolites. A recent study of vitamin D levels in clearly healthy elderly subjects in fact showed normal concentrations of this vitamin (30).

Studies of plasma calcitonin levels in subjects aged 20 to 80 years have shown a progressive decrease in basal levels with aging in both sexes (10). The response of calcitonin to calcium infusion was also inversely proportional to age, with a more marked reduction in women than in men. A decline with age in circulating levels of calcitonin could predispose to bone demineralization, as this hormone inhibits bone resorption.

PITUITARY-ADRENOCORTICAL AXIS

Advancing age does not alter plasma levels of cortisol (15). However, the cortisol degradation rate falls with age and is accompanied, secondarily, by a fall in glucocorticoid secretory rate. It is presumed that the latter change is simply a matter of negative feedback loop adjustment in endogenous adrenocorticotropine hormone (ACTH) release. The ability of the pituitary gland to release ACTH in response to stress (e.g., hypoglycemia) or to metyrapone is intact in older subjects (5,20), and it is clear that in man the response of the adrenal cortex to exogenous ACTH administration is intact through adult life. It has not been determined if the suppressibility of the pituitary-adrenal axis remains normal with advancing age. There is increasing interest in the validity of acute suppressibility of the pituitary-adrenal axis as a diagnostic test of the presence of depressive disorders (6). It is therefore important to establish if the administration of the potent glucocorticoid dexamethasone suppresses pituitary ACTH release as readily in older individuals as it does in young subjects.

In contrast to glucocorticoid secretion, important alterations in aldosterone release accompany normal aging. Although basal plasma aldosterone content (subject supine, dietary salt intake normal) is stable over the life span, stimulated levels of aldosterone (subject upright, dietary sodium restricted) are clearly decreased in older subjects, compared to the young. The response of plasma renin activity (PRA) to change in posture and dietary salt restriction or diuresis is also depressed in the elderly (24). It is not yet clear if the change in aldosterone secretory response is secondary, as one would suspect, to the change in PRA responsiveness. The biological significance of these alterations is not known. The clinical significance of such findings is twofold: (a) failure to appreciate that the renin-aldosterone axis is relatively unresponsive in the elderly can lead to the incorrect impression that selective hypoaldosteronism is present; and (b) the validity of the classification of "low-renin hypertension" is arguable in older patients (Chapter 4).

GONADAL FUNCTION

Inexorable decrease in ovarian function in middle-aged women and secondary increases in pituitary FSH and LH secretion are hallmarks of normal aging (Chapter 24). In rats, however, "senescent" ovaries may be returned to the functional state by pharmacological (and other) means (26). It is important to point out several other features of the aging pituitary-gonadal axis that occur in women in addition to decreases in secretion of estradiol, estrone, progesterone, and 17-hydroxyprogesterone and the enhancement of FSH and LH release. For example, the postmenopausal ovary continues to produce androgens (testosterone and androstenedione) (35). That the ovary is an important source of these steroids has been shown by comparing serum hormone profiles in spontaneously menopausal and ovariectomized women. Androstenedione may be converted in liver and adipose tissue to estrogen (estrone). Although androstenedione production rates decline with age, the peripheral conversion of this steroid to estrone may become two to four times more efficient over the life span (18), so that circulating levels of estrone fall less strikingly with age than do those of estradiol. Qualitative changes in circulating estrogen—loss of estradiol relative to estrone—may have clinical relevance if estrone proves to be a risk factor in gynecological cancer. The relationship of declining estrogen levels to osteoporosis is further considered in Chapter 24.

Pulsatile gonadotropin release is characteristic of the menopause. Both FSH and LH secretion become pulsatile in postmenopausal women—whereas during the intact menstrual cycle only LH is pulsatile—and pulse frequency is on a 1- to 2-hr basis in elderly women (37). The significance of these findings is unclear.

An inevitable decline with age in testosterone secretion by the testis is not observed (17), in contrast to the change in ovarian estrogen secretion. Although a number of earlier studies reported that serum testosterone levels fell with age in men, virtually all of these data originated from institutionalized males (geriatric hospitals). The recent data from Harman et al. (17) are drawn from a large population of healthy men and clearly document maintenance of serum testosterone content over the normal life span. There is general agreement, however, that circulating levels of FSH and LH in men increase with normal aging. If plasma levels of testosterone are intact over the life span in men but gonadotropin secretion increases, it must be concluded that end-organ response (Leydig cells in the testis) to gonadotropin decreases with aging. When tested directly, this appears to be the case in both men and animal models (17,32). The response of the pituitary gland to the administration of LH-releasing hormone (LHRH) is similar in old and young subjects (27). This contrasts with the observations described above relating to TRH administration and the pituitary-thyroid axis. Thus the feedback loop for sex hormone secretion is intact over the life span in men and women. A dramatic decrease in the capacity of the ovary to secrete estrogen leads to high circulating levels of gonadotropins; a modest decrease in testosterone secretory capacity in the aging testis requires that there be slight increases in LH to support normal circulating levels of androgen in men.

Androgen action on sexual tissue requires conversion of testosterone by target cells to 5α-dihydrotestosterone (DHT). Circulating DHT levels, derived in normal individuals primarily from extratesticular conversion of testosterone, may be relatively unchanged during the course of normal aging.

OTHER PITUITARY HORMONES

ADH

Age-related alterations in ADH secretion, heightened osmoreceptor sensitivity, and decreased responsiveness of the renal tubule to ADH are discussed in Chapter 7.

Growth Hormone

Secretion of growth hormone (GH) in response to stress (insulin-induced hypoglycemia) (22) and to dopaminergic stimulation (28) declines with age. This indicates a change in hypothalamic regulation of GH secretion, but the significance of the change and the functions of GH and somatomedins in the elderly remain to be defined.

Prolactin

The physiological role of prolactin (PRL) in men in general and in both elderly women and men is unknown. Basal serum PRL levels fall in women as a function of age (34), probably as a result of the decline in estrogen production as estrogen enhances PRL secretion. It is not yet clear what effects, if any, aging has on PRL production in men. TRH stimulates PRL release as well as TSH secretion. In contrast to the age-dependent change in TSH response to TRH described above, no age-related change occurs in PRL response to TRH administration (19).

CARBOHYDRATE METABOLISM

An extensive literature deals with age-dependent alterations in carbohydrate metabolism (3). For a variety of technical and other reasons, these studies have not, until recently, defined a consistent pattern of insulin physiology in older subjects. Currently, however, it is possible to draw a number of substantive conclusions about carbohydrate metabolism as a function of normal aging. These are:

1. Fasting blood sugar (FBS) content and fasting serum insulin concentration are unaffected by age. Thus the finding of an elevated FBS reflects seriously disturbed carbohydrate metabolism, regardless of patient age.
2. Blood sugar level responses in man to glucose loading ("glucose tolerance testing") are materially altered during the course of aging. National Diabetes Data Group (NDDG) criteria for establishing the diagnosis of diabetes—criteria published in 1979—do not specifically confront the issue of age-related change in carbohydrate tolerance. However, diagnostic 2-hr postprandial blood sugar values established by the NDDG are sufficiently high to minimize the risk of misdiagnosis of diabetes mellitus in the elderly.
3. The alteration in glucose handling with age in part depends on a change in the sensitivity of tissues to insulin action (9). This conclusion has been derived from studies in man utilizing the "glucose clamp" and "insulin clamp" techniques which permit, respectively, quantification of endogenous insulin release in response to various steady-state levels of blood glucose and of glucose disposal at steady-state levels of blood insulin (= insulin sensitivity). Although recent observations reveal that as much as a 30% decline in tissue sensitivity to insulin may occur over the life span (9), most of this change occurs between 20 and 50 years of age. It has not been clearly established whether this age-related change is insulin-receptor-mediated or de-

pends on a postreceptor mechanism. In addition to this change in insulin sensitivity, an alteration in β-cell sensitivity to hyperglycemia has also been described (3). Thus the rise in blood sugar content after glucose challenge evokes a smaller insulin response in older subjects (Chapter 5). If the blood sugar concentration in the course of a glucose clamp study is elevated and held above 300 mg/dl, however, resultant insulin secretion in old and young subjects is comparable. The apparent insensitivity of the β-cell to hyperglycemia after oral glucose loading may reflect relative unresponsiveness of the islet cell to one or more endogenous insulin secretogogues (1).

4. Glucagon secretion does not vary materially with aging. It has been reported that basal serum glucagon content increases slightly with age, but this change occurs principally over the third to fifth decades of life (4).

SUMMARY

From the foregoing it is obvious that the endocrinology of normal aging in man involves a variety of changes. None of these changes can be satisfactorily described as a determinant of the aging process, and aging itself does not result in the failure of any endocrine axis except for estrogen secretion. The "life support" endocrine axes (pituitary-adrenal and pituitary-thyroid) are, not unexpectedly, intact over the normal life span. Most of the other endocrine axes show changes in sensitivity, i.e., altered control of hormone secretion or altered target tissue responsiveness to hormone. Examples of such changes are the depressed response to stimuli of GH secretion and pituitary TSH secretion; the latter is sex-specific. Aging is characterized by decreased target tissue responsiveness to ADH and insulin, and in men by decreased gonadal response to LH.

It is not possible from these observations to define a common denominator which is "characteristic" of endocrine gland aging. For example, attempts to describe endocrine gland aging in global terms as a function of changed hormone feedback thresholds in the hypothalamus are at this point unconvincing with regard to human aging. It is tantalizing, however, to consider that changes in hormone responsiveness with age have a similar hormone receptor (or postreceptor) mechanism.

When caring for elderly patients, the physician should:

1. Be able to distinguish between pathological endocrine function and the effect of normal aging on endocrine physiology.
2. Know the laboratory tests of endocrine function which are unchanged by normal aging.
3. Recognize that, with the possible exception of ovarian failure, no age-dependent change in endocrine function mandates replacement hormone therapy.

REFERENCES

1. Andersen, D. K., Elahi, D., Brown, J. C., et al. Oral glucose augmentation of insulin secretion. *J. Clin. Invest.*, 62:152–161, 1978.
2. Andres, R. Aging and diabetes. *Med. Clin. North Am.*, 55:835–846, 1971.

3. Andres, R., and Tobin, J. D. Endocrine systems. In: *Handbook of the Biology of Aging*, edited by C. E. Finch and L. Hayflick, pp. 357–378. Van Nostrand Reinhold, New York, 1977.

4. Berger, D., Crowther, R. C., Floyd, J. C., Jr., et al. Effect of age on fasting plasma levels of pancreatic hormones in man. *J. Clin. Endocrinol. Metab.*, 47:1183–1189, 1978.

5. Blichert-Toft, M., and Hummer, L. Immunoreactive corticotrophin reserve in old age in man during and after surgical stress. *J. Gerontol.*, 31:539–545, 1976.

6. Carroll, B. J., Feinberg, M., Greden, J. F., et al. A specific laboratory test for the diagnosis of melancholia. *Arch. Gen. Psychiatry*, 38:15–22, 1981.

7. Davis, F. B., LaMantia, R. S., Spaulding, S. W., et al. Conventional therapy overtreats elderly hypothyroid patients. In: *Proceedings of the 62nd Annual Meeting of the Endocrine Society.* Washington, DC, 1980, abstract 33.

8. Davis, P. J., and Davis, F. B. Hyperthyroidism in patients over the age of 60 years. *Medicine*, 53:161–181, 1974.

9. DeFronzo, R. A. Glucose intolerance and aging: evidence for tissue insensitivity to insulin. *Diabetes*, 28:1095–1101, 1979.

10. Deftos, L. J., Weisman, M. H., Williams, G. W., et al. Influence of age and sex on plasma calcitonin in human beings. *N. Engl. J. Med.*, 302:1351–1353, 1980.

11. Gaffney, G. W., Gregerman, R. I., and Shock, N. W. Relationship of age to the thyroidal accumulation, renal excretion and distribution of radioiodine in euthyroid man. *J. Clin. Endocrinol. Metab.*, 22:784–794, 1962.

12. Gallagher, J. C., and Nordin, B. E. C. Treatment with oestrogens of primary hyperparathyroidism in post-menopausal women. *Lancet*, 1:503–507, 1972.

13. Gallagher, J. C., Riggs, B. L., and DeLuca, H. F. Effect of age on calcium absorption and serum 1,25(OH)₂D. *Clin. Res.*, 26:680A, 1978.

14. Gallagher, J. C., Riggs, B. L., Eisman, J., et al. Intestinal calcium absorption and serum vitamin D metabolites in normal subjects and osteoporotic patients. *J. Clin. Invest.*, 64:729–736, 1979.

15. Gherondache, C. N., Romanoff, L. P., and Pincus, G. Steroid hormones in aging men. In: *Endocrines and Aging*, edited by L. Gitman, pp. 76–101. Charles C Thomas, Springfield, IL, 1967.

16. Gregerman, R. I., Gaffney, G. W., and Shock, N. W. Thyroxine turnover in euthyroid man with special reference to changes with age. *J. Clin. Invest.*, 41:2065–2074, 1962.

17. Harman, S. M., and Tsitouras, P. D. Reproductive hormones in aging men. I. Measurement of sex steroids, basal luteinizing hormone, and Leydig cell response to human chorionic gonadotropin. *J. Clin. Endocrinol. Metab.*, 51:35–40, 1980.

18. Hemsell, D. L., Grodin, J. M., Brenner, P. F., et al. Plasma precursors of estrogen. II. Correlation of the extent of conversion of plasma androstenedione to estrone with age. *J. Clin. Endocrinol. Metab.*, 38:476–479, 1974.

19. Jacobs, L. S., Snyder, P. J., Utiger, R. D., et al. Prolactin response to thyrotropin-releasing hormone in normal subjects. *J. Clin. Endocrinol. Metab.*, 36:1069–1073, 1973.

20. Jensen, H. K., and Blichert-Toft, M. Pituitary-adrenal function in old age evaluated by the intravenous metyrapone test. *Acta Endocrinol. (Copenh.)*, 64:431–438, 1970.

21. Kempson, S., Marinetti, G. V., and Shaw, A. Hormone action at the membrane level. VII. Stimulation of dihydroalprenolol binding to beta-adrenergic receptors in isolated rat heart ventricle slices by triiodothyronine and thyroxine. *Biochim. Biophys. Acta*, 540:320–329, 1978.

22. Muggeo, M., Fedele, D., Tiengo, A., et al. Human growth hormone and cortisol response to insulin stimulation in aging. *J. Gerontol.*, 30:546–551, 1975.

23. Muller, H. Sex, age and hyperparathyroidism. *Lancet*, 1:449–450, 1969.

24. Noth, R. H., Lassman, M. N., Tan, S. Y., et al. Age and the renin-aldosterone system. *Arch. Intern. Med.*, 137:1414–1417, 1977.

25. Olsen, T., Laurberg, P., and Weeke, J. Low serum triiodothyronine and high serum reverse triiodothyronine in old age: an effect of disease not age. *J. Clin. Endocrinol. Metab.*, 47:1111–1115, 1978.

26. Quadri, S. K., Kledzik, G. S., and Meites, J. Reinitiation of estrous cycles in old constant-estrous rats by central-acting drugs. *Neuroendocrinology*, 11:248–255, 1973.

27. Rubens, R., Dhont, M., and Vermeulen, A. Further studies on Leydig cell function in old age. *J. Clin. Endocrinol. Metab.*, 39:40–45, 1974.

28. Sachar, E. J., Mushrush, G., Perlow, M., et al. Growth hormone response to L-DOPA in depressed patients. *Science*, 178:1304–1305, 1972.

29. Snyder, P. J., and Utiger, R. D. Response to thyrotropin releasing hormone (TRH) in normal man. *J. Clin. Endocrinol. Metab.*, 34:380–385, 1972.

30. Somerville, R. I., Lien, J. W. K., and Kaye, M. The calcium and vitamin D status in an elderly female population and their response to administered supplemental vitamin D₃. *J. Gerontol.*, 32:659–663, 1977.

31. Toss, G., Almqvist, S., Larsson, L., et al. Vitamin D deficiency in welfare institutions for the aged. *Acta Med. Scand.*, 208:87–89, 1980.

32. Tsitouras, P. D., Kowatch, M. A., and Harman, S. M. Age-related alterations of isolated rat Leydig cell function: gonadotropin receptors, adenosine 3′,5′-monophosphate response, and testosterone secretion. *J. Clin. Endocrinol. Metab.*, 105:1400–1405, 1979.

33. Tzankoff, S. P., and Norris, A. H. Effect of muscle mass decrease on age-related BMR changes. *J. Appl. Physiol.*, 43:1001–1006, 1977.

34. Vekemans, M., and Robyn, C. Influence of age on serum prolactin levels in women and men. *Br. Med. J.*, 4:738–739, 1975.

35. Vermeulen, A. The hormonal activity of the postmenopausal ovary. *J. Clin. Endocrinol. Metab.*, 42:247–253, 1976.

36. Wiske, P. S., Epstein, S., Bell, N. H., et al. Increases in immunoreactive parathyroid hormone with age. *N. Engl. J. Med.*, 300:1419–1421, 1979.

37. Yen, S. S. C., Tsai, C. C., Naftolin, F., et al. Pulsatile patterns of gonadotropin release in subjects with and without ovarian function. *J. Clin. Endocrinol. Metab.*, 34:671–675, 1972.

Fundamentals of Geriatric Medicine, edited by
Ronald D. T. Cape, Rodney M. Coe, and Isadore
Rossman, Raven Press, New York © 1983.

11

Age-Related Changes in Skin

Barbara A. Gilchrest

Skin is the interface between man and his environment which protects the other organs of the body against excessive temperature changes, mechanical injury, ultraviolet (UV) irradiation, toxic chemicals, and microbial pathogens. It is also a tactile organ through which man receives pleasurable stimuli and assesses his physical surroundings. With age, the skin performs each of these functions less well. Skin is also readily visible and hence of great psychological and social, as well as physiological, importance. For this reason the morphological changes in skin which accompany aging often affect an individual as much as the functional changes.

Consideration of age-induced changes in the skin is complicated by the fact that the skin is subjected to repeated and often cumulative environmental damage which is difficult to distinguish from true aging. For example, the public and many physicians consider actinically altered skin synonymous with old skin. In addition, portions of the skin and some of its appendages are very sensitive to hormonal stimulation, so that age-related hormonal shifts (e.g., puberty and menopause) may produce skin changes not directly attributable to aging itself.

The following sections review the morphological, physiological, and biochemical changes which occur in aging skin and discuss those changes specifically as they relate to altered frequency or clinical presentation of common skin disorders in the elderly.

MORPHOLOGICAL CHANGES

The major aging changes in gross morphology of the skin include "dryness" (by which is meant roughness), wrinkling, laxity, uneven pigmentation, and a variety of proliferative lesions (discussed below). Examination of cyanoacrylate skin surface impressions reveals slight disorganization and enlargement of the normally triangular cutaneous topographical pattern in old persons compared to young adults, although these age-related changes in the skin surface are dwarfed by those attributable to chronic sun exposure in the same individuals.

The histological features which have been associated with aging in human skin are listed in Table 1.

Epidermis and Dermis

The most striking and consistent change in biopsies of old skin is flattening of the dermoepidermal junction with effacement of both the dermal papillae and epidermal rete pegs (Fig. 1). This results in a much smaller interface between the two compartments and presumably less "communication" and nutrient transfer. A decrease in the density of enzymatically active melanocytes of approximately 10 to 20% of the remaining population per decade has been repeatedly documented. It is not known whether the cells truly disappear or simply become undetectable by ceasing to produce pigment; in either case, the body's protective barrier against UV light is reduced. The number of melanocytic nevi (moles) also decreases progressively with age beginning in the third or fourth decade.

Loss of dermal thickness is pronounced in elderly individuals and accounts for the paper-thin, sometimes nearly transparent quality of their skin. The remaining dermis is relatively acellular and avascular. The marked reduction of vascular bed and especially of the vertical capillary loops which occupy dermal papillae in young skin is believed to underlie many of the physiological alterations in old skin discussed in the following section. The marked reduction in the vascular network surrounding

TABLE 1. *Morphological features of aging human skin*

Epidermis	Dermis	Appendages
Flat dermoepidermal junction	Atrophy	Graying of hair
Variable thickness	Fewer fibroblasts	Loss of hair
Variable cell size	Fewer blood vessels	Conversion of terminal to vellus hair
Fewer Langerhans cells	Fewer mast cells	
Occasional nuclear atypia	Shortened capillary loops	Abnormal nailplates
Loss of melanocytes	Abnormal nerve endings	Fewer glands

FIG. 1. Histological changes associated with aging in normal human skin. Note flattening of the dermoepidermal junction and shortening of capillary loops in older skin. Variability in size and shape of epidermal cells, irregular stratum corneum, and loss of melanocytes are also apparent. Age-associated loss of dermal thickness and subcutaneous fat are not shown, as the diagram includes only the epidermis and superficial or papillary dermis. Normal epidermis is typically 0.1 to 0.2 mm thick; dermal thickness varies from 1 to 4 mm depending on body size. (From Gilchrest, B. Skin. In: *Health and Disease in Old Age*, edited by J. Rowe and R. Besdine, Little Brown, Boston, 1982.)

hair bulbs and eccrine, apocrine, and sebaceous glands may be responsible for their gradual atrophy and fibrosis with age.

Pacinian and Meisner's corpuscles, cutaneous end-organs responsible for pressure perception and light touch, display progressive disorganization and histological degeneration with age; free nerve endings appear not to change substantially.

Aging of Skin Appendages

Age-related changes in hair color, density, and distribution are widely recognized. Graying, which is pronounced in about half the population by age 50, is due to progressive and eventual total loss of melanocytes from the hair bulb. This process is believed to occur more rapidly in hair than in skin because melanocytes are called on to proliferate and manufacture melanin at maximal rates during the anagen, or growth, phase of the hair cycle, whereas epidermal melanocytes are relatively inactive throughout life. Similarly, scalp hair is believed to gray more rapidly than other body hair because its anagen:telogen (growth phase:resting phase) ratio is considerably greater than that of other body hair. Advancing age is also accompanied by a gradual decrease in the number of hair follicles over the entire body, with atrophy and fibrosis of many follicles.

Appreciable hair loss on the scalp, commonly called balding, results primarily from the androgen-dependent conversion of the relatively dark, thick scalp hairs to lightly pigmented, short, fine hairs similar to those on the ventral forearm. By age 50 the process is at least moderately advanced in approximately 60% of men and noticeable in perhaps 20% of women. As hair density must decrease by at least 50% to be clinically detectable, it is apparent that this loss of hair is substantial. Axillary hair is virtually absent in 30% of women and in 7% of men by age 60, and pubic hair also thins markedly. Remaining scalp and body hairs grow more slowly and may be smaller in diameter.

Eccrine, apocrine, and sebaceous glands become smaller, less numerous, and fibrotic throughout the skin, coincident with their reduced activity.

With age, fingernails and toenails develop longitudinal ridges (onychorrhexis), an expression of alternating hyperplasia and hypoplasia of the nail matrix, as well as generalized thinning. Frequently traumatized or relatively ischemic nails, usually on the feet, may thicken, as apparent overcompensation for the injury.

PHYSIOLOGICAL CHANGES

Table 2 lists the major functions of the skin which decline with age. Many of the entries are necessarily interrelated or overlapping.

An age-associated decrease in epidermal turnover rate of approximately 50% between the third and seventh decades has been documented by a study of desquamation rates for cells of the stratum corneum at selected body sites. Forty-five minutes after intradermal injection of ^{3}H-thymidine, the radiolabeled cells in the basal layer of the epidermis (site of production for all the cells destined to form the stratum corneum) averages 5.5% in adults aged 18 to 25 years but only 3% in

TABLE 2. *Physiological parameters in human skin which decline with age*

Growth rate
Injury response
Barrier function
Chemical clearance rates
Sensory perception
Resistance to infection
Vascular responsiveness
Thermoregulation
Sweat production
Sebum production

---

adults aged 71 to 86 years. Growth rates for hair and nails also slow considerably with age. Fingernail linear growth rates decrease approximately 0.5% annually from an average of 0.9 mm/week during the third decade to 0.5 mm/week during the tenth decade. Repair rate likewise declines with age, whether measured in terms of wound closure, regeneration of blister roofs (epidermal cell migration and mitosis), or excision of thymine dimers in UV-irradiated DNA of dermal fibroblasts. For example, comparison between adults below age 35 and those above age 65 reveals an approximately 50% prolongation in the average time required to re-epithelialize a deroofed skin blister site: from 3.5 to 5.5 weeks. In the only study to date that examines proliferative rates in diseased skin as a function of age, scale formation for patients with seborrheic dermatitis of the scalp (dandruff) was statistically significantly greater among young adults than among elderly adults with comparable clinical disease.

The time required for blister formation following topical application of irritant chemicals doubles between young and old adulthood, whereas the intensity of erythema (sunburn) following a standardized UV light exposure decreases, illustrating two other forms of compromised tissue response to injury (transudation and vasodilation).

An age-related decrease in the barrier function of intact stratum corneum has been documented by measuring percutaneous absorption of various substances. This increased permeability is accompanied by a decreased clearance of the absorbed materials from the dermis, probably due to alterations in the vascular bed and in the extracellular matrix. These combined changes render old skin quite susceptible to irritant and allergic reactions, both of which require local accumulation of the offending substance.

Decreased vascular responsiveness in the skin of older individuals has been documented by observing vasodilation after application of standardized irritants to young and old subjects. Compromised thermoregulation, which predisposes the elderly to heat stroke and hypothermia, may be due in part to reduced vasodilation or vasoconstriction of dermal arterioles, in part to decreased eccrine sweat production, and in part to loss of subcutaneous fat, all of which occur with advancing age. Central nervous mechanisms which control local reactions are also likely to be impaired.

The decrease in sebum production which accompanies advancing age in both men and women results in part from the concomitant decrease in production of gonadal androgen to which sebaceous glands are exquisitely sensitive. The clinical effects of decreased sebum production, if any, are unknown. There is no direct relationship to xerosis.

Both nerve conduction velocity and stimulation thresholds for cutaneous fibers and end-organs increase with age, undoubtedly contributing to the risk of mechanical or chemical injury to the skin.

Neoplasia of Skin

Benign Neoplasia

The numerous proliferative growths manifested in old skin (Table 3) are so nearly universal they might be considered part of the normal aging process. These lesions suggest that loss of modulation or control of growth in the skin may be even more characteristic of aging than is the simple decrease in proliferative capacity.

Malignant Neoplasia

The incidence of malignant neoplasms of the skin increases throughout adulthood and accounts for the majority of all malignancies over age 65 reported annually in the United States. Basal cell epitheliomas (by far the most common), squamous cell carcinomas, and lentigo maligna melanomas are all overwhelmingly lesions of sun-damaged skin. More than 90% arise on the head and neck, especially in fair-skinned individuals with extensive lifelong occupational or recreational sun exposure. In addition to UV light, other environmental carcinogens established as causes of cutaneous squamous cell carcinomas include x-irradiation, arsenic, soot, coal tar, and numerous industrial oils. Malignancies not attributable to environmental carcinogens are rare in all age groups. Because environmental carcinogens are usually present in small amounts over long time periods, and because induction time following adequate exposure is usually many years, it is not surprising that most cutaneous malignancies arise with disproportionate frequency in older indi-

TABLE 3. *Proliferative growths associated with aging in human skin*

Lesion	Participating cells or tissues
Acrochordon (skin tag)	Dermis, keratinocytes, melanocytes
Cherry angioma	Capillaries
Seborrheic keratosis	Dermis, keratinocytes, melanocytes
Lentigo	Melanocytes
Sebaceous hyperplasia	Sebaceous glands

viduals. In addition, there is evidence in rodents that older animals are more prone to develop skin cancers following a standardized challenge than are younger animals.

With respect to UV-induced carcinogenesis in man, two groups of investigators have reported an age-associated decline in the ability of dermal fibroblasts to repair DNA following *in vitro* exposure to non-ionizing radiation. DNA repair capacity in keratinocytes, the major target population for UV carcinogenesis, has not been examined as a function of age but appears in general to parallel that of dermal fibroblasts. The skin's progressive loss of functioning melanocytes may also render older skin more vulnerable to a given amount of sun exposure. Finally, decreased immunosurveillance in the elderly may be especially pertinent to cutaneous carcinogenesis, as UV exposure itself in mice has been demonstrated to induce tolerance toward otherwise highly antigenic UV-induced tumors.

BIOCHEMICAL CHANGES

The numerous investigations in the area of biochemical changes have been restricted to consideration of the dermis. Changes that occur during fetal development and early childhood are much greater than those which occur after maturity. However, they reflect growth and development rather than aging and therefore are not reviewed here.

Collagen constitutes 70 to 80% of dermal dry weight. With advancing age, collagen fibers are believed to become progressively cross-linked; they are certainly less soluble and less hydrated. These biochemical changes are accompanied by a decrease in extensibility and an increase in isometric tension. Elastin, which constitutes approximately 2% of dermal dry weight, increases nearly threefold with age, and elastin fibers become progressively cross linked and may calcify. These combined changes in collagen and elastin are responsible for the laxity and inelasticity of old skin.

The nonfibrous matrix of the dermis, the ground substance, is a hydrated gel composed of mucopolysaccharides and proteins. Numerous, sometimes contradictory studies have revealed little if any change in its composition, although the ratio of ground substance to collagen decreases with age, undoubtedly affecting tissue turgor.

Total water content of human skin has not been found to decrease with age, contradicting the popular image of "dry skin" in old age.

SUMMARY

There are age-related morphological, physiological, and biochemical changes in normal skin that decrease function and may predispose to certain diseases. Morphological changes in the skin may decrease protection against UV light and reduce vascular responsiveness. Hair color, density, and distribution are also affected by age; fingernails and toenails become ridged and thinner. Physiological alterations decrease the rapidity of tissue repair and the degree to which the skin reacts to irritants and potential allergens. Thermoregulation is also less efficient in the elderly.

Skin cancer is very common, probably due to a combination of lifelong exposure to UV and other carcinogens and to decreased immune surveillance. Biochemical changes account for the skin's loss of elasticity. Contrary to popular belief, the aging human skin does not lose its water content, and so the "dry skin" of the elderly is a myth.

When caring for elderly patients, the physician should consider the important age-related changes that take place in morphology, physiology, and biochemistry of the skin and that these changes may affect the expression of both dermatologic and systemic disorders.

SUGGESTED READING

Christophers, E., and Kligman, A. M. Percutaneous absorption in aged skin. In: *Advances in Biology of Skin, Vol. IV: Aging*, edited by W. Montagna, pp. 163–175. Pergamon Press, Oxford, 1965.

Gilchrest, B. A. Some gerontologic considerations in the practice of dermatology. *Arch. Dermatol.*, 115:1343–1346, 1979.

Gilchrest, B. A. Age-associated changes in the skin: Overview and clinical relevance. *J. Am. Geriatr. Soc.*, 30:139–143, 1982.

Lavker, R. M., Kwong, P., and Kligman, A. M. Changes in skin surface patterns with age. *J. Gerontol.*, 35:348–354, 1980.

Leyden, J. J., McGinley, K. J., and Grove, G. L. Age-related differences in the rate of desquamation of skin surface cells. In: *Pharmacological Intervention in the Aging Process*, edited by R. D. Adelman, J. Roberts, and V. J. Cristofalo, pp. 297–298. Plenum Press, New York, 1978.

Montagna, W., Kligman, A. M., Wuepper, K. D., and Bentley, J. P. Special issue on aging. *J. Invest. Dermatol.*, 73:1–134, 1979.

Selmanowitz, V. J., Rizer, R. L., and Orentreich, N. Aging of the skin and its appendages. In: *Handbook of the Biology of Aging*, edited by C. E. Finch and L. Hayflick, pp. 496–509. Van Nostrand Reinhold, New York, 1977.

Tindall, J. P. Skin changes and lesions in our senior citizens: incidences. *Cutis*, 18:359–362, 1976.

Fundamentals of Geriatric Medicine, edited by
Ronald D. T. Cape, Rodney M. Coe, and Isadore
Rossman, Raven Press, New York © 1983.

Questions for Self-Assessment

DIRECTIONS: In questions 1–20, only *one* alternative is correct. Select the one
best answer and blacken the corresponding lettered box on the
answer sheet.

1. The primary effect of aging is:

   (A) A reduction in adaptive capacity
   (B) Increased fatigability
   (C) Increased number of physical complaints
   (D) Loss of memory
   (E) Impaired hearing

2. The endocrine axis in which target tissue sensitivity is intact over the life
   span is:

   (A) Insulin-responsive tissues
   (B) Testicular response to gonadotropins
   (C) Thyroid gland response to TSH
   (D) Pituitary growth hormone secretion in response to dopaminergic stim-
   ulation
   (E) Distal renal tubule response to ADH

3. In response to acute reduction in salt intake, an elderly person without renal
   disease:

   (A) Conserves sodium as well and as quickly as a young patient
   (B) Cannot conserve sodium as well as a young patient
   (C) Conserves sodium as well as a young patient, but the response is delayed
   (D) Will have no change in urinary sodium output regardless of intake
   (E) None of the above

4. Factors associated with excess antidiuretic hormone (ADH) secretion in elderly patients include:

    (A)   Stroke
    (B)   Pneumonia
    (C)   Chlorpropamide administration
    (D)   General anesthesia and surgery
    (E)   All of the above

5. With increasing age:

    (A)   The ability of the pancreas to produce insulin is markedly reduced
    (B)   Glucose tolerance is reduced
    (C)   Glucose absorption is reduced
    (D)   The sensitivity of tissues to insulin is increased
    (E)   Glucose turnover is increased

6. The normal serum creatinine value (mg/100 ml) for a healthy 80-year-old man is:

    (A)   1.2
    (B)   4.0
    (C)   2.0
    (D)   2.5
    (E)   3.0

7. Normal creatinine clearance for a healthy 80-year-old man compared with that of a 30-year-old is:

    (A)   The same
    (B)   10% less
    (C)   20% less
    (D)   30% less
    (E)   45% less

8. Measurement of adrenocortical function in elderly patients shows:

    (A)   Reduced 8 a.m. cortisol and decreased response to metyrapone
    (B)   Increased aldosterone response to diuresis
    (C)   Normal cortisol levels and decreased response to metyrapone
    (D)   Normal response to stress and normal cortisol levels
    (E)   Increased glucocorticoid secretory rate

9. Altered glucose handling in elderly subjects is primarily due to:

    (A)   Decreased tissue sensitivity to insulin
    (B)   Increased insulin release in response to a glucose load

    (C)   Increased tissue sensitivity to insulin
    (D)   Decreased glucagon secretion
    (E)   Increased growth hormone levels

10.   An elderly patient recovering from surgical repair of a fractured hip has a seizure and is found to have a serum sodium concentration of 105 mEq/L. The appropriate immediate management includes:

    (A)   Thiazide diuretics
    (B)   Normal saline (0.9%) infusion
    (C)   Hypertonic (3%) saline infusion
    (D)   Lactated Ringer's solution infusion
    (E)   Dimethylchlortetracycline

11.   One way in which normal aging affects the pituitary-adrenocortical axis is:

    (A)   Decreased cortisol degradation and secretion rates, with maintenance of circulating levels of cortisol similar to those in young adult subjects
    (B)   Sluggish ACTH responsiveness to stress
    (C)   Increased secretion of adrenal androgens
    (D)   Increased secretion of aldosterone

12.   The principal reason for difficulty in establishing the causes of biological changes associated with aging is the:

    (A)   Plethora of physiological decrements that occur
    (B)   Unavailability of old experimental animals
    (C)   Difficulty in designing adequate experiments to test theories
    (D)   Inability to distinguish a particular effect from a more fundamental cause
    (E)   Absence of an adequate animal model

13.   Aging:

    (A)   Accelerates at about the age of 65 years in most people
    (B)   Impairs coordination of activities of different organ systems
    (C)   Affects the cardiovascular system to a greater extent than the respiratory system
    (D)   Is the principal cause of death in persons over 65
    (E)   Can be delayed by administering medications

14.   Increased gonadotropin levels found in elderly men result from:

    (A)   Increased conversion of androgens to estrogens
    (B)   Decreased estrogen synthesis in the adrenals
    (C)   Decreased end-organ responsiveness to gonadotropins
    (D)   Increased prolactin concentrations

(E)   Increased end-organ responsiveness to gonadotropins

15.   Changes in the renin-angiotensin-aldosterone system with age include:

(A)   No change in plasma renin or aldosterone levels
(B)   Decrease in both renin and aldosterone levels
(C)   No change in renin and a decrease in aldosterone
(D)   Decrease in renin and no change in aldosterone
(E)   Increase in both renin and aldosterone

16.   During the period immediately following major surgery, elderly patients are at risk for the development of:

(A)   Acidosis
(B)   Alkalosis
(C)   Hyponatremia
(D)   Hypernatremia
(E)   Hyperchloremia

17.   Aging:

(A)   Affects most organ systems to about the same extent
(B)   Begins at about age 65 in most people
(C)   Is a complex process that affects people at different rates
(D)   Is an inevitable disease
(E)   Is a unitary process

18.   In a healthy 73-year-old man, typical thyroid function test results would be:

(A)   Low serum total T_4 and low serum total T_3 levels
(B)   Low serum total T_3 level and increased TSH response to TRH
(C)   Increased T_4 turnover rate and elevated thyroidal radioiodine uptake
(D)   Elevated serum TBG levels due to increased conversion of androgen to estrogen
(E)   Normal serum total T_4, free T_4, and T_3 concentrations

19.   Aging is associated with:

(A)   Slowing in the rate of recovery from physiological stress
(B)   Reduced rate of oxygen utilization at the cellular level
(C)   Reduced activity of most cellular enzymes
(D)   Increased caloric intake
(E)   Reduced interindividual variance

20.   Genetic theories of aging are based on the fact that:

(A)   Random errors are known to occur in information-containing molecules

(B)   The genetic apparatus is the fundamental reservoir of biological information

(C)   The genetic apparatus is uniquely susceptible to environmental influences

(D)   Genes control all known aging processes

(E)   Radiation accelerates aging

DIRECTIONS: In questions 21–33, *one or more* of the alternatives may be correct. You are to respond either *yes* (Y) or *no* (N) to each of the alternatives. For every alternative you think is correct, blacken the corresponding lettered box on the answer sheet in the column labeled "Y". For every alternative you think is incorrect, blacken the corresponding lettered box in the column labeled "N".

21.   Compared with young persons, elderly persons who exercise have a greater:

(A)   Increase in systolic blood pressures

(B)   Increase in diastolic blood pressures

(C)   Increase in heart rates

(D)   Delay in the return of their systolic blood pressures to pre-exercise levels

(E)   Incidence of left ventricular dysfunction

22.   The consequences of decreased ventricular compliance with impairment of ventricular filling in elderly persons include:

(A)   Increased incidence of systolic hypertension

(B)   Increased incidence of S4 gallop sounds

(C)   Higher left ventricular filling pressures at rest

(D)   Higher right ventricular filling pressures during exercise

(E)   Increased coronary blood flow

23.   Primary functions of normal skin include:

(A)   Protection against infrared radiation

(B)   Protection against ultraviolet radiation

(C)   Mechanical protection of internal organs

(D)   Assessment of physical environment

(E)   Excretion of toxic chemicals

24.   Metazoan cells that age include:

(A)   Hematopoietic cells

(B)   Germ cell precursors

(C)   Epithelial lining of the gut

(D)   Serially transplantable cancer cells

(E)   Dermal cells

25. Changes in myocardial function with aging include:

   (A)   Prolongation of the ejection period
   (B)   Shortening of the diastole
   (C)   Decrease in the maximum rate of rise in the left ventricular pressure
   (D)   Decrease in the reactive capacity to acetylcholine
   (E)   Decrease in the reactive capacity to catecholamines

26. Orthostatic hypotension is common in aged adults. Baroreceptors that are most important in the maintenance of blood pressure in all body positions are located in the:

   (A)   Descending thoracic aorta
   (B)   Carotid sinus
   (C)   Atria
   (D)   Aortic arch
   (E)   Coronary sinus

27. Age-associated biochemical changes in normal skin include:

   (A)   Decreased water content
   (B)   Loss of collagen and elastin fibers
   (C)   Alteration of collagen and elastin fibers
   (D)   Decreased ratio of dermal ground substance to collagen
   (E)   Deposition of amyloid

28. Age-associated morphological changes in normal skin include:

   (A)   Hyperplasia of the epidermis
   (B)   Atrophy of the dermis
   (C)   Increased pigmentation
   (D)   Increased vascularity
   (E)   Disorganization of the nerve endings

29. Age-associated physiological changes in normal skin include:

   (A)   Decreased turnover rates for cells in the epidermis
   (B)   Increased clearance rates for substance introduced into the dermis
   (C)   Increased inflammatory response to irritant chemicals
   (D)   Impaired thermoregulatory function
   (E)   Decreased sebum excretion

30. Decreased sensitivity of the baroreceptor reflexes with aging is an important

factor in the development of orthostatic hypotension. Other important contributing factors in elderly persons include:

(A) Febrile illness
(B) Use of diuretics
(C) Use of digitalis preparations
(D) Prolonged hot baths
(E) Excessive intake of salt

31. Cutaneous neoplasms in elderly patients:

(A) Are demonstrated in more than 90% of patients
(B) Are usually malignant
(C) Account for the majority of malignancies reported in this age group
(D) Usually occur on sun-protected areas
(E) Are usually of dermal origin

32. Factors contributing to atrial arrhythmias in elderly persons include:

(A) Decreased automaticity of the sinoatrial node
(B) Fibrosis and dilatation of the atria with damage to the atrial muscle
(C) Increase of fibrotic tissue in the intranodal tracts
(D) Increased ventricular compliance
(E) Decreased sensitivity of the heart to acetylcholine and catecholamines

33. The immunological theory of aging is based on the:

(A) Reduction of quantity of antibody formation with age
(B) Production of antibody to self cells
(C) Presence of an immune system in all animals that age
(D) Reduction of quality of antibody formation with age
(E) Fact that all nonaccidental deaths during old age have an immunological etiology

Diagnosis

Fundamentals of Geriatric Medicine, edited by
Ronald D. T. Cape, Rodney M. Coe, and Isadore
Rossman, Raven Press, New York © 1983.

12

Overview

Philip J. Henschke

Illness in the very old is a deterring rather than a challenging experience for
many physicians. This is so for several reasons. Illness episodes are typically less
acute in the older patient and usually occur against a background of previous
disabilities and therapies. Therapeutic success may be modest and is often evident
only to the patient and those to whom previous performance levels are known.
Illness during old age often produces symptoms that do not point to any particular
organ system but rather to a general failure of a number of body systems. The
possible needs for continuing care of the patient and slow-tempo rehabilitation deter
many doctors from involvement with the multiple problems of the older patient.
Hemoptysis and chest pain are excellent passwords for entering the hospital system,
but mental confusion, immobility, or falling tend to be viewed negatively—as
undeserving of careful medical analysis.

Many studies have confirmed that loss of mobility, mental confusion, incontinence, and homeostatic breakdown are four of the most common problems in elderly
people (Chapter 2). These are not diagnoses but clinical problems. They stem largely
from aspects of brain failure which become increasingly common as the patient
ages and are aggravated by a wide variety of associated conditions. Effective
measures to prevent cerebral deterioration are not yet available. Impaired cerebral
function is the key predisposing factor in the initiation of these four problems. To
them, we must add iatrogenic disease. In our anxiety to make some effort to help
clinical situations, we enthusiastically employ a number of agents to treat the heart
failure, infections, metabolic upsets, cancer, or other associated pathology, forgetting that increasing numbers of drugs and excessive dosages mean a greater risk
of adverse reactions.

Falling, confusion, incontinence, homeostatic disturbance, and iatrogenic illness
form a geriatric quintet which is found separately or together in almost every acute

or long-term illness of an elderly person. They constitute an interrelated complex of old age syndromes that are the essence of clinical geriatric medicine. The older the patient, the more common are the problems. The interlinking rings of this "O-complex" (Fig. 1) emphasize the close relationship between the problems and their common association in the individual patient. The symbol represents the hard core of clinical problems unique to the medical care of the very old. The key to solving the problems of the O complex lies in the brain. Cerebral cellular metabolism holds the answer, and further understanding of its mechanisms will do more to help the old to maintain their independence than anything else.

At the present time the rewards of accurate medical diagnosis and response to treatment are as satisfying in the old as in the young. On the other hand, many elderly quietly endure their remediable misfortunes because of a fatalistic acceptance of a gradual loss of independence or a belief that little can be done for the ailments of later life. Fear of hospitalization, investigation, and the thought of a one-way street to institutional care deter others. Lack of access to manageable transportation and reduced personal concern arising from social isolation, depression, other forms of psychopathology, or dementing illness cause many to delay seeking help. Others who are ultimately propelled into the health services system already have far-advanced pathology and attendant social problems.

Williamson and his colleagues in Scotland (2) elegantly demonstrated that if one studies a random group of old people one could uncover a variety of significant diseases and disabilities which the patients did not bring to the attention of their physicians. In that Edinburgh study, there were more than twice as many disabilities unknown to the physician as there were conditions duly documented. It would be foolish to attempt such thorough probing in all cases, and there are undoubtedly many situations which can safely be left uninvestigated. However, somewhere between accepting concealment by the old person and overenthusiastic investigation by physicians, there must surely be a balance.

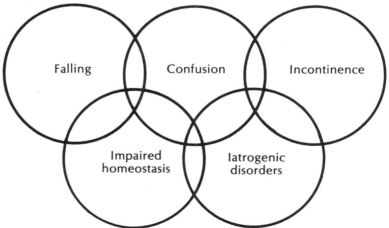

FIG. 1. The O complex of geriatric medicine. (From ref. 1.)

The problems the physician encounters while seeking to diagnose his elderly patients can be discussed under the following headings: altered presentation of disease in the elderly, documentation of the history, physical examination, and the need for investigation.

ALTERED PRESENTATION OF DISEASE IN THE ELDERLY

In the early literature promoting geriatric medicine as an area worthy of study, much was made of differing clinical presentations among the elderly. Atypical and silent myocardial infarction and oligosymptomatic hyperthyroidism are notable examples. Although such situations arise more frequently in the elderly, they may be seen in patients of all ages. What is more typical of elderly patients is the vagueness of their complaints. Good examples are weakness and tiredness, symptoms which are difficult to describe and perhaps even more difficult to evaluate but which are common complaints of the geriatric patient. Weakness of the legs is responsible for reducing mobility and causing increased liability to fall, sometimes setting up a vicious circle. The expression "inactivity debility" somehow explains and describes a not uncommon situation in elderly people, particularly those over 80. A variety of factors—sometimes disease, sometimes prescribed medication, and sometimes overenthusiastic self-medication—may produce states in which the old person feels weak and tired and not interested in doing things. Isolated elderly persons may be particularly prone to this, although individuals with an active family who pamper them may also suffer from these complaints, their family preventing them from undertaking the numerous minor chores of daily living which serve to maintain an adequate level of muscular activity in legs and arms. Whatever the cause, this symptom insidiously increases in severity over a period of weeks or months and almost always culminates in one or two falls, resulting in the old person literally taking to bed.

Altered presentation of illness in the elderly may thus arise in the following ways: (a) It is often the summation of the effects of multiple pathology producing problems in daily living. (b) Physical reactions to illness such as fever, pain response, and tachycardia are often blunted. (c) Nonspecific features such as mental confusion, "slowing up," altered behavior, apathy, and self-neglect are observed rather than volunteered phenomena. These are clues to aid in diagnosis. Changes in the pattern, severity, or character of symptoms arising from previously determined pathology or disabilities should excite diagnostic interest and the possibility of adverse drug effects.

DOCUMENTATION OF THE HISTORY

Documenting the history is commonly a difficult task which is made more time-consuming by the need for a complete profile of past and present problems. It often requires consultation with relatives, friends, or neighbors. Thirty percent of older people suffer from significant hearing loss. If the physician positions himself or herself in front of the patient and speaks slowly and clearly, with a moderate increase in loudness, even the patient with mild to moderate deafness in most instances will be able to hear. Shouting in the ear, in contrast, accentuates vowel sounds and diminishes the high tone consonants the elderly patient has most difficulty in hearing.

The physician should convey a sense of unhurried concern early in the interview. Many elderly patients in their anxiety not to forget items of importance unburden themselves by reeling off a long list of symptoms. It is good policy to allow the patient free rein when this happens and then retrace one's steps over the list with the patient. Direct questions are usually discouraged in history taking, but in the elderly they are often required in order to establish the significance of complaints. Old persons are frequently unable to establish accurately the duration of their complaint. It is helpful to refer to significant events, such as "How were you feeling last Chirstmas?" "Did you rake the leaves last fall?" In the hospital setting it should be remembered that the sequence of ambulance travel, emergency room, preadmitting investigations, and ward admission leaves most elderly patients exhausted. A complete exploration of immediate and past history can often be deferred until the next day.

Mental confusion is common but often reversible. Simple testing by a mental status questionnaire should be an early routine in the history taking of older patients, particularly when the patient's story is rambling and circumstantial. Perseveration and confabulation are employed as "time buying" maneuvers by patients with defective memory. Hypochondriasis, on the other hand, is commonly due to a neurotic personality but may be a feature of the agitated depressive individual, particularly when collateral inquiry can establish this as a recent trait. It is generally wise to avoid interviewing the patient and relatives together for the initial data collection, but checking the story is an essential confirmatory step.

In summary, history taking is often difficult. Much can be gathered in unhurried dialogue with the patient and, when appropriate, with family, spouse, and close contacts. The patient should be instructed to present all medication containers for review at the time of his initial interview, as this is the only reliable check on the drugs being taken.

PHYSICAL EXAMINATION

The physical examination of the older patient differs little from that carried out in a younger adult. The examiner should bear in mind, however, that a number of disorders occur more commonly in those of advanced age.

When examining the head and neck, palpation of temporal arteries for tenderness or thickening and auscultation for cervicocranial bruits are indicated in persons with a history of vascular disease. Examination of the auditory canal for wax occlusion should not be omitted in those with a hearing defect. Many older folks spend little time outdoors, and skin pallor should be checked against the color of the conjunctiva and mucous membranes. Pernicious anemia presents in a variety of ways, and routine examination of the tongue mucosa for atrophy is wise in all patients. The state of the patient's dentition should not be ignored. The presence of a goiter or neck scar should be looked for in all patients, as thyroid disorders in the elderly are commonly overlooked. Examination of the ocular fundus is made difficult in the elderly by lens sclerosis and the small pupillary size. Neck stiffness, due to osteoarthrosis, is commonly encountered, making the determination of meningitic irritation difficult.

Systolic murmurs are common in the elderly; their frequency increases from about 30% in persons who are 65 years of age to nearly 60% in those age 80. The typical benign murmur of aortic sclerosis is short, early peaking, grade 1/6 to 2/6 at the base, and radiates poorly into the carotids. Clinically significant aortic stenosis is present in approximately 5% of elderly patients with such murmurs. A late-peaking, grade 2/6 to 5/6 long-lasting ejection murmur with a slowly rising carotid pulse and a diminished aortic second component are findings in this disorder. Many systolic murmurs in the aged, even those with ejection characteristics, are associated with abnormalities of the mitral valve and may closely mimic aortic stenosis or sclerosis in the elderly. It should be remembered that postural hypotension without apparent cause occurs in about 20% of persons over 75 years of age (Chapter 8). Many drugs prescribed for the elderly compromise standing blood pressure. A standing or sitting blood pressure record is advisable in all elderly patients. The detection of bronchial breathing or adventitious sounds in the elderly patient by auscultation may be difficult, as basal lung expansion is often weak due to poor musculature and costovertebral joint disease.

The neurological examination of healthy elderly individuals may reveal limitation of upward gaze and poor ocular convergence. In addition, absent ankle reflexes, diminished or absent vibration sense at the foot level, and minor wasting of hand musculature are sometimes found even in the absence of disease. A palmomental reflex may be present without pointing to diffuse cerebral disease. Normal aging is associated with reduced stride length and a tendency to body flexion which may suggest parkinsonism.

Rectal and pelvic examinations and percussion for a full bladder are advisable in the mentally confused patient, where an incomplete history is usual. Examination of the patient's underclothing may reveal evidence of fecal or urinary incontinence or unnoticed rectal or vaginal bleeding or discharge.

Inspection of the patient's home can provide a valuable insight into a patient's nutritional state (e.g., accounts unpaid for many months, spoiled food lying about the kitchen) or may confirm suspected incontinence (soaked bedding or newspapers on lounge chairs).

THE NEED FOR INVESTIGATION

The investigation of any patient should be directed toward confirming or rejecting a reasonable diagnostic formulation of the cause of that patient's problem. Confirmation of a diagnosis in the elderly is not mandatory unless subsequent therapy directed at the finding is planned to improve the patient's lot. Investigation not directed at this goal in many instances is simply medical voyeurism. On the other hand, the more accurate the diagnosis, the better will be the management program, whether it is aimed at cure or palliation. The level of discomfort to the patient during the investigation is another factor to be taken into account, including the ability of the elderly patient to cooperate or comprehend the nature of the planned procedure.

A common diagnostic problem in the elderly is mental confusion. Before any investigations are planned, the most important question is: "How long has the patient been confused?" A patient who has been dementing for a number of years is unlikely to benefit from extensive investigations. Where a dementing process has been present for this length of time, a careful history rarely fails to establish the etiology. A stereotyped approach to the investigation of dementia is unjustified. Although the relevance of thyroid function and vitamin B_{12} status, cerebral mass lesions, and hydrocephalus should be borne in mind, routine screening is unjustified unless other clinical features support this action. Many clinicians adopt a knee jerk approach for dementia with routine referral for cerebral scanning. This approach is often logistically difficult and unjustifiable on a cost-benefit basis unless atypical or accompanying clinical features suggest that such pathology is likely.

Baseline blood, biochemical, electrocardiographic, and chest radiographic studies are advisable and valuable for the elderly patient entering institutional care, as they provide baselines for interpreting abnormalities subsequently unearthed.

A healthy skepticism about diagnoses already reported and excessive drug regimens should be encouraged. Where doubt exists about the need for medications, phased withdrawal or cessation is generally successful. Investigations to this end should be encouraged.

The time dimension is one of the least used and most appropriate strategies when investigating the elderly patient whose diagnosis remains obscure after an initial diagnostic thrust. A rewarding policy often neglected is to return to the patient at a later date, retaking and re-examining the evidence in the light of clinical progress.

REFERENCES

1. Cape, R. D. T. *Aging: Its Complex Management.* Harper & Row, Hagerstown, MD, 1978.
2. Williamson, J., Stokoe, I. H., Gray, S., Fisher, M., Smith, A., and Stephenson, E. Old people at home, their unreported needs. *Lancet*, 1:1117–1123, 1964.

SUGGESTED READING

Brocklehurst, J. C. *Textbook of Geriatric Medicine and Gerontology.* Churchill-Livingstone, New York, 1978.

Caird, F. I., and Judge, T. G. *Assessment of the Elderly Patient.* Pitman, London, 1974.

Coni, N., Davison, W., and Webster, S. *Lecture Notes on Geriatrics.* Blackwell Scientific Publications, London, 1977.

Rossman, I., editor. *Clinical Geriatrics*, 2nd ed. Lippincott, Philadelphia, 1979.

Von Hahn, H. B., editor. *Practical Greiatrics.* Karger, New York, 1975.

Fundamentals of Geriatric Medicine, edited by
Ronald D. T. Cape, Rodney M. Coe, and Isadore
Rossman, Raven Press, New York © 1983.

13

Falls by the Aged

Manuel Rodstein

Falling is the most common manifestation of "accident liability" in the aged. Accident liability is a comprehensive term which encompasses all personal factors that contribute to the occurrence of accidents, including the effects of the aging process, acute and chronic illness, psychological characteristics, and medications. Despite their high frequency—falls are everyday events in any institution for the aged—there remains much room for their scientific study. Even in the best of circumstances, the reason for a particular fall may not be determinable and the weight of any particular fall hard to assess. It is nonetheless important to do a differential diagnosis when someone has had a fall in order to avoid missing such correctible factors as anemia or dysrhythmia. This chapter incorporates observations and opinions derived from long experience in an institution for the aged where there has been an ongoing interest in the problem of falls.

Falls in the aged often differ markedly from falls in younger individuals. In the elderly they occur as a gentle slumping or collapse to the floor which is often asymptomatic, unobserved, and not recalled. Most often they are due to "patient factors" and not "environmental factors," e.g., tripping over a hazardous rug. For this reason falls that occur in institutions are often reported as "incidents" rather than "accidents." The principal reasons the aged give for falling are loss of balance, dizziness, poor vision, and the knees giving way.

In the United States in 1977 falls accounted for 1,997 deaths among persons 65 to 74 years of age and 8,123 deaths among those 75 and over; this translated to death rates of 14/100,000 persons 65 to 74 years of age and 93/100,000 for those 75 and over. The 10,120 deaths from falls among the approximately 11% of the population which is 65 years of age and over constituted approximately 72% of the total of 14,136 for the entire population of the United States (1).

Falls in the aged thus account for a disproportionate number of disabling injuries and hospitalizations, as well as prolonged stays in hospitals and other institutions. Yet these serious falls represent only a small percentage of the total number of falls sustained by the aged. The majority of falls, about 90% in persons over 75, do not result in significant injury. Because predisposing factors tend to be recurrent or ongoing, repeated falls by the same individual are common.

PATIENT FACTORS

Osteoporosis and Fractures

The most common serious consequence of falling is fracture, which in the aged is related to the degree of osteoporosis present at the time of the fall. This is particularly true for fractures of the hip, wrist, and spine, which are almost invariably associated with osteopenia; a fall resulting in hip fracture is not uncommonly preceded by a long history of falling without injury. A minor fall or slip to the floor without obvious cause may result in a hip fracture if the osteoporosis has become sufficiently advanced. Largely for this reason, there is a 500% increase in hip fractures among females aged 70 to 79 years compared with those 50 to 59 years of age.

Psychological Factors

Depression, apathy, and confusion are among the patient factors that contribute to an increased prevalence of falls. Denial of the limitations imposed by alterations in gait, coordination, vision, etc. together with a tendency to hoard things, causing a crowded and hazardous environment, all contribute to falls. An unfamiliar environment has similar effects, and the increased frequency of falls when the elderly are first transferred to an institution is a well-recognized hazard.

Vision

The impairment of vision which accompanies aging also increases the liability of accidents. The impairments include a loss of visual acuity, a decrease in the lateral fields of vision, a need for increased illumination for optimal vision, a decreased tolerance of glare, loss of night vision, and the development of cataracts. Glaucoma, diabetic retinopathy, and macular degeneration cause progressive loss of vision, and these conditions increase in frequency and severity with aging. These impairments of vision increase the likelihood of falling on stairways or tripping over unseen or misjudged objects.

In the differential diagnosis of falls due to nervous system disease, a loss of balance when the eyes are closed is indicative of a loss of proprioceptive sensation, as in pernicious anemia, a combined-system disease. Among hemiplegics, homonymous hemianopsia is a fairly frequent contributor to impaired vision and resultant falls.

Orthostatic Hypotension

The increased tendency to orthostatic hypotension in the aged is a significant contributory factor to falls (Chapter 8 and Overview to this section). There is impaired efficiency of the vasomotor reflexes involved in arterial and venous constriction and an increased heart rate on standing, which in younger individuals maintain venous return and prevent a decline in blood pressure and cardiac output. Furthermore, the decreased strength of muscular contraction in the lower extremities on standing may contribute to the failure of the compensatory mechanisms. The incidence of orthostatism appears to be increased by large varicose veins, diabetic neuritis, anemia, and central nervous and spinal cord disease. It occurs more commonly on arising after periods of bed rest.

Orthostatic hypotension is exaggerated and often precipitated by medications commonly used by the aged. These include many of the antihypertensive drugs (e.g., guanethidine), the ataractics (e.g., tricyclic antidepressants), and nitroglycerine sublingual tablets.

Vertigo and Dizziness

Vertigo and dizziness are frequent causes of falls in the aged consequent to degenerative or vascular changes in the vestibular apparatus. Any movement of the head in space may be accompanied by an illusion of rotary motion, a sense of unsteadiness, a loss of balance, and falling. The patient may describe any sensation from faintness to rotary vertigo.

In addition, in the presence of arteriosclerotic narrowing of the carotid and vertebral arteries, lateral movements of the head may compress the carotid arteries, and extension of the head may compress the vertebral arteries enough to yield cerebral ischemia and a fall. Such falls typically occur while performing such activities as looking into side-view mirrors while driving, adjusting drapes, or changing ceiling bulbs.

Drop Attacks

The aged are subject to a particular form of fall which occurs when the antigravity muscles suddenly become weak and flaccid. There is no loss of consciousness. This may occur as a consequence of the vertebrobasilar arterial insufficiency described above and has also been attributed to paroxysmal ischemia of the midbrain.

Impaired Gait in the Aged

A variety of changes—neuromuscular, collagenic, arthritic—impair the gait of aging individuals and increase the risk of falling. Often superimposed diseases (e.g., parkinsonism) greatly increase this risk as well. The aged have greater difficulty initiating and stopping movement and thus must expend greater energy to do so. The center of gravity shifts forward, causing knee flexion to keep a support base directly below the center of gravity. This results in a crouch and a forward leaning posture, which, together with decreased resistance to the forces of inertia and gravity, causes difficulty in thrusting the foot out fast enough to regain balance. As a result, the aged individual's gait becomes a shuffle—slow, halting, and short-stepped—with the feet lifted only a small distance from the floor.

Magnetic Apraxia

In a more advanced phase, the aged individual's feet may only slide on the floor. When asked to walk he may stand as if rooted to the spot for varying lengths of time before moving, and then advance each foot, a few inches at a time, by sliding them across the floor. This is known as magnetic apraxia. It is associated with lurching, unsteadiness, and grasping for support while walking. Thus for these persons every irregularity or minor obstacle in their path—thresholds, rug edges, electrical cords, uneven sidewalks, curbs—becomes a potential cause of falls.

Hypokinetic-Hypertonic Syndrome

In the hypokinetic-hypertonic syndrome, which has been attributed to extrapyramidal dysfunction, there is muscle rigidity and immobility. Movements are slow and deliberate with a shuffling gait, the head and neck thrust forward, the upper trunk bowed, the upper limbs carried in flexion at elbows and wrists, and the knees bent. This resembles parkinsonism but without cogwheel rigidity and the alternating, resting tremor.

Marche à Petit Pas

In marche à petit pas the toes are advanced only an inch or two at a time, often rapidly, with exaggerated swinging movements of the arms. When the individual with this disorder attempts to start or turn, he takes a number of tiny, rapid, step-like movements of the feet while remaining in the same spot or turning in the desired direction.

Muscle Weakness and Arthritis

Muscle weakness and wasting with arthritic changes at the joints which limit the use of subserving muscles contribute to a slow, cautious, unsteady walk with waddling and difficulty in climbing stairs.

Hemiplegia, Parkinsonism, and Lues

The impaired gait of the hemiplegic with wide swinging out of the affected limb, the slow, cautious gait with propulsion of the parkinsonian, and the impaired gait of luetic central nervous system disease are familiar to the physician and need no further description. They all exaggerate and increase accident liability in the aged.

Proprioception

Proprioceptive sense together with vestibular and visual function are needed for spatial orientation when standing and walking. Many of the aged have impaired proprioceptive function demonstrable by a diminution or loss of vibratory sensation, especially in the feet. In some cases this may be the result of a form of peripheral neuritis. A decreased appreciation of slow or subtle movements of the great toes and a cautious gait result, with a tendency to watch the feet when walking and frequent missteps; hence there is an increased liability to falls.

Intercurrent Illness

Because of diminished reactivity, acute disease may be unappreciated by the elderly, particularly those of advanced age with some degree of dementia. Contributing factors are a decreased appreciation of pain, diminished febrile response, and the effects of psychotropic medications. Ambulation continues, however, and a fall may occur. This is known as a *premonitory accident*. A variety of disease conditions have been implicated, including febrile conditions (e.g., pneumonia), acute blood loss, hypoglycemia, and various causes of cerebral ischemia including cardiac dysrhythmias.

Cerebral Ischemia

Cerebral ischemia as a cause of falls in the aged is of multifactorial origin. Small cerebral thrombi, compression of the carotid and/or vertebral arteries by head movements, a hypotensive episode due to excess diuresis or antihypertensive or ataractic medication, anemia, polycythemia, and cardiac emboli particularly from atherosclerotic plaques with ulceration of the carotid arteries must be considered. When these are ruled out, a significant number of falls will be found to be due to cardiac dysrhythmias. With 24-hr or longer periods of continuous cardiac monitoring, it has been shown that a significant percentage of transient cerebral ischemic attacks and unexplained episodes of dizziness or syncope are due to episodes of cardiac dysrhythmia. These produce cerebral ischemia through a final common pathway of reduced cardiac output and pressure. The episodes may be of short duration and unaccompanied by palpitation. They are most common with significant organic heart disease of arteriosclerotic and hypertensive origin and calcific aortic stenosis.

Conditions which have been described include paroxysmal atrial fibrillation and flutter, frequent ventricular extrasystoles, second- or third-degree heart block, paroxysmal supraventricular tachycardias, short episodes of asystole, and marked sinus bradycardia with a ventricular rate below 40 accompanied by sinus arrests and sinoatrial blocks. The sick sinus syndrome manifests as sinus bradycardia with sinus arrests and/or numerous premature atrial beats, at times with alternating rapid atrial and occasionally ventricular escape rhythms. There may be a period of asystole of several seconds' duration at the end of the escape rhythms. Although the aged can tolerate a sinus rate of as low as 40 beats per minute without impaired cardiac output, any irregularity may have an adverse effect.

Chronic Illness

The depression, apathy, and sense of detachment from the environment which so often are seen with the aged, especially among those with chronic illness, are associated with an increase in falls due to lessened alertness and decreased self-care.

Medications

The polypharmacy resulting from the multiple diseases and disabilities of the aged together with their increased susceptibility to drug toxicity from such drugs as digitalis, barbiturates, phenothiazines, the tricyclic antidepressants, and the benzodiazapines lead to poor coordination, confusion, and cardiac dysrhythmias, with an increased liability to falls. This risk is increased by the frequency with which the aged make errors of omission and commission in taking prescribed medications as well as a tendency to self-medication.

ENVIRONMENTAL FACTORS

Hospital

The hospitalized aged are particularly susceptible to falls. As many as 90% of all hospital accidents among the aged are falls, more than half of which are falls out of bed. In addition to the many intrinsic accident hazards inherent to the hospital environment and the appreciable number due to staff negligence, many age-related factors increase accident liability. Risk factors include an impaired ability to adjust to new surroundings; decreased sensory acuity; irritability; poor memory, amnesia, and intransigence; night wandering; insomnia and night confusion; increased sensitivity to and a multiplicity of medications; multiple and severe chronic disease states resulting in decreased awareness of the environment and mental capacity; impairment of gait and loss of strength; prolonged bed rest with decreased efficiency of the circulatory system and muscle weakness; the unappreciated onset of acute illness; and osteoporosis with lessened bony resistance to fracture.

Long-Term Care Institutions

Falls are a major problem in long-term care institutions with populations who average over 80 years of age and who have a high prevalence of chronic disease, prior hip fractures, strokes, and senile dementias. Most falls occur in the bathroom, bedroom, dining room, corridors, and from wheelchairs. The majority of falls result in little or no injury and are due to inherent patient factors rather than environmental factors.

Home

All of the factors associated with falls in institutions may also precipitate falls in the home. Risks associated with furniture, thresholds, icy doorsteps and driveways, clutter, and poor illumination may be especially great.

DEATHS DUE TO FALLS

Deaths attributed to falls in the aged most often are due to the aggravation of pre-existing disease such as heart failure, pneumonia exacerbated by bed rest, nosocomial infections, and the effects of surgery and anesthesia.

SUMMARY AND CONCLUSIONS

Falling, which increases in severity with advancing age, is a major cause of disability and death in the elderly. Falling is a symptom, not a diagnosis, and it demands a thorough evaluation of psychological, psychiatric, medical, and drug-induced factors.

Special attention should be given to the detection of patient factors which lead to increased liability to falls. These include such conditions as acute intercurrent illness, chronic illness, orthostatic hypotension, osteoporosis, vestibular disease, disorders of gait, and cerebral ischemia.

The discovery and differentiation of factors that cause increased patient liability to falls and of the environmental hazards leading to accidental falls can initiate appropriate measures which will reduce the incidence of disabling and fatal falls among the aged.

When caring for elderly patients, the physician should:
1. Know that their increased risk for accidents is the principal factor in their falls.
2. Know that falls in elderly persons are indications for comprehensive evaluation of physical and mental status, including assessment of the possibility of acute or chronic illness and assessment of the contribution of normal age-related processes.
3. Know how increased risk of falls in the aged may depend on factors involving the cerebrum, peripheral nervous system, musculoskeletal system, cardiovascular system, special senses, effects of drugs, and environment.

REFERENCE

1. National Safety Council. *Home Accident Facts*. National Safety Council, Chicago, 1978.

SUGGESTED READING

Barron, R. D. Disorder of gait related to the aging nervous system. *Geriatrics*, 22:113–120, 1967.

Brain, R. Some unsolved problems of cervical spondylosis. *Br. Med. J.*, 1:771–777, 1963.

Gordon, M. Occult cardiac arrhythmias associated with falls and dizziness in the elderly. *J. Am. Geriatr. Soc.*, 26:418–423, 1978.

Rodstein, M. Accidents among the aged: incidence, causes and prevention. *J. Chronic Dis.*, 17:515–526, 1964.

Rodstein, M. Accidents among the aged. In: *Clinical Aspects of Aging*, edited by W. Reichel. Williams & Wilkins, Baltimore, 1978.

Rodstein, M., and Camus, A. S. Interrelations of heart disease and accidents. *Geriatrics*, 28:87–96, 1973.

Rodstein, M., and Zeman, F. D. Postural blood pressure changes in the elderly. *J. Chronic Dis.*, 6:581–588, 1957.

Steinberg, F. U. Gait disorders in old age. *Geriatrics*, 22:134–143, 1966.

Walter, P. F., Reid, S. D., and Wenger, N. K. Transient cerebral ischemia due to arrhythmia. *Ann. Intern. Med.*, 72:471–474, 1979.

Fundamentals of Geriatric Medicine, edited by
Ronald D. T. Cape, Rodney M. Coe, and Isadore
Rossman, Raven Press, New York © 1983.

14

Urinary Incontinence and the Significance of Nocturia and Frequency

F. L. Willington

The emphasis of this chapter is on the elucidation of the common causes of incontinence and the significance of the various symptoms which indicate that it is likely to occur. Detailed information on the subject is available in the "Suggested Reading" and is not dealt with here.

In order to understand the difficulties and complexities of the problem of incontinence, it is necessary to view it from the broadest standpoint. This is best achieved by considering the normal first.

CONTINENCE

Ninety-nine percent of normally developed children have achieved a socially acceptable level of control of their bodily evacuations by the age of 4.5 to 5 years. This is the skill of continence. It is not wholly inborn but is partly based on training. The failure of this skill is termed incontinence—a symptom, not a disease—the cause of which must be diagnosed. Continence has the following characteristics:

1. *A bladder reflex.* The reflex arc depends on an afferent link from stretch sensors in the bladder, an efferent link through the efferent fibers of the autonomic fibers of the sacral outflow, and an intact spinal cord up to the level of L2. This reflex is present at birth in the normal child and enables periodic evacuation of the bladder or bowel to take place without any intended alteration.
2. *Ability to postpone micturition (or defecation).* This is not present at birth but develops from about 2 years onward by endeavor, modified by parental or social influences and mediated from the cerebral cortex. It requires, in ad-

dition, an intact spinal cord and peripheral nerve connection, as well as functioning sympathetic and paraympathetic nervous systems.

The ability to postpone appears to diminish frequently during old age, and neuronal loss from the cortex must be considered a contributory factor. The duration of postponement may become so short that no warning at all is given before evacuation occurs. The ability may be severely affected, often by a dominant lobe cardiovascular accident (CVA).

3. *Ability to micturate or defecate voluntarily.* The ability to micturate or defecate, without the sensory stimulus to do so, is based on operant or conditioned reflex training principles. It is dependent on an intact neuronal mechanism, including spinal cord connection with the cerebral cortex. It is extremely difficult to train patients with a dominant lobe CVA. This part of the skill of continence remains unaltered for life. It seems to be endangered or altered by psychological stress or trauma at any age. It is through this faculty that the whole nursing procedure of "bladder training" is based.

ESSENTIAL ANATOMY

The bladder is a hollow viscus with its open end pointing downward. The urethra is angulated to the axis of the trigone at an angle of 80° to 90°. This angulation is maintained at rest by contraction of the constrictor urethra muscle, pulling toward the pubis.

Muscles

The wall of the bladder fundus is surrounded by smooth muscle fibers (the detrusor muscle) which are concentrated in the trigone area and at the outlet of the bladder. They also extend downward, ensheathing the proximal part of the urethra. This downward extension forms the internal sphincter. It is arranged with internal longitudinal fibers and outer circular fibers. There is also a dense stroma of collagenous and elastic fibers interspersed with the muscular fibers. Surrounding the mid and distal part of the urethra are striated muscle fibers. The external sphincter is a component of the urogenital diaphragm, the principal support structure of the bladder, uterus, and rectum. The muscles of the diaphragm are all striated and include the levator ani as the principal support muscle.

Innervation

The innervation is complex and in the normal adult is under the overall control of the cerebral cortex. It is conveniently considered under the headings of "central" and "local" tracts. An adequate understanding of these is necessary in order to diagnose incontinence.

Central tracts: The highest center for control is in the premotor area of the cortex proximal to the cyngulate gyrus. Other centers of activity have been located in the hypothalamus, midbrain, and pons, especially in the reticular substance. It has been found that the cerebral cortex is the principal area for suppression of the desire to micturate. The areas involved appear to be arranged alternatively as inhibitory and excitatory.

Local tracts: The motor impulses are transmitted by the corticospinal tracts to synapse in the pudendal nucleus for voluntary muscular activity. The involuntary motor impulses pass down the lateral columns in close proximity to the central canal and synapse with the sacral gray matter.

Peripheral nerves: The autonomic efferent nerves supply the motor impulses to the detrusor muscle. The pudendal nerve supplies the motor impulses to the striated muscle of the external sphincter.

Sensory supply: The fundus of the bladder is mainly sensitive to stretch and to a lesser extent to touch and pain. The stretch receptors are also concentrated at the trigone and bladder outlet. Their impulses pass through the afferent nerves of the sympathetic nervous system to the posterior horn and then to the lateral columns, eventually passing to the brainstem.

PHYSIOLOGY

During normal filling there is a pressure gradient between the intraluminal pressure in the urethra and the bladder cavity. The intraurethral pressure is higher than the intravesicular pressure, so long as the detrusor muscle does not contract. Provided the gradient exists, urine cannot flow. Contraction of the detrusor in response to stimulation of stretch receptors, in addition to causing contraction of the fundus, causes contraction of the trigone of the bladder. This has the effect of straightening out the angulation between it and the urethra; it also causes contraction of the internal sphincter, which has two further actions: (a) it shortens the urethra, and (b) it opens the proximal posterior portion of the urethra. This reduces the pressure gradient, and some urine passes into the proximal urethra. The evacuation reflex then operates.

The structural features which maintain continence are: (a) the resting tone of the internal sphincter producing the pressure gradient between the urethra and bladder; (b) the satisfactory support of the urogenital diaphragm, which ensures the support of the bladder base and the urethra; (c) the angulation of the urethra on the trigone axis, which has the effect of diverting the gravitational weight of urine from the urethra; (d) the length of the urethra, which is adequate for maintaining the pressure gradient; and (e) the internal softness of the urethral mucosa and probably the submucous connective tissue matrix, which ensures close apposition by forming a water-tight plug.

DIAGNOSIS OF INCONTINENCE

Failure of the complex action of containment and evacuation is often multifactorial in the elderly. In general, as age increases the more likely it is that there will be neurological causes for failure. Elucidation of the etiology is often complex, and multiple pathology may be present.

History

The history is probably the most important part of the diagnosis. The increased time taken to produce a comprehensive history in a case of incontinence is repaid in terms of the clarity of diagnosis, and it forms an essential part in the rehabilitation of the patient. Essential questions and subsidiary questions are shown in Table 1. Table 2 shows the significance of the individual symptoms.

Once the history had been taken, it should be possible to relate the symptom and history to failure of a particular muscle group. Thus if incontinence occurs during the filling phase (passive incontinence), it is likely that the sphincters are at fault. If it occurs during the phase of postponement (active incontinence), the detrusor action is faulty. This serves as a preliminary diagnosis but deserves more explanation.

TABLE 1. *Essential points to be established in history taking*

History of continence
  1. If the degree of continence is personally and socially acceptable
  2. Age of attainment of continence
  3. Previous history of enuresis
  4. History of "weak bladder"
  5. Family history of incontinence

Evidence of psychological effect
  1. History of depression, confusion, anxiety, or fear: nature of any effects on micturition
  2. If there was incontinence, the emotional reactions to it

Evidence of failure of supporting structures
  1. If incontinence occurs on first standing upright; if so, amount of urine passed
  2. If there is leakage on straining, sneezing, coughing, etc.

Micturition analysis
  1. Amount normally voided
  2. Postponement
      a. Ability to postpone desire to micturate
      b. Length of time (urgency when < 2 min)
      c. Incontinence from delay (urge incontinence)
  3. Frequency
      Night
      a. Nocturia (> twice nightly)
      b. Amount voided each time
      Day
      c. Frequency of micturition
  4. Uninhibited neurogenic incontinence
      a. Incontinence without warning
  5. Obstruction
      a. Difficulty on commencement
      b. Alteration in stream
      c. Sudden cessation of stream on voiding
      d. Straining required to void
  6. Inflammation
      a. Scalding or pain on voiding
      b. Strangury present
  7. Completeness
      a. If there is satisfaction from voiding

TABLE 2. *Significance of leading symptoms*

Symptom	Significance
Daytime frequency	Indication of hyper-reflexia or overflow retention. Hyperreflexia due to detrusor instability, or inflammation from another cause, e.g., idiopathic uninhibited neurogenic bladder, obstructive states, urinary tract infection, or involutional incontinence.
Nocturia	Prime symptom of impending incontinence; twice nightly acceptable in the elderly; mechanism uncertain; possibly present in chronic urinary retention due to redistribution of weight of urinary mass in the bladder when lying down. When present with small contracted hyperreflexive bladder is a symptom of minimal bladder distention from any cause.
Urgency	The reduction of the normal interval of postponement before irresistable evacuation occurs produces urgency. A symptom of failure of cortical inhibition. Complete failure leading to uninhibited neurogenic contractions. Sensory urgency reflects intense sensory stimulation without consequent motor activity.
Dysuria	Usually means difficulty rather than pain; present in obstructive states from any cause, e.g., prostatic or bladder outlet obstruction, or urethral stricture from any cause. Changes in texture of urethral mucous membranes or submucous layers can cause dysuria without evidence of stricture formation.
Scalding	Pain receptors and prostaglandin receptors in trigone, bladder outlet, and urethra give rise to scalding, painful sensation in the presence of inflammation, ulceration, and mechanical irritation from lithiasis.

Clearly, if material leakage occurs during the filling phase, a full bladder is not likely, and the patient will be constantly wet unless sitting in a chair when the pressure on the perineum closes the bladder outlet until the position is changed. If the detrusor muscle is at fault, sufficient urine must accumulate in the bladder to trigger the micturition reflex, so incontinence must be intermittent and confined to the time of the evacuation. This is too simplistic but is useful because it focuses attention on the functional failure that requires further investigation to produce a final diagnosis.

It often happens that the detrusor becomes so hyperactive that the bladder evacuates only a small amount frequently (e.g., less than 10 ml); this situation must be carefully distinguished from passive incontinence. Incontinence due to stress falls between these two groups and indicates a failure of the support systems as a result of primary trauma (e.g., difficult birth) or secondary trauma (e.g., stretching of the tissues from gross obesity or a large scrotal hernia). In the majority of cases, the history and clinical examination reveal the presence of stress incontinence.

Clinical Examination

A general physical examination is often not revealing, and an examination of the central nervous system is essential. It is important to test sensation in the corda equina distribution, as well as that of the limbs. It is also essential to establish that the pyramidal tracts are intact, and a test should be made of the cauda equina reflexes (Table 3). The external genitalia should of course be examined carefully. A rectal examination is essential in every male and a gynecological examination in every female.

Residual Urine

An estimate of the efficiency of bladder emptying is necessary, so an estimate of the residual urine is required at some stage of the investigation. This is performed by passing a catheter after evacuation. It is often convenient for this investigation to be left until the catheter has been passed for urodynamic investigation. As the bladder floor may be prolapsed and may not empty when the patient is prone, the estimation should be done in two stages: prone and in full flexion.

Examination of the Urine

This is a convenient time to assess the question of urinary tract infection; hence the urine evacuated should be examined macroscopically and microscopically. Both a bacterial and a cellular count are required.

Urinary Tract Infection

The position about bacteriuria, cellular content, and relevant symptoms requires clarification. A great deal of work has been done with regard to the significance in terms of renal damage and bacterial infection. The question here is if either of these findings, separately or in combination, produces symptoms of incontinence. The symptoms involved are frequency, urgency, and scalding.

It has been shown that there is a statistically significant relationship between acute infection and incontinence but not with long-term bacteriuria. Moreover, it has been shown that there is a statistical relationship between urgency and dysuria and bacterial infection in females only. The presence of white blood cells may be an indication of inflammatory reaction, but they have also been shown to be present when no bacteria can be cultured. Thus the point is reached that the same symptoms may occur independently in any bladder infection. The combination of a significant bacterial count plus more than 15 leukocytes per high power field is probably an indication of a reaction to bacteria likely to cause symptoms; the presence of a significant bacterial count without cellular increase is unlikely to affect the symptomatology.

TABLE 3. *Cauda equina reflexes*

Reflex	Stimulation	Result
Anal	Pinching mucosa or pricking	Contraction of sphincter
Bulbocavernosus	Squeezing of glans penis	Contraction of anal sphincter

If a definite diagnosis is to be made, some form of cystometric examination and an estimate of the urethral flow rate are necessary. The former can be carried out simply and adequately, but the latter requires specialized equipment.

It may become necessary for the patient to have a full urodynamic examination, but in the elderly this may be counterproductive as it can cause anxiety and sometimes confusion.

The salient points to be found in the principal groups of incontinent patients are now given as a guide to the likely results obtained from the procedures discussed.

ACTIVE INCONTINENCE

Active incontinence occurs during the phase of postponement, when detrusor action is faulty.

Defective Development of Continence

Defective development of continence may be obvious in a "graduate" who had spent time in an institution with subnormality or with a congenital defect, e.g., spina bifida. However, in the elderly the most common finding may be termed family-induced incontinence.

The history shows a late development of continence, with enuresis, and sometimes daytime incontinence with defective postponement. Continence may never have been fully attained or may break down under stress, the episodes being termed "weak bladder." The maternal and sometimes the paternal history of continence is often defective. The dominant symptoms are anxiety and frequency. Physical examination is negative.

Dementia and Confusion

Persons with dementia or in a confusional state who are incontinent comprise a large group. The pattern of incontinence may involve defective postponement and defective voluntary micturition. Memory is short. Enuresis is common. It is important to distinguish reversible from irreversible confusional states. The outlook for recovery from incontinence is much better in those whose state is reversible. Depressed patients sometimes present as incontinent, confused patients who recover dramatically when treated correctly. Many patients have a diminished degree of continence, and an episode of acute urinary tract infection that leads to incontinence may cause them to become distressed and subsequently confused.

Obstructive Incontinence

Obstruction usually develops slowly. In the bladder outlet an obstruction gives rise to dysuria (difficulty in micturating), frequency during the day, and especially nocturia. Other complaints are poor stream, postmicturition dribbling (in men with prostatic enlargement), and a feeling that the bladder is not empty after the micturition. The general effect is on the detrusor, which overacts. The sphincter is also affected owing to the changes at the bladder outlet. Thus urgency and urge incontinence are common.

The most common cause is prostatic obstruction in men and bladder neck obstruction in women. Stricture formation in both sexes leads to distention of the bladder in which a large amount of residual urine is not a dominant feature. The eventual situation is overflow incontinence.

It should be noted that an unstable reaction of the detrusor may precede the obstruction or may occur because of it, with the result that removal of the prostate has no appreciable benefit. The essential criterion is constant, poor urethral flow.

Involutional Incontinence

The changes in the female tract in the older age groups are very important, and reference to the "Suggested Reading" list is recommended. Briefly, changes in the vagina and atrophy of the external genitalia are well known. It should be noted that the base of the bladder is an estrogenic area, and inflammation is common and presents as "bladder infection."

The urethra is also affected. The mucous membrane becomes atrophic, and there is cellular infiltration of the submucous layers with accompanying edema. This produces dysuria because of the changes in the urethra, but with scalding on micturition due to cracking of the urethral mucous membrane. The combined effect is to produce an unstable detrusor reaction, with frequency, urgency, urge incontinence, and marked nocturia. The urethral flow may be almost obstructed because of the changes in the bladder outlet, or strictures may form due to prolapse of the urethra at the orifice, where it shows as a red ring which may ulcerate.

Neurogenic Incontinence

Neurogenic incontinence is commonly divided into four types or categories: (a) uninhibited neurogenic, in which the neurological defect is usually central (cerebral); (b) accelerated neurogenic (spinal reflex bladder), with the defect in the upper spinal cord above L2; (c) atonic, caused by a sensory deficiency with consequent reflex failure, e.g., diabetic, tabetic, peripheral neuropathy; and (d) autonomous, caused by destruction of afferent and efferent nerves of the corda equina. This is called "autonomous" because defective contraction still occurs.

The effect of the first two types is interference with postponement: Detrusor activity is increased, leading to incontinence during the postponement phase of the cycle—active incontinence. This is common with strokes, multiple sclerosis, and disc lesions. Uninhibited neurogenic incontinence is the most common cause of neurogenic incontinence and, in fact, of all incontinence in the elderly.

Cystometric investigation is necessary to demonstrate the nature of bladder function. This is usually a hyperreflexic bladder action with a small bladder, slow to relax after a contraction, and minimal evidence of cortical inhibition. The predominant symptoms are urgency, often extreme; urge incontinence; uninhibited neurogenic contractions; marked nocturia; daytime frequency and some residual urine;

small bladder capacity. It can be idiopathic, associated with involutional incontinence or obstructive incontinence.

A subgroup of this type shows a large bladder, hyporeflexic with a large amount of residual urine, and poor detrusor contractions, passing a large amount of urine at frequent intervals. On cystometry it is found that detrusor instability occurs only after there is about 200 ml in the bladder.

It should always be remembered that chronic constipation is the most common cause of urinary incontinence, presenting usually as an unstable bladder but sometimes as urinary retention.

PASSIVE INCONTINENCE

Passive incontinence occurs during the filling phase and is likely to be due to failure of the sphincters.

Neurogenic Incontinence

The two relevant classes of neurogenic incontinence involved are concerned with lesions below L2 and with the peripheral nerves. This may result in defective sphincter action, either alone or combined with defective action of the sphincter and detrusor muscles.

Atonic Bladder

The term "atonic bladder" indicates the presence of a large bladder due to the initiating stimulus being lost because of damage to the afferent nerves (e.g., tabes dorsalis or diabetic neuropathy). The result is defective action, causing distention. In obstructive conditions the final state of overflow incontinence—a large, distended bladder—is similar except that the primary damage is done to the muscles because of the obstruction, not because of nerve damage.

Autonomous Bladder

The term "autonomous bladder" is used to describe the situation in which there are no nervous connections with the bladder because the corda equina has been damaged from trauma, neoplasia, etc. There is a built-in neurological connection in the bladder wall, however, so some contractions still take place, although they are erratic and incomplete. In general there is a large atonic bladder, and manual pressure may be required to empty it. Sensations are absent.

Traumatic Bladder Syndromes

The traumatic bladder syndromes include postprostatectomy incontinence, which is usually due to sphincter damage. Leakage is therefore continuous in this type of disorder. Also included in this group is incontinence following hysterectomy and severe lumbar osteoarthropathy. Scars and a history of central nervous system changes are apparent on examination. Rectal examination reveals a loss of sphincter tone.

The trauma due to parturition may give rise to "stress incontinence." The history is characteristic and gynecological examination usually confirms the diagnosis, although occasionally more sophisticated urodynamic methods are required. Stress incontinence can also occur in men with defective pelvic floor musculature. Rectal examination may reveal a gaping of the anus and prolapse of the perineum on straining.

IATROGENIC INCONTINENCE

It should never be forgotten that many cases of incontinence in the elderly are the result of therapy. The role of hypnotics and fast-acting diuretics is well known. It is not always realized that fast-acting diuretics give rise to sensory urgency and not just the simple effect of rapid filling of the bladder.

Care should be taken to exclude the use of benzodiazepines when continence is impaired. Diazepam, especially, gives rise to reduced muscle tone and may result in sphincter weakness.

The principal agents likely to alter the adrenergic/cholinergic balance are hypotensive agents and drugs for cardiac dysrhythmias, causing α-adrenergic blockade, β-blockade, ganglion blockade, etc. To this important group must be added the phenothiazines, which have the effect of reducing α-adrenergic stimuli and which also result in failure to recognize the "bladder cues" due to their central effect.

CONCLUSION

If the normal sequence of clinical procedures is followed as outlined above, but with a shift in emphasis toward bladder function, a diagnosis of incontinence can usually be made with reasonable accuracy, enabling appropriate treatment to be initiated.

When caring for elderly patients, the physician should:

1. Have a systematic procedure for the assessment of the elderly person who has incontinence, including appropriate use of standard diagnostic procedures.
2. Know how the common pathological and psychological conditions causing incontinence may present and which historical data are most useful in the differential diagnosis.
3. Know how the symptoms demonstrated in incontinent patients vary with the cause.
4. Know how relatively simple and standard diagnostic procedures can obviate the need for high-technology interventions, with the indications for the latter.

SUGGESTED READING

Willington, F. L., editor. *Urinary Incontinence in the Elderly*. Academic Press, London, 1976.

Willington, F. L. *Urinary incontinence and urgency. Practitioner*, 220:739–747, 1978.

Willington, F. L. Urinary incontinence: a practical approach. *Geriatrics*, 35:41–43, 47–48, 1980.

Fundamentals of Geriatric Medicine, edited by
Ronald D. T. Cape, Rodney M. Coe, and Isadore
Rossman, Raven Press, New York © 1983.

15

Functional Psychiatric Disorders

James T. Moore and Alan D. Whanger

Most psychiatric illnesses are first seen and treated by primary care physicians. Extremely common in general medical practice, most of these disorders are treatable, although unfortunately many are missed. In a 1964 survey of elderly patients in the United Kingdom, Williamson and his colleagues (7) found that 71% of depressions and 61% of neuroses had not been diagnosed by the primary physician.

Functional psychopathology in the elderly is even more difficult to recognize than in younger patients for at least three reasons: (a) Atypical presentations of psychiatric disease are common so that depression, for example, frequently does not conform to the standard presentation seen in younger patients. (b) Functional psychiatric illness can present with predominantly physical symptoms (e.g., depression may present as hypochondriasis). (c) The high incidence of multiple physical problems and their associated symptoms often covers psychopathology.

In this chapter we discuss some of the more common functional psychiatric disorders, e.g., affective disorders, anxiety and neurotic disorders, paranoid states, and hypochondriasis.

AFFECTIVE DISORDERS

Depression

Although depression is undoubtedly the most common psychiatric problem of elderly patients, estimates of incidence vary depending on the criteria used to define depression as well as on the selection of subjects to be surveyed. Williamson (7) found 5.4% of a random community sample and 14% of persons referred to a geriatric consultative clinic in Edinburgh to be depressed. In the Duke University longitudinal studies of independently living elderly, the proportion of persons considered depressed remained constant at 25% throughout the study, and 70% of persons examined a minimum of seven times had at least one episode of depression. Depression was the major disorder in over 50% of geriatric admissions to the university psychiatry service (4).

Social, psychological, and biological factors play a role in the increased incidence of depression in the elderly. Social factors frequently associated with depression include isolation secondary to decreased mobility, unavailable transportation, and loss of employment.

Of all psychological factors associated with depression, loss plays the greatest role in the elderly. Busse and co-workers (1,2) noted that the loss of one's physical health appears to be the most stressful loss, at least for males, and that loss of financial security plays a central role for females. Busse contrasted the psychodynamics of depression in the elderly with that in younger persons. Anger and guilt are major factors in the psychodynamics of depression in younger persons, whereas they play a relatively less significant role in the elderly, as loss becomes more important.

Biological factors predisposing the elderly to depression are based on recent discoveries about the role of catecholamine neurotransmitters in depression. Depression is associated with deficits in the catecholamine neurotransmitter systems (particularly norepinephrine and serotonin). The enzyme monoamine oxidase plays an important role in the metabolism of these neurotransmitters. There is an increase in platelet and brain monoamine oxidase activity with age which might partially explain the increased incidence of depression in the elderly. Some investigators have also noted a decrease in catecholamine neurotransmitters in elderly suicide victims.

It is important to note that depression may present differently in elderly persons than in younger individuals. Table 1 summarizes features of depression in the elderly. There is likely to be an emphasis on somatic rather than psychological complaints. In elderly patients symptoms of apathy and withdrawal are likely to predominate. The elderly are less likely to manifest guilt as a major symptom, and they are often reluctant to admit feelings of dysphoric mood, thus making it difficult to use the standard criteria for diagnosis of depression. This makes it important to use behavioral observations rather than relying completely on the patient's report of symptoms.

TABLE 1. *Depression in the elderly*

Common characteristics
    Somatic complaints likely to predominate over psychological
    Apathy and withdrawal
    Guilt rare
    Loss of self-esteem prominent
    Dysphoric mood often denied
    Inability to concentrate, with resultant memory impairment common

Atypical presentations
    "Pseudodementia"
    Alcoholism
    Hypochondriasis
    Pain

Depression in the elderly frequently presents with symptoms of organic brain syndrome (e.g., agitation, memory impairment, emotional lability). Wells has used the term "pseudodementia" to describe this phenomenon (6). It is frequently difficult to distinguish depression from dementia. Table 2 summarizes clinical features that help make the distinction between depression and dementia (Chapter 6).

Another atypical presentation of depression in the elderly is alcoholism. Any elderly individual with a relatively short history of alcoholism should be investigated for depression. This is particularly important if the onset of alcoholism coincides with a significant loss, e.g., the death of a spouse.

Hypochondriasis in the elderly may also be a symptom of depression. As with alcoholism, special attention should be given to the patient with a relatively short history of hypochondriasis. De Alarcón (3) reported a series of 152 depressed elderly patients, more than half of whom had prominent hypochondriacal symptoms.

It is not uncommon for atypical pain to be the major, if not the only, symptoms of depression in the elderly. Such pain has been called a "depressive equivalent" and responds to treatment for depression. Persistent, atypical pain which does not fit a diagnostic category should raise the suspicion of depression.

Suicide

Suicide is one of the 10 leading causes of death of adults in the United States. More than one-third of the suicides are by older persons (who make up less than one-eighth of the population), and the vast majority of these are associated with depression. Many studies have shown that most persons who commit suicide were seen by a physician shortly before their death. Several factors have been shown to be associated with an increased risk of suicide. Lack of social support, isolation, feelings of hopelessness, and the presence of definite suicide plans are perhaps the highest risk factors. Although some physicians feel concerned that they will "give the patient ideas" if they ask about suicide directly, there is no reason to believe this is the case; it is imperative that any patient who shows symptoms of depression be asked about suicide. Questions such as the following are helpful in assessing suicide potential:

"Have you ever felt life wasn't worth living?"
"Have you ever wanted to go to sleep and not wake up?"
"When you had those feelings, have you ever thought how you might do it?"

The decision of whether to hospitalize a patient with depression is often difficult and is influenced by medical and social considerations. Can the individual promise that "no matter how bad it gets" he/she will not act on suicidal impulses for at least some minimum time (until the next visit to the physician's office)? Are there good social supports including friends and family who will treat the person at home? Is there a history of drug abuse, alcoholism, or impulsive behavior which increases suicide risk? It is also important to remember that the suicide risk of many people increases as they improve with treatment. During the early phase, they may have

TABLE 2. *Major clinical features differentiating pseudodementia from dementia*

Pseudodementia	Dementia
Clinical course and history	
Family always aware of dysfunction and its severity.	Family often unaware of dysfunction and its severity.
Onset can be dated with some precision.	Onset can be dated only within broad limits.
Symptoms of short duration before medical help is sought.	Symptoms usually of long duration before medical help is sought.
Rapid progression of symptoms after onset.	Slow progression of symptoms throughout course.
History of previous psychiatric dysfunction common.	History of previous psychiatric dysfunction unusual.
Complaints and clinical behavior	
Patients usually complain of cognitive loss.	Patients usually complain little of cognitive loss.
Patients' complaints of cognitive dysfunction usually detailed.	Patients' complaints of cognitive dysfunction usually vague.
Patients emphasize disability.	Patients conceal disability.
Patients highlight failures.	Patients delight in accomplishments, however trivial.
Patients make little effort to perform even simple tasks.	Patients struggle to perform tasks.
Patients do not try to keep up.	Patients rely on notes, calendars, etc. to keep up.
Patients usually communicate strong sense of distress.	Patients often appear unconcerned.
Affective change often pervasive.	Affect labile and shallow.
Loss of social skills often early and prominent.	Social skills often retained.
Behavior often incongruent with severity of cognitive dysfunction	Behavior usually compatible with severity of cognitive dysfunction.
Nocturnal accentuation of dysfunction uncommon.	Nocturnal accentuation of dysfunction common.
Clinical features related to memory, cognitive, and intellectual dysfunctions	
Attention and concentration often well preserved.	Attention and concentration usually faulty.
"Don't know" answers typical.	Near-miss answers frequent.
On tests of orientation, patients often give "don't know" answers.	On tests of orientation, patients often mistake unusual for usual.
Memory loss for recent and remote events usually equally severe.	Memory loss for recent events usually more severe than for remote events.
Memory gaps for specific periods or events common.	Memory gaps for specific periods unusual.
Marked variability in performance on tasks of similar difficulty.	Consistently poor performance on tasks of similar difficulty.

From Wells, C. E. Pseudodementia. *Am. J. Psychiatry*, 136:895–900, 1979.

so little energy that they cannot act on their suicidal feelings, but as they improve with treatment their energy might improve while the mood is still depressed enough to make suicide a serious risk.

Depression and Physical Disease

Depression may be the first symptom of physical disease. Early dementia and cancer of the pancreas are two diseases in which depression may be the first symptom. The bradykinesia, rigidity, and expressionless facies of Parkinson's disease can be confused with depression. The emotional lability and crying spells accompanying multi-infarct dementia can also be mistaken for depression. Many diseases can have a nonspecific presentation, including weight loss, decreased energy, and fatigability, and their presence should always raise the question of occult malignancy or, indeed, benign and treatable disease, e.g., gastric ulcer.

Drug-Related Depression

Many drugs commonly used in the elderly can cause depression. Consequently, a careful drug history is always important in depressed patients. The best way to obtain this history is to ask the patient to bring all his/her medicines to the office. Antihypertensive drugs (e.g., reserpine, methyldopa, guanethidine) are the drugs most often associated with depression, but other drugs which inhibit sympathetic activity may also be implicated (e.g., propranolol). Alcohol is a commonly used drug which can produce depression, and a pattern of mild depression resulting in increased alcohol consumption leading to more severe depression is not uncommon. As noted elsewhere in this chapter, alcoholism is a common presentation of depression in the elderly. Stimulants such as amphetamines are rarely prescribed today, but they formerly were used quite frequently in the elderly, and abrupt cessation of such drugs is very often associated with depression.

Mania

Although much less common than depression, mania may also occur in elderly individuals. It has been estimated that between 5 and 13% of elderly patients with an affective disorder are manic. Mania frequently has a different symptomatic picture in the elderly and is consequently easily missed. Increased activity might be less striking than in younger patients, paranoid delusions are common, and the affect is often more irritable and angry than elated. Patients also frequently show mild organic brain syndrome. These differences are summarized in Table 3. Manic episodes generally require psychiatric hospitalization, as compliance with treatment is poor and the risk of injury to self or others is significant. The treatment of choice

TABLE 3. *Clinical presentation of mania*

Symptom category	Younger patients	Older patients
Activity	Increased	Likely to appear agitated
Mood	Elated	Angry, irritable
Affect	Elated, grandiose	Suspicious, paranoid
Thought	Flight of ideas; distractable	Circumstantial
		Can appear as organic brain syndrome

for mania is lithium. Care must be used in evaluating cardiovascular, thyroid, and renal function before initiating treatment.

ANXIETY AND NEUROTIC DISORDERS

Anxiety is the primary symptom of neurotic disorders and has both psychological and physical signs and symptoms. Psychological symptoms include a sense of fear or dread without a specific source. Physiological accompaniments of anxiety are generally related to autonomic activity and include muscle tension, tachycardia, and increased sweating. Sources of anxiety include intrapsychic conflict over unacceptable impulses, overwhelming stress, and anticipated loss of support with a resulting sense of helplessness. In general, the latter two factors are most important in the elderly (i.e., stress and anticipated loss of supports). Anxiety and neurosis during late life may be residual from earlier chronic conditions or they may be new problems arising for the first time in an individual's life.

In a community survey in the United Kingdom, Kay et al. (5) identified neurotic illness in 12% of persons surveyed and found that about 5% of persons were suffering from an illness that began after age 60.

Studies from the United Kingdom suggest that impairment in physical health (especially in the cardiovascular and gastrointestinal systems) are frequently associated with neurosis, as are loneliness and difficulty in self-care.

Evaluation of the patient with anxiety should include a history, physical examination, and judicious use of laboratory tests. The history should include a careful drug history, including medicines stopped as well as those presently taken, as abrupt cessation of many drugs can cause anxiety. Similar questions about personal habits such as coffee intake are important as caffeinism can cause anxiety. Patients often use psychological defenses to avoid recognizing the cause of anxiety. For example, an elderly woman might complain of feeling anxiety since the preceding Christmas but deny any stress in her life. However, when asked about what was going on in her life last Christmas, she might report that her children suggested she sell her home and move to a smaller apartment near one of them (all of whom live long distances from her).

Because many physical diseases can present with nervousness, tachycardia, and other symptoms of anxiety, a careful medical history and physical examination are mandatory. Furthermore, physical illness can itself increase anxiety as noted above. Laboratory tests should not be used indiscriminately to replace the history and examination but should supplement them. Because, for example, thyroid disease can cause symptoms of anxiety in the absence of more classic physical symptoms, thyroid function studies are sometimes useful. Other laboratory studies of similar value and the problems they can help identify include complete blood counts (anemia), serum calcium and phosphorus (parathyroid disease), and serum electrolytes (hypokalemia).

Because prognosis and treatment are related to the type of anxiety, it is useful to identify symptoms of anxiety in one of three major groups: (a) acute anxiety (usually stress-related); (b) chronic anxiety (often associated with long-standing personality traits); and (c) anxiety-depression.

Acute anxiety is associated with a traumatic experience such as bereavement, relocation, or retirement. These disorders are generally self-limited and respond well to supportive intervention using a crisis-intervention model. Short-term use of anxiolytic agents (e.g., benzodiazepines) is often helpful. Counseling focuses on helping the patient cope with the environmental stress and might emphasize replacement of losses, change in the patient's behavior, or changing the environment where stress is especially high.

Chronic neurotic anxiety is more difficult and has a less favorable prognosis. In general, benzodiazepines are to be avoided in these patients, who frequently are predisposed to drug dependence. If medication is necessary, major tranquilizers may be preferred. Many of these patients also have elements of hypochondriasis which complicate management.

Anxiety is frequently combined with elements of depression. In general, these patients respond more favorably to treatment which focuses on the depressive element rather than treatment which focuses on the anxiety element.

PARANOIA

Like depression and dementia, paranoia is not always obvious. This is because the disorder exists on a continuum from mild suspiciousness to severe psychosis. Tolerance of the paranoid individual's environment may be as important as the severity of symptoms in determining who comes to professional attention.

As many as 17% of a community sample of elderly have been identified as showing suspiciousness to a symptomatic degree. Approximately 10% of all psychotic patients admitted to psychogeriatric units in the United Kingdom suffer primarily from a form of paranoid psychosis.

Diagnosis

Paranoid disorders have been classified in many ways. A clinically useful system is to describe them in terms of severity of symptoms.

Suspiciousness is the mildest form of paranoia and may exist in as many as 11% of elderly persons living independently in the community. Although some of these individuals may have a life-long history of suspiciousness, the social isolation of old age, incipient mental impairment, and use of projection as a psychological defense mechanism make the elderly increasingly at risk for mild forms of paranoia. For example, if an individual is having some degree of memory loss and cannot find his glasses in the morning, it might be less threatening to assume someone took them than to face the fact that he cannot remember where he left them. As aging individuals lose control over their environment, it is understandable that the environment would be perceived as increasingly hostile and threatening. Sensory loss (especially hearing) has also been noted to play a major role in the development of suspiciousness.

Paranoid hallucinosis is a more severe disorder than suspiciousness. The individual may present with a focused complaint, and both visual and auditory hallucinations may be present.

Paraphrenia or *schizophreniform syndrome* includes delusions of theft, poisoning, being observed, etc. Visual and auditory hallucinations may also be present. Although these individuals often look schizophrenic, their symptoms can be explained as exaggerations and misinterpretations of a threatening environment. The symptoms also improve when the individual is removed from his environment.

Paranoid schizophrenia is the most severe form of suspiciousness seen in the elderly. The question of whether this disorder is different from paranoid schizophrenia in younger persons is not yet resolved. It is often difficult to distinguish schizophrenics from paraphrenics; however, schizophrenics exhibit Schneider's first-rank symptoms (e.g., the auditory hallucinations discuss the individual in the third person). Unlike paraphrenia, symptoms characteristically do not improve on changing the environment.

Treatment

Evaluating and treating the paranoid patient is difficult, as the physician must maintain sympathy for the patient's distress without challenging or supporting the delusions. The first step in evaluating the paranoid patient is to identify factors which strengthen the suspicions. Sometimes, in fact, what appear to be delusions are true. More commonly, well-meaning family and staff interact in such a way as to reinforce the elderly person's suspicions. For example, one elderly woman who lived with her daughter, son-in-law, and teen-aged granddaughter was quite suspicious of her family. One factor contributory to this was the fact that the patient's daughter was allowing the granddaughter to use the patient's car without consulting the patient. The overall family situation was much improved when the daughter returned control of the car to the patient.

After identification of contributory factors from persons in the patient's environment, it is generally useful to minimize conversation about the delusions. Attempts to convince the patient to give up the delusions are usually counterproductive. It is preferable to reinforce any conversation that is not related to the delusions.

Although paranoia is frequently the major disorder, it often is associated with other illnesses—most notably depression and dementia. When other diseases accompany the paranoid symptoms they must of course be treated as specifically as possible.

When caring for elderly patients, the physician should:

1. Know how social, psychological, and biological factors contribute to depression in elderly persons.
2. Know six ways in which depression may be manifested in elderly persons that do not fall within the classical description of depression.
3. Know four atypical presentations of depression in elderly persons.

4. Know two or more drugs that commonly produce depression in elderly persons.
5. Know four or more ways in which the clinical history or interview can be used to differentiate depression from dementia.
6. Be aware of the revised categorization of paranoid disorders, as proposed in the Diagnostic Statistical Manual (DSM III, 1980).
7. Know how sensory deficits contribute to suspiciousness in elderly persons.

REFERENCES

1. Busse, E. W., and Blazer, D., (editors). *Handbook of Geropsychiatry.* Van Nostrand Reinhold, New York, 1980.
2. Busse, E. W., and Pfeiffer, E. *Behavior and Adaptation in Late Life.* Little Brown, Boston, 1975.
3. De Alarcón, R. Hypochondriasis and depression in the aged. *Gerontol. Clin.,* 6:266–277, 1964.
4. Gianturco, D. T., and Busse, E. W. Psychiatric problems encountered during a long term study of normal aging volunteers. In: *Studies in Geriatric Psychiatry,* edited by A. D. Isaacs and F. Post. Wiley, New York, 1978.
5. Kay, D. W. K., Beamish, P., and Roth, M. Old age mental disorders in Newcastle upon Tyne. I. A study of prevalence. *Br. J. Psychiatry,* 110:146–158, 1964.
6. Wells, C. E. Pseudodementia. *Am. J. Psychiatry,* 136:895–900, 1979.
7. Williamson, J., Stokoe, I. H., Gray, S., Fisher, M., Smith, A., McGhee, A., and Stephenson, E. Old people at home: their unreported needs. *Lancet,* 1:1117–1120, 1964.

SUGGESTED READING

Blazer, D. *Psychopathology of Aging.* American Academy of Family Physicians, Kansas City, MO, 1977.

Diagnostic and Statistical Manual of Mental Disorders. American Psychiatric Association, Washington, DC, 1980.

Isaacs, A. D., and Post, F. *Studies in Geriatric Psychiatry.* Wiley, New York, 1978.

Pitt, B. *Psychogeriatrics: An Introduction to the Psychiatry of Old Age.* Churchill Livingstone, Edinburgh, 1974.

Post, F. *Persistent Persecutory States of the Elderly.* Pergamon, London, 1966.

Wang, H. S. Diagnostic procedures. In: *Handbook of Geropsychiatry,* edited by E. W. Busse and D. G. Blazer. Van Nostrand Reinhold, New York, 1980.

Whanger, A. D. Paranoid syndromes of the senium. In: *Psychopharmacology in the Aging,* edited by W. E. Fann and C. Eisdorfer. Plenum Press, New York, 1973.

Whanger, A. D., and Verwoerdt, A. Management of affective disorders. In: *Clinical Geropsychiatry,* 2nd ed. edited by A. Verwoedt. Williams & Wilkins, Baltimore, *(in press).*

Fundamentals of Geriatric Medicine, edited by
Ronald D. T. Cape, Rodney M. Coe, and Isadore
Rossman, Raven Press, New York © 1983.

16

Organic Brain Syndromes, Other Nonfunctional Psychiatric Disorders, and Pseudodementia

Alvin J. Levenson

Nonfunctional psychiatric disorders are psychopathological states which have an organic etiology. These states are not part of normal aging, and so when they occur they require the same evaluation they would in a younger population.

ORGANIC BRAIN SYNDROME

The most commonly occurring late-life nonfunctional state is the organic brain syndrome (OBS), of which there are two major classes: chronic (irreversible) and acute (potentially reversible).

An OBS is a disorder manifested by cognitive/intellectual and memory dysfunction. The diagnosis is made on the basis of clinical signs and not laboratory values. The presence of any one or more of the following findings indicates the presence of an OBS: partial or total disorientation to person, place, or time; impaired recent memory (recall to two objects at approximately 2 min); impaired digit retention (greater than a two-digit gap between the number of single digits that the patient can remember forward versus reversed); impaired intellectual function (reduced fund of general information, e.g., as the first or current President of the United States, as well as an inability to perform simple calculations, e.g., 100 minus 5); and concrete thinking (inability to abstract proverbs such as "Don't count your chickens before they hatch" or "People who live in glass houses shouldn't throw stones").

In addition to purely cognitive and memory dysfunctional states, an OBS may present with its logical extensions, i.e., additional psychiatric abnormalities which are caused by the same insult that caused the OBS. These logical extensions include lability of affect (an excessive emotional response to minimal or no provocation);

stereotypy (repetitive, redundant, and illogical speech and other motor activities, e.g., perseveration); pathological resistance; frightening delusions and hallucinations; purely visual hallucinations and/or tactile, kinesthetic, gustatory, or olfactory hallucinations. Importantly, OBSs, with or without their logical extensions, can be accompanied by any functional psychiatric state and therefore are unrelated etiologically. The functional psychopathological concomitants arise by one of several routes. First, they may have preceded the OBS. Second, the OBS may be stressful and hence evoke the appearance of stress-related psychopathology in predisposed individuals (usually the individual with strong obsessive-compulsive personality traits). Third, the OBS may provoke the surfacing of previously submerged psychopathology via a poorly understood frontal lobe releasing mechanism. Regardless, the concomitant functional states must not be regarded as organic equivalents.

OBSs are caused by an insult of sufficient magnitude to disrupt function in critical areas of the cerebral cortex, primarily the frontal lobes, which control cognitive and intellectual function as well as stability of affect, and the temporal lobes, which control memory and the emotions. Consequently, regardless of the insult, the OBS presents in the same way depending on the area of the cortex affected. The insult itself, however, determines accessory clinical findings. For example, a hypothyroidism-induced OBS will be accompanied by the clinical manifestations of thyroid insufficiency. A tumor large enough to encompass the prefrontal and motor strip areas of the frontal lobes will present as an OBS accompanied by contralateral motor dysfunction.

Chronic OBS

Chronic OBSs, also referred to as "dementia," are of two main types, based on cause.

Primary Neuronal Degenerative States

The first subdivision is the primary neuronal degenerative state. In this state, the initial pathogenetic events are believed to occur within the neuron itself, exclusive of such extraneous factors as cerebral blood flow, followed by neuronal hypofunction and death. This subdivision is represented by diseases such as Alzheimer's disease, senile degenerative brain disease, Pick's disease, Jacob-Creutzfeldt disease, and Huntington's chorea. The most commonly occurring primary neuronal degenerative state causing an OBS in the elderly is a combination of the senile degenerative and Alzheimer types; many refer to this combination as senile dementia of the Alzheimer's type (or SDAT). The exact cause(s) of these conditions is largely unknown. For some there may be a genetic basis, although the link between that and the process of degeneration itself is enigmatic. Regardless, they all present with the progressive onset of an OBS, although there are generally some distinguishing histopathological and clinical features which assist in the diagnosis.

Histopathologically, there are some distinct differences. Alzheimer's disease affects neurons from all six layers of the cortex in every lobe of the brain. Affected neurons manifest senile plaques (affecting intrasynaptic function), neurofibrillary tangles (potentially affecting intraneuronal activity), and granulovacuolar degeneration. One question is whether Alzheimer's disease represents a more severe form of senile degenerative brain disease, or a pathological progression of normal aging, as nondemented subjects and those with senile degenerative brain disease possess all of the above-mentioned cellular characteristics. There is, however, a marked quantitative difference, sufferers from SDAT having many more plaques and tangles than subjects exhibiting aging per se.

Pick's disease possesses neither the neuronal characteristics nor the extensiveness of Alzheimer's disease. It usually affects only the top three cortical layers, predominantly in the frontal and temporal lobes. A genetic predisposition has been identified in Alzheimer's disease, and a dominant mode of transmission is currently accepted in Pick's disease. An autosomal dominant transmission occurs in Huntington's chorea, a disease which predominantly affects the middle and deeper layers of the cortex, especially in the frontal lobes. There is derangement of the cellular architecture of involved structures due to neuronal loss and replacement gliosis. Those cells which remain are in varying states of chronic cell change. Although it is unclear, there seems to be a small genetic-related incidence of the autosomal dominant mode (approximately 9%) in Jacob-Creutzfeldt disease. Of all the irreversible OBSs, this illness is the only one in which a slow virus has definitely been implicated. Some workers suspect that a virus may also be involved in the etiology of SDAT, although there is not yet satisfactory evidence of this. Jacob-Creutzfeldt disease is a rapidly progressive, fatal central nervous system disease of middle life. It is mentioned here because of its uniqueness (slow virus) and for the sake of completeness.

Clinical differences between these entities are variable and in some cases dramatic. Huntington's chorea and Jacob-Creutzfeldt disease generally have their onset during midlife, as may Pick's and Alzheimer's diseases, although this is variable for the latter. Senile degenerative brain disease usually has its onset during the seventies. Jacob-Creutzfeldt disease and Huntington's chorea tend to affect the sexes equally; the other dementing diseases are somewhat more common in women. Jacob-Creutzfeldt disease and Huntington's chorea are manifested by signs of basal ganglia dysfunction, in addition to the OBS. Jacob-Creutzfeldt disease has a fulminating course, with death occurring 1 to 2 years from onset. Alzheimer's disease tends to run a course of approximately 2 to 5 years, and Pick's 5 to 15 years to death. The life expectancy in patients with senile degenerative brain disease is generally not well elucidated in the literature; however, it is not known to be rapidly progressive. Certainly, irreversible OBS tends to shorten life expectancy.

Vascular OBS

The second subdivision of irreversible OBS is the secondary neuronal degenerative state (i.e., causes extraneous to the neuron), specifically cerebrovascular disease. The major representatives of this category are stroke and multi-infarct-induced OBS due to cerebrovascular atherosclerosis.

For a long time, cerebrovascular atherosclerosis was thought to be the major cause of late-life OBS. Furthermore, until recently it had been thought that there was a decrease in cerebral blood flow, an increase in cerebrovascular resistance, and a decrease in cerebral neuronal oxygen metabolism in all elderly individuals.

Current thought, based on recent experimental investigation, holds that there is no essential difference between the normal young and elderly subjects in cerebral blood flow and cerebral metabolic consumption of oxygen. Because of raised systolic blood pressures in the elderly, there may be a slight increase in cerebrovascular resistance, but this is considered normal and essential to adequate tissue perfusion. Therefore, any reduction of cerebral blood flow or cerebral oxygen metabolic rate is a pathological state. In the primary neuronal degenerative states described above, reduced cerebral blood flow is not the primary event but, rather, a secondary and compensatory phenomenon in response to lower metabolic demand (manifested in part by a lower oxygen and metabolic rate). In vascular OBS reduced blood flow is the primary event, and a reduced oxygen and metabolic rate follows.

There are believed to be at least two possible mechanisms by which cerebrovascular disease produces an OBS. The first is via numerous, ischemia-induced multiple infarcts known as "multi-infarct" dementia or a lacunar state (état lacunae). These lesions occur in the gray and white matter in the watershed areas of the brain (areas of the terminal distribution of the cerebral arterial vessels). The second is via a more generalized infarction which destroys at least 50 to 100 cc of brain tissue. Both may, and probably do, occur in the same person and cause encephalomalacia. Either of the above types of intracerebral lesion may be produced by thrombotic or embolic induced vascular occlusion or hemorrhage due to hypertension. Hypertension and atherosclerosis are the major contributing factors in cerebrovascular disease.

Of all elderly with irreversible OBS, autopsy studies have revealed the following causes: atherosclerosis (definite in 12%, probable in 6%), SDAT (50%), and mixed SDAT and multi-infarct or atherosclerosis (18%). It is believed that no greater than 7% of all elderly have irreversible OBS. Thus, it is not a normal part of aging. Further, ten to thirty percent of all OBSs that occur during late life may be potentially reversible.

Acute OBS

The general classes of reversible etiologies and typical examples of acute OBS are as follows.

Iatrogenic Factors

Iatrogenic acute OBS may be due to compounds such as prescription and over-the-counter medications, illicit drugs (e.g., opiates), ethanol, and heavy metals. Medications are frequently implicated in the production of reversible OBS. These agents have been repeatedly demonstrated to inadvertently produce untoward psychiatric states, with the elderly considerably more predisposed than their younger counterparts. Prescription acquisitions of the elderly have been shown to be greater than twice those of younger groups and are believed to represent approximately 50% of their total health care budget. Complicating the elderly's increased predisposition to iatrogenic psychiatric illness is the fact that the use of over-the-counter medications constitute an essential part of their lives.

Regardless of the biogenesis, there are three main types of adverse drug reaction. The most common is the pharmacodynamic type. These reactions are due simply to an extension of the known pharmacological effects of the drug, either secondary to age-inappropriate excess dosage or interactions with other drugs having similar effects. The second and least common adverse reactions are those due to allergic hypersensitivity reactions with the individual. The third type are those which might be considered "idiosyncratic," presumably due to some physiological peculiarity in the individual.

Almost any drug that crosses the blood-brain barrier or impairs cerebrocortical functions by virtue of peripheral effects has the potential for causing an OBS for any one of the reasons mentioned above. Those specific classes which have been implicated include, among others: antibiotics, cardiovascular-active drugs (e.g., cardiac glycosides, antihypertensives, diuretics, and antiarrhythmics), psychotropic agents and hypnotics, antiparkinsonian agents, analgesics and antipyretics, steroids, antidiabetic agents, laxatives and cathartics, and cancer chemotherapeutic agents.

There are only scant reports of opiate use in the elderly. Approximately 1% of opiate addicts are 60 years of age and older, and it is believed that most of them have been addicted since their early years. Additional sources of toxic etiology are the heavy metals, e.g., lead, aluminum, magnesium, mercury. The individual is affected owing to excessive exposure to these agents in work situations or by virtue of their proximity to certain industrial plants.

In regard to substance abuse, alcohol is most commonly implicated. There are two groups of elderly alcoholics, those who developed the illness previously and continue on into later life and those who develop the problem for the first time during the geriatric years (usually in response to stress). Regardless, 12% of males 65 and older who were admitted to mental hospitals in 1968 were there because of alcoholism; in 1969 it was 11%. Although the majority of aged alcoholics are males, the percentage of affected women increases considerably after age 60. Alcoholism is believed to be a strong contributing factor to crimes committed by the elderly.

Infections

Infections, primarily of the lung or kidney, with or without bacteremia, often produce acute confusional states. Even low-grade pneumonias with relatively little fever and clinically inapparent may cause an OBS. Pyogenic meningitis often presents atypically during old age without the classic findings of high fever and headache. It may mimic stroke or present as a brain syndrome with apathy.

Nonfunctional psychopathology due to syphilis may not be apparent until the geriatric years if the primary infection has occurred during midlife. It may begin as epilepsy of late onset, tremor, dysarthria, and/or psychopathology.

Nutritional and Metabolic Factors

Apart from the obvious role of certain foodstuffs, minerals, and vitamins in physiological homeostasis (including cerebral function), little is conclusively known about nutritional effects on brain function in the elderly. It is believed that, in general, the nutritional needs of the reasonably healthy elderly person are not significantly different from those of younger populations. Old persons retain the capacity to build new body tissues, but only if they have adequately nutritious diets. Furthermore, malnutrition has been repeatedly demonstrated to be a known cause of nonfunctional psychopathology, notably OBS, as evidenced by numerous reports of improvement or recovery upon correction of such states as dehydration, electrolyte imbalance, and deficiencies of folic acid and vitamin B_{12} (pernicious anemia and subacute combined degeneration), thiamine (alcohol-induced Wernicke's and Korsakoff's syndromes), and niacin (the characteristic pellagra triad of diarrhea, dermatitis, and dementia) (Chapter 30).

Diabetes mellitus is another relevant metabolic disorder. The complications of this illness (e.g., atherosclerosis of the cerebral arterial vasculature and diabetic ketoacidosis) may contribute to the etiology of OBS, rather than the direct effect of hyperglycemia on cerebrocortical function. Hypoglycemia may produce an acute reversible brain syndrome. Under ordinary circumstances the principal fuel for the brain is carbohydrate. However, stores of glucose and glycogen in the brain are so limited they can meet metabolic requirements for less than 1 min. Therefore the brain must constantly withdraw glucose from the circulation for use as fuel. If the supply of glucose in the blood falls below a critical level, the brain breaks down its own structural proteins and lipids to use as substitute fuels for brain metabolism. The exact mechanisms by which these deficiencies are converted into aberrant cerebral processes are largely unknown; however, the major manifestation of hypoglycemia in humans is abnormal cerebral function. These symptoms and signs resemble those of any other metabolic encephalopathy, beginning with loss of high mental functions, followed by behavioral abnormalities and other psychiatric deviations.

Three major possible etiological considerations of hypoglycemia in the elderly include oral or parenteral (insulin) antidiabetic agents (in prevalent usage among this population), malnutrition, and, less likely, an insulin-secreting pancreatic islet cell tumor. Regardless, any acutely developing neuropsychiatric symptoms or signs in a diabetic individual on antidiabetic treatment should be evaluated immediately for evidence of hypoglycemia.

Thyroid disease, especially hypothyroidism, should also receive consideration. It has been noted that during late life there is a reduction in pituitary function; serum triiodothyronine (T_3) is lowered, although the T_4 level is relatively normal. It is not implied from the foregoing data that every old person has hypothyroidism. However, the elderly patient manifesting signs of OBS accompanied by one or more of the classical signs of hypothyroidism [low T_3 resin uptake, serum T_3, serum T_4, free thyroxine index (FTI), effective thyroxine ratio (ETR), and ^{131}I uptake] are candidates for etiological evaluation and appropriate treatment for hypothyroidism. Etiological considerations in the elderly include autoimmune thyroiditis (Hashimoto's disease), overtreatment of previous hyperthyroidism, primary pituitary dysfunction (rare in the elderly), and thyroid neoplasia among others.

Hyperthyroidism, including its extreme state (thyrotoxicosis), is a definite potential etiology of acute OBS. The exact mechanisms by which cerebrocortical function is impaired are unknown; however, one might conjecture that it is a state akin to schizophrenia, where rapid input of stimuli (secondary to the hypermetabolic state) precludes adequate central neuronal integration and processing. This question is further confounded by the occasional elderly hyperthyroid patient who presents with apathy and lethargy. (Many a thyrotoxic patient has been initially suspected of having myxedema.) There appear to be no known age-related physiological predispositions or correlates to a hyperthyroid state, as with hypothyroidism. The clinical complex of hyperthyroidism in the elderly is not believed to be significantly different from that in younger persons, save for the more commonly occurring atypical presentation. There seems to be no dispute that hyperthyroidism is more common in women, but there is some debate as to its incidence during late life. Regardless, should the patient present with the classical or even atypical signs of hyperthyroidism, appropriate evaluation and treatment should ensue.

In that light, two major points should be mentioned. First, if cognitive or memory impairment are absent, one must not overlook another key sign of organicity, lability of affect, which may be the only presenting sign of the hyperthyroid state. The second point is that, as with hypothyroidism, this state has its abnormal physiological equivalents as well, which may either contribute to or directly affect cerebrocortical function; among others, these are cardiac arrhythmias, notably atrial fibrillation and tachyarrhythmias, both of which affect cerebral perfusion, as well as diarrhea (affecting fluid and electrolyte balance).

It is not within the scope of this chapter to discuss every possible metabolically based illness predisposing to or causing nonfunctional psychiatric states. Many of the more common ones have been mentioned. For the sake of completeness, other potential metabolic etiologies are: congestive heart failure, hypoparathyroidism (an age-related decrease in blood parathyroid hormone noted), hyper- and hypomagnesemia, cerebral anoxia (presenting much the same clinical picture as hypoglycemia), Addison's disease, as well as water, electrolyte (primarily Na^+ and K^+), and acid–base imbalance states due to other causes such as improper diet, renal disease, and iatrogenic problems (drug-induced, e.g., diuretics).

Trauma

The most important sequel of head trauma in the elderly is subdural hematoma; however, the aged individual is susceptible to other forms of trauma to the brain, e.g., subarachnoid hemorrhage, epidural hematoma, concussions, and uncomplicated contusions. Naturally, extracerebral trauma can have intracerebral consequences, e.g., emboli or hypoperfusion with consequent cerebral hypoxia secondary to peripheral blood loss. It must be remembered that the memory loss effects of head trauma can cloud the history of the actual traumatic event. Consequently, this etiology must always receive strong consideration, even in the absence of supporting history. Falls due to age-related fragile musculoskeletal structures, inadvertent hypotensive episodes due to medications (e.g., diuretics and alpha-blocking agents), poor vision and audition, as well as normal age-related decline in the effectiveness of peripheral baroreceptors account for the majority of head traumas.

Neoplasia

The most common nonmalignant tumor arising in the aged brain is the meningioma. It tends to be more common in females and has its peak incidence during the fifth and sixth decades. It is found usually in the frontal and temporal lobes.

Vascular Problems

Vascular factors in cerebrovascular disease include such entities as arteriovenous malformations, aneurysms, and collagen vascular disease. Generally, however, these are relatively rare in the geriatric population. This fact, however, should not by any means undermine their significance. Arteriovenous malformations may grow large enough to impinge on critical cognitive/memory function areas. Because of low resistance, they may also be responsible for pooling, with the subsequent production of cerebral ischemia; they may also rupture and bleed, usually producing a subarachnoid hemorrhage. Cerebrovascular aneurysms, most commonly occurring in the anterior half of the circle of Willis (important to frontal and temporal lobe arterial blood supply), are especially vulnerable to rupture (especially in the face of hypertension) with the consequent production of primary (nontraumatic) subarachnoid hemorrhage.

Hydrocephalus

The hydrocephalus which is potentially reversible is the normal-pressure type (NPH). It is due most commonly to some process causing a cerebrospinal fluid (CSF) outflow obstruction (e.g., previous subarachnoid hemorrhage or chronic meningitis), although an idiopathic type has been identified.

NPH's characteristic clinical triad consists of an OBS, gait spasticity, and urinary incontinence. Importantly, these clinical findings can be seen with OBSs that have other causes, notably the primary neuronal degenerative states. Furthermore, ventricular dilatation [on computed tomographic (CT) scan] is present in both NPH and the primary neuronal degenerative state. The dilatation in NPH is due to obstruction. Ventricular enlargement in the primary neuronal degenerative state is due to a relative and compensatory increase in ventricular size secondary to an atrophy-induced reduction in brain mass (hydrocephalus ex vacuo).

Laboratory screening beyond the CT scan is generally necessary to differentiate obstructive from compensatory dilatation. In NPH the pneumoencephalogram reveals little or no air over the cerebral convexities, and the RISA scan manifests an obstructive pattern.

The most commonly utilized treatment for NPH is the ventriculoperitoneal shunt. Treatment results have been mixed. There are numerous reports in the literature of recovery or significant improvement. Success seems to depend greatly on the condition's duration, a longer time predisposing to excessive impingement on critical cerebral areas and consequent neuronal death.

OTHER NONFUNCTIONAL STATES

OBS is only one of several nonfunctional psychiatric states. Certain depressions (Chapter 5), frightening delusions and hallucinations, or the other entities listed as "logical extensions" of OBS may and often do occur in the absence of cognitive/intellectual or memory disturbances. These are nonfunctional states nevertheless. They may be caused by *any* of the reversible etiologies mentioned earlier, but they are caused most commonly by the toxic-metabolic factors.

CLINICAL APPROACH

The initial clinical approach to patients presenting states resembling nonfunctional psychopathology is a thorough physiological evaluation to determine the presence of a reversible organic etiology. If the practitioner assumes automatically and arbitrarily that such states in the elderly are irreversible, sufficient and often preventable neuronal death may render an otherwise reversible state irreversible, a self-fulfilling prophecy.

Therefore, in addition to a careful history and physical examination, baseline laboratory studies should include the following: CBC with differential, BUN, creatinine, electrolytes, FBS, serum glutamic oxalic transaminase (SGOT), SGPT, total and direct bilirubin, LE preparation, ANA, VDRL, vitamin B_{12} and folic acid levels; T_3/T_4/FTI, uric acid, urine for drug and heavy metal screens, electrocardiogram, electroencephalogram, and a CT scan of the head. Questionable or abnormal values on any of the above suggests the need for appropriate additional examinations or consultations.

The treatment of choice for nonfunctional states is etiological reversal where possible. If a reversible cause cannot be found, the clinician may deploy the appropriate modalities where not contraindicated (Chapter 23).

PSEUDODEMENTIA

Organic etiologies can mimic or produce a syndrome or entity resembling a functional psychiatric state. Likewise, functional entities can produce a state resembling a nonfunctional entity. The most common of the latter type is the pure OBS (cognitive/intellectual and memory deficits). The most commonly implicated functional state in the elderly is the retarded depression. However, other functional states may be implicated, e.g., schizophrenia and agitation or agitated depressions.

Pseudodementia is believed to be a functional state, and so there is no organic etiology or link. Patients present a clinical picture compatible with a pure OBS. For example, schizophrenia, agitation, and agitated depressions may depict a seeming cognitive disorganization. The patient with a retarded depression manifested largely by excessive reductions in energy, motility, and motivation sometimes finds it extremely difficult or impossible to answer questions testing cognition and memory.

There is no reliable way to confirm the presence of pseudodementia with a clinical interview. Many have attempted to do so via clinical trials with antidepressant medication and electroconvulsive therapy (ECT).

It is the author's contention that any patient presenting with symptoms or signs of a nonfunctional nature must be evaluated thoroughly to determine the presence or absence of an organic cause. If there is no organic component, a functional state can be inferred and treated appropriately. Antidepressants and ECT (assuming they are indicated at all) used to rule out an organic condition may cloud and worsen an existing clinical organic state.

SUMMARY

The most common nonfunctional psychiatric disorder in elderly persons is the organic brain syndrome. OBSs may have irreversible and reversible causes. It is vital to the patient for the physician to be able to distinguish between the two.

Other nonfunctional states are seen in the elderly as well. The clinical approach to such disorders is to determine their physiological basis. This is done via laboratory testing.

Pseudodementia must be considered as well. Although believed to be a functional state, pseudodementia has no apparent organic etiology. These patients mimic those with pure OBS.

When caring for elderly patients, the physician should:
1. Know the cardinal signs of nonfunctional psychopathology.
2. Have a logical and orderly approach to the differentiation of nonfunctional psychopathology from a functional psychiatric disturbance, even when they occur together.
3. Know which common causes of nonfunctional psychopathology are reversible and which are not, and their relative frequencies.

SUGGESTED READING

Eaton, M. T., and Peterson, M. H. *Psychiatry, Medical Outline Series*. Medical Examination Publishing Co., Flushing, NY, 1969.

Levenson, A. J., editor. *The Neuropsychiatric Side Effects of Drugs in the Elderly*. Raven Press, New York, 1979.

Levenson, A. J., editor. *Psychiatric Manifestations in Physical Illness in the Elderly*. Raven Press, New York, 1980.

Smith, W. L., and Kinsbourne, M. *Aging and Dementia*. Spectrum Publications, New York, 1977.

Verwoerdt, A. *Clinical Geropsychiatry*. Williams & Wilkins, Baltimore, 1976.

Wells, C. E. Editorial: role of stroke in dementia. *Stroke*, 9:1–3, 1978.

Fundamentals of Geriatric Medicine, edited by
Ronald D. T. Cape, Rodney M. Coe, and Isadore
Rossman, Raven Press, New York © 1983.

17

Cerebrovascular Disease

James C. Grotta and William S. Fields

"Stroke" is a commonly used but nonspecific term which includes any neurological deficit caused by cerebral infarction or hemorrhage. A better general term is cerebrovascular disease (CVD), which includes cerebral infarction due to thrombosis or embolism and cerebral hemorrhage due to bleeding into either the parenchyma of the brain (intracerebral hemorrhage) or the subarachnoid space (subarachnoid hemorrhage).

The incidence of stroke in the United States has shown a gratifying decline during recent years, but CVD is still a major cause of disability in individuals over age 65. In 1976, 414,000 Americans suffered an acute stroke. The overall incidence of stroke in patients 55 to 64 years of age was 4/1,000 per year, and in the 65- to 74-year-old age group it approached 10/1,000 per year. Approximately 40% of patients with their first stroke suffer death or a permanent disabling functional deficit, and this rate increases to 80% for those with multiple infarctions. Total costs due to stroke are approximately $7.36 billion per year, and 55% of this amount, or $4.1 billion, is in lost earnings due to disability or death. Stroke is therefore an important disease in the geriatric age group. Moreover, because CVD rarely occurs in younger individuals, most published information about its cause and treatment is applicable to the elderly.

CEREBROVASCULAR ANATOMY AND PHYSIOLOGY

An understanding of cerebrovascular disease is based on a knowledge of the vascular anatomy of the brain. There are four major arteries supplying the brain: the right and left internal carotid arteries which arise at the bifurcation of the common carotid arteries in the neck, and the two vertebral arteries which travel through the vertebral canal in the cervical vertebrae and unite just above the foramen magnum of the skull to form the basilar artery. These vessels are interconnected at the base of the brain through the circle of Willis. It is by means of these arterial channels that blood from one of the major vessels may travel to supply branches of another major vessel through which there is insufficient flow.

Cerebral Arteries

There are three paired cerebral arteries—the anterior, middle, and posterior—which arise from the circle of Willis and supply most of the cerebral cortex. Occlusion of one of these arteries, usually by an embolus from the heart or from an atherosclerotic plaque in the carotid, basilar, or vertebral artery, produces distinct clinical syndromes the nature of which depends on the part of the cortex involved. These are summarized in Table 1.

The cortical areas supplied by these vessels overlap to a certain extent. When one of them becomes occluded, blood flow from the most distal branches of an adjacent artery often provides some flow to the ischemic region by traveling in a retrograde fashion down the distal branches of the occluded vessel. This "collateral" flow is sometimes very rich, particularly when the occlusion is slow in developing. The adequacy of the collateral flow often accounts for the difference between a minor and a disabling clinical deficit. Elderly individuals, especially those with diffuse atherosclerotic narrowing of small intracranial vessels, usually have inadequate collateral circulation, and when infarction occurs these patients suffer severe clinical deficits which seldom improve with treatment.

Other Arteries

Another group of arteries arise from the circle of Willis and supply the deep gray nuclei, internal capsule, thalamus, diencephalon, and brainstem. These small-caliber perforating vessels may also be affected by atherosclerosis. Occlusion of these vessels is common in elderly hypertensive individuals, but because each perforating artery supplies a very small region, with minimal overlap of an adjacent region, the lesions are clinically silent ("lacunar" infarcts). What symptoms these infarcts do produce are usually mild and often reversible.

Small aneurysms, first described by Charcot and Bouchard in 1868, can also occur on these perforating arteries and result in weakness in the vessel wall. Because the high perfusion pressure in the circle of Willis and major intracranial arteries is

TABLE 1. *Results of occlusion of the cerebral arteries*

Artery	Area supplied	Results of occlusion
Anterior cerebral	Anterior part of frontal lobe Parasagittal parts of frontal and parietal lobes	Personality change Weakness and sensory loss in leg and to a lesser extent in arm
Middle cerebral	Temporal lobe Lateral aspect of frontal and parietal lobes	Contralateral face and arm weakness Sensory loss Language impairment (if infarct is in dominant hemisphere) Spatial disorientation (if infarct is in non-dominant hemisphere)
Posterior cerebral	Posterior temporal and parietal lobes Visual cortex of the occipital lobe	Contralateral homonymous hemianopia

transferred directly to these small-caliber, thin-walled branches, the latter frequently rupture. Events of this kind are particularly common in hypertensive individuals. This accounts for the classical location of hypertensive intracerebral hemorrhages in the putamen, thalamus, and brainstem.

Autoregulation

Certain physiological properties of the cerebral circulation are significantly altered in cerebral ischemia and may play a role in the ultimate outcome of a stroke. Normally, cerebral blood flow (CBF) is maintained at a constant level despite wide fluctuations in blood pressure. This phenomenon, known as autoregulation, is the result of changes in cerebrovascular resistance in response to changes in systemic blood pressure. The ability of the cerebral vessels to autoregulate is lost in regions of ischemia, so that CBF becomes passively related to perfusion pressure. Thus hypotension as an accompaniment of cerebral infarction can further reduce CBF and increase the insult. Hypertension, on the other hand, may increase CBF, but at the same time this increase may result in cerebral edema and even hemorrhage when there has been ischemic injury to the vessel wall.

CLINICOPATHOLOGICAL CORRELATIONS IN CVD

It is difficult to distinguish the various types of CVD on a clinical basis alone, and in most patients laboratory investigations are necessary to understand the pathophysiological mechanism underlying their illness. Modern diagnostic techniques, particularly computed tomography (CT), have demonstrated that what we might previously have thought on clinical grounds to be a "classic" cerebral infarct may in fact be an intracerebral hematoma. These techniques have provided us with precise anatomical diagnosis, and still newer methods promise a fuller understanding of physiological and metabolic changes in CVD.

Thrombotic Cerebral Infarction

Thrombosis of a major artery supplying the brain accounts for 50 to 60% of patients with CVD. Pathologically, thrombosis tends to occur in large arteries (e.g., the internal carotid or basilar) in anatomical association with an atherosclerotic plaque. Our present understanding is that hemorrhage may occur in the vessel wall beneath the base of the plaque, causing the atherosclerotic lesion to enlarge and produce an even greater degree of narrowing (stenosis). The enlarging atheroma then causes turbulence in the bloodstream, resulting in the formation of a thrombus on the plaque. In this fashion the vessel becomes occluded.

Thrombotic infarction is frequently associated with hypertension, diabetes, and evidence of atherosclerotic disease elsewhere in the arterial system. It may also occur in patients with coagulopathy, especially young women on birth control pills. Prolonged vasospasm associated with migraine or subarachnoid hemorrhage may also induce cerebral thrombosis. Other less-frequent causes include hyperviscosity states (e.g., paraproteinemia and polycythemia) and inflammatory disorders of the cerebral arteries. Giant cell arteritis commonly seen in temporal arteries characteristically affects the ophthalmic artery but may also affect other intracranial vessels; it occurs more often in elderly individuals.

Thrombotic infarcts were once thought to have a characteristic onset, often occurring at night during sleep and having a "stuttering" or stepwise progression over 12 to 24 hr. However, the application of cerebral angiography and our improved ability to correlate the clinical picture with the arterial lesion has shown that the clinical deficit caused by these lesions may appear abruptly or may even be slowly progressive over days.

Individuals with internal carotid artery thrombosis usually have a deficit similar in distribution to that of a middle cerebral artery occlusion, but the clinical manifestations may be quite mild if there is good collateral circulation. Basilar artery thrombosis, on the other hand, is usually devastating owing to the coincident obstruction of the perforating vessels which arise directly from the basilar artery and which supply vital brainstem structures. Vertigo, disorders of eye movement, dysarthria, cerebellar dysfunction, visual loss, and loss of consciousness are characteristic of vertebrobasilar lesions.

Lacunar infarcts due to obstruction of individual perforating arteries are also considered thrombotic infarcts and are an incidental finding in a large percentage of elderly hypertensive individuals coming to postmortem examination. These are the cause of most "minor" strokes and may produce a characteristic clinical picture depending on the cerebral structures supplied by the vessel. Clinically apparent lacunar infarcts usually occur in the internal capsule (hemiparesis or hemisensory loss) or the brainstem (hemiparesis and/or sensory loss associated with cranial nerve and/or cerebellar dysfunction).

Multiple lacunar infarcts may result clinically in a progressive dementia with focal neurological signs and dysarthria. This syndrome is not common, but it is important to emphasize that multiple cerebral infarction is the only well documented cause of dementia related to cerebrovascular disease (Chapter 16). Dementia does not occur as a result of reduced CBF caused by "cerebral arteriosclerosis." Although there may be a slight drop in CBF with increasing age in some clinically normal individuals and an even greater decline in those who are demented, this reduction is secondary to reduced metabolic demand rather than arterial obstruction. Even in patients with severe atherosclerosis of the cerebral circulation, CBF remains well above the levels required to supply the metabolic demands of the brain. Most of what was once considered "arteriosclerotic dementia" is really dementia due to primary neuronal degeneration (Alzheimer's disease).

Embolic Cerebral Infarction

Approximately 30% of patients with CVD have infarction due to embolization to one of the intracranial arteries. Cerebral emboli consist of an aggregation of platelets, fibrin, and red blood cells, although microemboli may be composed of only small platelet clumps or atherosclerotic debris. Most emboli are formed in the heart chambers, on the heart valves (especially the mitral valve), or on atherosclerotic lesions, most frequently at the carotid bifurcation or along the vertebral or basilar arteries. When emboli arise in the heart, it is often in association with myocardial infarction or cardiac arrhythmia, especially atrial fibrillation. These embolic fragments travel distally and usually lodge in one of the major cerebral arteries or one of their large branches. Because of the sudden occlusion, collateral circulation usually has insufficient time to develop as is the case with a gradual thrombosis, and this may result in a more severe clinical deficit. However, the embolus frequently fragments, and the fragments move distally into the smaller intracerebral branches, enabling blood flow to the ischemic region to be restored and the deficit to resolve. Recently the term "reversible ischemic neurological deficit" (RIND) has been applied to such events, and these differ from transient ischemic attacks in that the deficit lasts longer (more than 24 hr) and some tissue infarction probably occurs.

Cerebral embolism produces the sudden onset of a clinical deficit which is maximal immediately, although repetitive embolization into the same vascular territory may produce a deficit that is progressive in a stepwise fashion. Transient ischemic attacks, most likely due to microemboli, occur prior to embolic infarction in up to 20% of cases.

When emboli fragment and blood flow is re-established to an infarcted area in which there are injured vessel walls, some hemorrhage into the infarcted area is likely to occur. This becomes a real danger in patients who are hypertensive or who have been anticoagulated in order to prevent further embolization. Up to 1,000 red blood cells per cubic millimeter may often be seen in the CSF following embolic infarction.

Transient Ischemic Attacks

Transient ischemic attacks (TIAs) are brief reversible neurological deficits secondary to a temporary focal decrease in CBF. The clinical onset is usually sudden and the deficit lasts minutes to a few hours. Most TIAs resolve by 6 hr, and by definition all resolve within 24 hr, with the patient returning to the preattack status.

TIAs may occur on a hemodynamic basis secondary to high-grade stenosis or occlusion of the carotid or vertebrobasilar system coupled with a transient drop in perfusion pressure. More often, however, TIAs are due to microemboli which arise from an upstream atherosclerotic plaque or from the heart. Roughly 70% of patients who develop cerebral infarction have had TIAs on the basis of one of these mechanisms. Approximately 35% of patients with TIAs will go on to have a cerebral infarct within the next 5 years (i.e., 7% per year). Therefore the occurrence of a TIA is an important sign of threatened cerebral infarction, and appropriate therapy may prevent a severe neurological deficit.

The initial clinical manifestations of a TIA closely resemble those of cerebral infarction. Other forms of TIA may occur, however, such as transient monocular blindness (amaurosis fugax), which is due to ophthalmic artery ischemia. Vertebrobasilar artery ischemia (VBI) is very common, particularly in elderly patients with orthostatic hypotension and atherosclerotic narrowing of the vertebral and/or basilar arteries. Such patients may present with vertigo, dysarthria, blurred or double vision, drop attacks, or loss of consciousness. When the attacks occur in association with extreme rotation or extension of the neck, degenerative arthritis of the cervical spine is probably present, resulting in compression of the vertebral arteries in the vertebral canal.

Intracerebral Hemorrhage

Hemorrhage into the parenchyma of the brain accounts for 10% of patients with clinically evident CVD. Most hemorrhages occur in patients with longstanding hypertension and are due to rupture of small penetrating vessels arising directly from the circle of Willis or its major branches. Pathological changes in these vessels that predispose them to rupture have already been discussed.

The widespread use of computed tomography in acute CVD has revealed that many patients who were thought on clinical grounds to have had a cerebral infarct have in fact had a cerebral hemorrhage. These are sometimes not in the typical location of hypertensive hemorrhages, and their etiology may at first be unclear. Impaired coagulation, often iatrogenic (due to the use of anticoagulants or agents affecting the bone marrow), is a rapidly increasing cause of hemorrhage. Rupture of a vascular malformation, hemorrhage into an embolic infarction, hemorrhage into a tumor, and trauma are other causes of intracerebral hemorrhage.

Hypertensive hemorrhages are usually associated with an extensive neurological deficit, and up to 60% of these patients are comatose on admission. One reason is that the usual location of this type of hemorrhage is near critical areas, e.g., the internal capsule or the brainstem. Furthermore, the mass effect of the clot frequently results in transtentorial or central herniation of the brain if the hemorrhage is supratentorial or direct pressure on the brainstem if the bleeding is in the cerebellum. Because autoregulation is lost in the injured region, CBF is passively dependent on perfusion pressure, which is equal to the difference between the mean arterial blood pressure and the intracranial pressure. Therefore a marked increase in intracranial pressure due to the massive hemorrhage will result in decreased cerebral perfusion, and this may also play a role in depressing the level of consciousness.

The onset of clinical symptoms due to hemorrhage is usually very rapid, and 50% of patients complain initially of severe headache. Vomiting is also frequent. However, there is no bedside method for distinguishing in intracerebral hemorrhage from infarction.

The long-term morbidity and mortality of hypertensive hemorrhage remains high. Patients with smaller hematomas, on the other hand, particularly those limited to the lobes of the brain rather than those located in the central regions, often make excellent recoveries, as the blood tends to dissect between fiber tracts and may not produce much parenchymal destruction.

Subarachnoid Hemorrhage

Bleeding into the subarachnoid space occurs in 5 to 10% of patients with CVD and if not related to trauma is almost always due to spontaneous rupture of a saccular aneurysm or arteriovenous malformation (AVM). Of all the varieties of CVD, this is the only one which is not more common among the geriatric population.

Aneurysms are due to abnormalities in the internal elastic membrane of the large intracranial vessels. They are usually located on the carotid or basilar arteries, along the circle of Willis, or on the proximal few millimeters of the major cerebral arteries at or adjacent to the origin of branches.

The major immediate morbidity of subarachnoid hemorrhage (SAH) is due to the abrupt rise in intracranial pressure caused by the bleeding. Cardiac arrhythmias and reflex pulmonary edema may also develop acutely. Over the following few days or weeks, delayed complications may occur, including rebleeding, the accumulation of an intra- or extracerebral blood clot, arterial spasm producing decreased blood flow and possibly infarction, and hydropcephalus.

The onset of SAH is almost always associated with a very severe headache. Coma develops acutely in 25% of patients, many of whom die before reaching the hospital. SAH is one neurological cause of "sudden death."

Twenty to thirty percent of patients reaching the hospital with SAH die the first day and another 20 to 30% die between days 1 and 60. Earlier studies have shown that 20 to 30% of patients surviving the first day will rebleed during the first month, with a maximum incidence between the seventh and tenth days; newer forms of therapy (e.g., the use of antifibrinolytic agents), however, have resulted in a gratifying reduction of the rebleeding rate. Overall, only 50% of all patients with SAH survive 2 years. However, the clinical outcome is clearly dependent on the patient's clinical condition at the time of admission.

DIAGNOSTIC TESTS IN CVD

It is usually not difficult to diagnose CVD, but it is impossible to be certain about the underlying pathology from the history and physical examination alone. A history of previous TIAs makes the diagnosis of infarction more likely, and a carotid bruit or a cardiac arrhythmia suggests an embolic basis. On the other hand, a severe headache and vomiting suggest hemorrhage, and papilledema or retinal hemorrhages are confirmatory physical findings.

The most important functions of the history in CVD are to: (a) determine the course of the disease (i.e., if the process is progressing, a more aggressive approach to therapy may be indicated); (b) determine the presence of CVD risk factors which when identified and eliminated may reduce the risk of future strokes. Chief among these risk factors, in addition to family history, are smoking and hypertension.

CT Scan

The laboratory evaluation of CVD should include a computed tomography (CT) scan with contrast enhancement. This is the most valuable tool available to differentiate infarction from hemorrhage. With the exception of the larger ones with associated cerebral edema, most infarcts cannot be seen on CT during the first 48 hr. Hemorrhages, on the other hand, are readily identified due to the attenuation of the x-ray beam by blood. Furthermore, the pattern of infarction seen on CT can assist in distinguishing between a lacunar infarct and an embolic infarct.

Lumbar Puncture

CSF examination by lumbar puncture is no longer considered a routine diagnostic procedure unless the patient has positive serology or signs and symptoms of an inflammatory process (meningitis) or SAH.

Cerebral Angiography

The place and timing of cerebral angiography in patients with cerebral ischemia remains controversial, but angiography is the only technique by which one can accurately delineate the nature of a vascular occlusion or the extent and nature of extracranial vascular disease. The test is usually performed as part of the evaluation of patients with TIAs or minor infarctions who would be candidates for endarterectomy if an accessible major artery obstruction or source of embolism could be demonstrated. Angiography should also be considered in any patient who has an incomplete or worsening acute deficit. This procedure is also the definitive means of identifying an aneurysm or other source of bleeding in patients with intracerebral or subarachnoid hemorrhage.

Angiography in the hands of experienced operators has a very low incidence of mortality but an associated morbidity which approaches 4% in some centers. This morbidity includes stroke, which becomes more likely the more extensive the atherosclerosis in the vessels and the more time spent performing the examination. In the older patient, these risks of morbidity are increased.

Brain Scan

Although radionuclide brain scanning has largely been replaced by CT, the dynamic flow study may provide a clue to the existence of a carotid stenosis by showing asymmetry in the rate of isotope uptake on the two sides.

Noninvasive Studies

Noninvasive carotid studies are used as screening tests in patients with symptoms of cerebral ischemia. *Phonoangiography* analyzes carotid bruits, which often cannot be heard with the stethoscope. This test can help distinguish between bruits which are transmitted from the lower neck or upper thorax and those which might be produced by carotid bifurcation atheroma. *Oculoplethysmography* and *periorbital directional Doppler studies* utilize the ophthalmic and periorbital pulses originating from the internal carotid artery to determine the presence of a hemodynamically significant stenosis in the internal carotid system. These tests are without risk or discomfort and can detect a 70% or greater carotid stenosis with an accuracy approaching 90%, but they *cannot* detect nonobstructing plaques which may be associated with cerebral emboli. Newer techniques to image the bifurcation by ultrasonography and by intravenous injection of dye are presently being developed.

If cerebral embolism is suspected, the patient should have a thorough cardiac evaluation with Holter monitoring of the cardiac rate and rhythm and an echocardiogram if a murmur is heard. A cardiac examination is necessary in all patients with CVD, as most deaths during the 5 years following cerebral infarction are due to cardiac and not neurological events.

The extent of the diagnostic evaluation of the patient with CVD depends of course on the age of the patient and the presence of other complicating medical problems. However, there is no arbitrary age cutoff beyond which thorough investigation of CVD aimed at possible surgical therapy should be excluded. This decision must be individualized and is a particular challenge in the elderly in whom medical and social complexities make thorough investigation and therapy more difficult.

THERAPY IN CVD

General supportive measures and nursing care are particularly important in patients with CVD, as a gratifying recovery may follow an initial period of severe disability. Because swallowing is often impaired for the first several days, one should proceed very slowly in feeding patients, withholding liquids in particular until competent swallowing is achieved. Bedside physical therapy should be instituted as early as feasible, as a rehabilitation program promotes a positive attitude on the part of the patient. Long-term rehabilitative regimens are particularly important in patients with major deficits, as improvement may be delayed for up to 8 weeks after the acute stroke.

Blood pressure elevation is a common problem in patients with cerebral infarction and hemorrhage. It is rarely necessary to administer potent antihypertensive drugs during the first few hours of hospitalization. Blood pressure in many patients will return to acceptable levels with bed rest and prompt attention to any airway obstruction or a distended bladder. In addition, some patients with increased intracranial pressure may have elevated blood pressure because of the need to maintain adequate CBF. This group is treated most effectively by antiedema agents or other means aimed at reducing intracranial pressure. If the blood pressure remains alarmingly high for 12 to 24 hr and there is no marked elevation in intracranial pressure, the blood pressure can be cautiously reduced by employing antihypertensive agents.

Patients with large infarcts or hemorrhages, especially those with concomitant increased intracranial pressure, can be treated with medications to reduce cerebral edema such as osmotic agents (mannitol, glycerol) and glucocorticoids. Neither therapy has been shown in clinical trials to be invariably effective in patients with cerebral infarction.

If the patient has an incomplete neurological deficit (e.g., a mild paresis or mild dysphasia), if there are recurring TIAs, or if there is evidence of a progressive worsening of the deficit either due to recurrent cerebral emboli or progressing thrombosis, some neurologists treat the patient with intravenous heparin for several days, accepting the small risk of turning an infarct into a hemorrhage. Of course one would have to conclusively rule out hemorrhage with a CT scan and/or CSF examination before embarking on a course of anticoagulation.

If the patient has TIAs or a permanent deficit on an embolic basis, long-term therapy aimed at suppressing platelet aggregation is indicated. Aspirin, 600 mg b.i.d., has been shown to reduce the incidence of cerebral infarcts in patients with TIAs, but currently much smaller doses (300 mg and less) are being advocated. After a cerebral infarct or TIA, elective carotid endarterectomy should be considered if there is an angiographically proved source of embolism or a high-grade stenosis in the cervical carotid artery. The patient should have some residual function in the affected hemisphere, and the surgery should be performed no sooner than 2 weeks postinfarction.

Emergency endarterectomy following an acute infarction is a controversial issue. There is no role for carotid endarterectomy in completed carotid occlusion. Emergency surgery for a high-grade stenosis or a fresh occlusion is sometimes indicated during the first few hours following an infarct if the patient has only a minor deficit, as there may be further embolization from the distal end of the clot or propagation of the clot into the middle cerebral artery.

If a surgically inaccessible stenosis exists in the carotid siphon or intracranially in TIA patients, or if the carotid is completely occluded, some surgeons recommend a superficial temporal artery to middle cerebral artery anastomosis. This procedure is still investigational, and its clinical utility remains to be proved. A cooperative study comparing it to nonsurgical therapy is presently under way.

Aggressive nonsurgical methods to manage increased intracranial pressure should be tried before clot evacuation in patients with a deeply situated intracerebral hematoma. Methods to control intracranial pressure include antiedema agents, hyperventilation, ventricular drainage, and barbiturate coma. The intracranial pressure can be accurately monitored by a ventricular catheter.

The treatment of subarachnoid hemorrhage is quite complex and aimed at preventing rebleeding first by administering epsilon-aminocaproic acid (Amicar®), which stabilizes the clot formed around the aneurysm, and later by surgically clipping the neck of the aneurysm. Because of the many complications and the high morbidity and mortality, these patients are best managed in a neurological intensive care unit.

Obviously the best therapy for CVD is prevention. This is already occurring in the general population due to better control of blood pressure and attention to other risk factors for atherosclerosis. In addition, the incidence of embolic and thrombotic infarcts might be further reduced by careful attention to symptoms suggestive of TIA and proper therapy of underlying conditions, e.g., cardiac arrhythmia and carotid atheroma. This includes a thorough evaluation of asymptomatic individuals with carotid bruits.

SUMMARY

Diagnosis and treatment of CVD depends on the physician being familiar with the cerebrovascular anatomy and physiology, as well as the pathophysiological mechanisms that underlie this disease. These are reviewed in this chapter.

Laboratory investigation is necessary to adequately determine the cerebrovascular problem. Computed tomography has greatly advanced our diagnostic capabilities, but a careful history lays the foundation to proper diagnosis.

Therapy may be surgical or nonsurgical, but general supportive measures and good nursing care are very important to the elderly patient with CVD. Treatment is of course individual, depending on the particular patient's needs.

When caring for elderly patients, the physician should:

1. Know the basic anatomy of the cerebrovascular system and how collateral circulation may help reduce the extent of cerebral infarction in case of embolism or thrombosis.
2. Know the basic pathophysiological mechanisms underlying cerebral thrombosis, cerebral embolism, TIAs, intracerebral hemorrhage, and subarachnoid hemorrhage.
3. Understand the indications for an aggressive approach to diagnosis as well as the indications for surgery in patients who have CVD.
4. Understand the role of anticoagulation and other nonsurgical methods of treatment in CVD.

SUGGESTED READING

Canadian Cooperative Study Group. A randomized trial of aspirin and sulfinpyrazone in threatened stroke. *N. Engl. J. Med.*, 299:53–59, 1978.

Fields, W. S., Lemak, N. A., Frankowski, R. S., et al. Controlled trial of aspirin in cerebral ischemia. *Stroke*, 8:301–315, 1977.

Fisher, C. M. Lacunes: small deep cerebral infarcts. *Neurology*, 15:774–784, 1965.

Hutchinson, E. C., and Acheson, E. J. *Strokes: Natural History, Pathology and Surgical Treatment.* Saunders, Philadelphia, 1975.

Mohr, J. P., Caplan, L. R., Melski, J. W., et al. The Harvard cooperative stroke registry: a prospective registry. *Neurology*, 28:754–762, 1978.

Toole, J. F., Truscott, B. L., Anderson, W. W., et al. Report of the joint committee for stroke facilities. VII. Medical and surgical management of stroke. *Stroke*, 4:270–320, 1973.

Toole, J. F., and Patel, A. N. *Cerebrovascular Disorders*, 2nd ed. McGraw-Hill New York, 1974.

Toole, J. F., Yuson, C. P., Janeway, R., et al. Transient ischemic attacks: a prospective study of 225 patients. *Neurology*, 28:746–753, 1978.

Whisnant, J. P., Anderson, E. M., Aronson, S. M., et al. Report of the joint committee for stroke facilities. V. Clinical prevention of stroke. *Stroke*, 3:804–825, 1972.

Williams, D., and Wilson, T. G. The diagnosis of the major and minor syndromes of basilar insufficiency. *Brain*, 85:741–774, 1962.

Fundamentals of Geriatric Medicine, edited by
Ronald D. T. Cape, Rodney M. Coe, and Isadore
Rossman, Raven Press, New York © 1983.

18

Complaints Related to the Spine

Leonard P. Seimon

The purpose of this chapter is to give the reader a logical, practical approach to the diagnosis and management of spine-related symptoms in the elderly. It is as easy to disregard symptoms as trivial as it is to overinvestigate what is relatively unimportant. In order to investigate and treat appropriately, the doctor must have some insight about the possible etiology of the patient's symptoms. As pain is far and away the most common symptom, much of the ensuing discussion relates to it. Stiffness, paraesthesia, and changes in posture are less frequent complaints. Backache may arise from a multitude of causes, but the incidence of specific conditions varies with the age of the patient. For example, acute disc prolapse is more common in those under age 50, whereas pathological fracture of vertebral bodies is much more common in older persons.

HISTORY

Correlation of the history and physical findings coupled with a basic knowledge of anatomy and pathology puts matters in their right perspective. To approach it in this way, nothing is more important than spending 15 to 20 min taking an accurate history from the patient. The following items are relevant:

1. *Onset.* How did the pain start? Was it sudden or gradual in onset, or was there an aggravation of pre-existing milder symptoms? Was injury a possible precipitating factor? Did the patient have a fall, move furniture, lift a weight, bend over acutely, or sustain a sudden jarring movement such as occurs with sneezing or coughing?
2. *Variability.* What aggravates the pain? Is it worse when sitting, standing, walking, or lying down? Is it aggravated by change of position, e.g., getting out of bed or getting up from a chair? Is the pain worse at night, or does it disappear in recumbency? Does turning over in bed aggravate the symptoms? What relieves the pain: sitting, standing, walking, recumbency, change of position, analgesics? For symptoms in the cervical region, how many pillows does the patient prefer to use?

163

3. *Radiation.* Is the pain predominantly in the back (neck, thoracic, or lumbar regions), or does it radiate into the limbs or around the torso, or up the neck into the occipital region? If it radiates, which is worse, the pain in the spinal region or that in the area of radiation? Is there a feeling of paresthesia in the referred regions, e.g., pins and needles, numbness, coldness?

4. *Other factors.* The history is particularly important. Is there any history of back (or neck) symptoms, even if many years previously? Has the patient had any major illnesses or operations with special attention to blood dyscrasias, malignancy, or endocrine problems? Is the patient on prolonged medication, e.g., adrenal corticosteroids? Has there been a change in the patient's posture; e.g., has the patient's spine become more rounded (kyphotic); have any local midline bumps become evident (gibbus); has there been a loss in height? The latter is a not infrequent complaint.

During the course of eliciting the history, observe the patient's emotional status, especially if there is any suggestion of depression. If necessary, question the patient about emotional problems and also if the symptoms vary with the emotional state.

The last phase of the history-taking relates to the various systems. Complaints such as occipital headaches, increasing fatigability, cough and abdominal or genitourinary symptoms are particularly noteworthy.

PHYSICAL EXAMINATION

The physical examination begins the moment the patient walks into the office. Watch how he walks, sits, and gets up from a chair. Let him undress and remain standing for the first part of the examination. This avoids unnecessary getting on and off the couch, which can be very distressing. Check that posture is normal and look for any evidence of kyphosis, scoliosis, or a localized gibbus. Ask the patient to indicate where most of the pain is felt. It takes only a minute or two to test movements in all regions of the spine. If restricted, check whether this is due to pain or stiffness. Note if there are any masses (not forgetting to palpate the front of the neck) or areas of spasm. Feel for areas of localized tenderness. Ask the patient to walk on tiptoe and also on the heels, as this is an excellent way of detecting early evidence of weakness in the calf and dorsiflexor muscles, respectively.

At this point, have the patient lie down and take note if difficulty is encountered when he climbs onto the examination couch. Conduct a neurological examination looking for evidence of wasting, loss of power, increased tone, sensory impairment, and reflex activity. Finally, do a general examination of the head and neck, thorax, and abdomen, not forgetting to palpate the peripheral pulses and lymph nodes. Especially in cases of chronic low back symptoms, carry out a rectal examination. With practice, this interview and examination should be completed within approximately 20 to 25 min. It should determine how much further investigation is required.

CAUSES OF SPINAL SYMPTOMS

Muscle Pain

The vertebrae are clothed from top to bottom by muscles and ligaments, which are subject to the same injuries and diseases as muscles and ligaments elsewhere in the body. If there has been an acute strain or direct blow, with damage to a muscle or ligament, the patient will complain of pain at the site, and localized tenderness will be elicited. Active and passive movements will be restricted because of pain. The history and the clinical findings will suggest the diagnosis, and generally simple analgesics and gradual increasing mobilization of the painful area are all that are necessary. For simple mild back strain, one should not routinely send an elderly patient off to a physiotherapist for frequent treatments. The patient may experience increased discomfort traveling to and from the physiotherapist and will be much happier to remain at home.

Osteoarthritis

The vertebrae are joined anteriorly by the intervertebral disc and posteriorly by the synovia-lined facet joints. The disc is firm and rubbery. If for any reason the disc narrows, the vertebral bodies will come closer together anteriorly and the facet joints at the back will begin to override. If they do not fit congruously, osteoarthritic changes will begin to develop, as with synovial joints elsewhere in the body. This is no different from the osteoarthritis which might occur in the hip, knee, or any other synovial joint. The symptoms likewise are very similar. Patients with osteoarthritic hips frequently state that so long as they are active they feel relatively comfortable. It is on getting out of bed in the morning or getting up from a chair after resting that the hip feels stiff and aches. After moving about for a short period the symptoms ease. Osteoarthritic facet joints in the spine also produce aching on arising in the morning and discomfort when getting up from a chair. After walking for a short while the symptoms ease, but with too much walking the symptoms become progressively worse. These patients prefer to keep moving and frequently change position when resting. It is on mobilizing after resting that the symptoms are most pronounced. Frequently restriction of movements are evident on examination, especially if the cervical spine is affected. It must be remembered that in this region there are additional synovial joints at the sides of the vertebral bodies (joints of Luschke). These too can become osteoarthritic.

Symptoms arising from osteoarthritis frequently disappear for several months at a time. This is seen in the hip and other joints as well. Patients who present with such a history should be treated symptomatically with simple analgesics and simple exercises. They should keep mobile, walking being an excellent exercise. With this typical picture, there is no need for special investigations, and one can wait to see the response to simple measures. A basic fact is that the majority of elderly patients, if examined by x-ray show evidence of osteoarthrosis, but most have no symptoms. X-ray examination is therefore generally not important.

Disc Changes

If there is gradual loss of the disc spaces, the vertebrae draw closer together. There is a normal kyphosis in the thoracic area, and this is aggravated if the disc spaces narrow. As the kyphosis increases, the ligaments between the spinous processes are chronically stretched, and this in turn causes aching. When we relax while sitting we tend to slump forward slightly, which further increases the kyphosis. Tenderness may be elicited along the spinous processes and over ligaments between them. These patients are completely relieved of pain in recumbency and usually feel much better when walking about.

This is a difficult problem to treat. Exercising the extensor muscles of the back is beneficial but is not easy for older persons to perform. Encourage them to sit in a reclining chair when watching television, rather than in a soft easy chair. Some of these patients complain more of loss of height than of the associated pain, but the cause is the same. In the cervical region the pain frequently refers down to the shoulder or scapular area on one or the other side. If the pain is very acute, prescribe a simple cervical collar and analgesics, but as soon as possible the patient should be encouraged to begin active exercises and discard the collar.

Herniated Disc

Instead of gradually narrowing, a disc may suddenly rupture posteriorly. When this occurs, disc material protrudes into the spinal canal and may impinge on a nerve root. The patient experiences severe pain in the distribution of the affected nerve, and there may be other associated neurological signs. Edema may aggravate the pressure on the nerve root. Disc prolapse is not common in the elderly, but it does occur. Patients frequently have difficulty finding a comfortable position even in bed. Symptoms tend to be increased by specific movements which increase the pressure on the nerve; coughing and sneezing may also cause discomfort by further increasing the pressure within the spinal canal.

Treatment is symptomatic. Analgesics should be prescribed, and the affected part should be put to rest to allow the edema to subside and the extruded disc material to shrivel up. To the extent possible, the patient is advised to exercise both upper and lower limbs, and to do frequent breathing exercises. If pain remains pronounced at rest, it is feasible to apply cervical traction for cervical disc problems and pelvic traction for the lumbar region. A large soft pillow behind the knees is a great help. After the acute symptoms subside, the patient should wear a cervical collar or lumbar corset for a few weeks, and then begin gradual active mobilization of the affected region without the appliance. Allowing free movement too soon may result in a relapse. When neurological signs and symptoms are more marked, or if the patient does not respond to a simple conservative regimen, referral to either an orthopedist or a neurosurgeon should be considered. Symptoms eventually resolve in most patients. Persistence of sensory loss or mild weakness is not important provided the pain disappears or is minimal. A small percentage of these elderly patients do not improve satisfactorily. If symptoms remain distressing and unremitting, and do not respond to the usual conservative measures, surgical treatment must be considered. At this stage either myelography or a computed tomographic (CT) scan is necessary to verify the diagnosis. Spinal surgery should not be lightly undertaken in the elderly, but neither should it be summarily discounted.

Spondylolisthesis

Spondylolisthesis is a condition in which one vertebra slides forward on the vertebra below it. It is not an uncommon condition in the elderly. The patients generally have no discomfort at rest, either sitting or recumbent, but change of position aggravates symptoms. Bending is the biggest problem, accompanied by as much difficulty when resuming the erect position as when bending down. Pain frequently radiates down one or the other thigh but not usually below knee level. The back symptoms are always worse than those in the limb unless there is an associated disc rupture. If symptoms are mild, the patient should be advised to avoid the movements or activities which aggravate discomfort. A lumbosacral corset frequently affords considerable relief. If symptoms are persistent or severe, the patient should be referred to an orthopedist to decide what further investigation or treatment is necessary.

Spinal Stenosis

Any disorder which causes relative narrowing of the spinal canal diminishes the space available for the neural tissue. The problem may arise as a late sequel to spinal surgery, in some cases of spondylolisthesis, and when there are anatomical variations in the size and shape of the canal. The neural structures in a narrow spinal canal can be readily compromised should there be encroachment, e.g., when a hard, degenerate disc bulges into it. These patients present with low back discomfort that radiates into both buttocks and thighs while walking. Symptoms disappear on bending forward or sitting down for a short period, only to recur when walking is resumed. The symptoms are highly suggestive of vascular claudication. Examination may reveal no physical abnormality, and it is the history which suggests the diagnosis. CT scans are of tremendous diagnostic value in these cases, sometimes supplemented by myelography.

Symptoms do not usually respond to simple conservative measures, as etiological factors remain unchanged, and so conservative therapy is often disappointing. Physiotherapy does not help, and a surgical corset only occasionally affords some relief. Considerable time must be spent explaining the problem to the patient. Although many are content to adjust their activities to their symptoms, others are quite desperate because of the unrelenting decrease in their functional activity; the latter are quite prepared to undergo surgical treatment. Generally this entails excision of laminae, thereby relieving the pressure in the spinal canal. For example, one 79-year-old woman presented with progressive symptoms over a period of 16 years. She was quite desperate as no form of conservative treatment had succeeded in halting the progression. She was able to walk only 40 to 50 yards before having to rest for a few minutes. Two days after decompressive laminectomy she was up and about, free of the complaint.

Compression Fracture

The most important group of conditions causing spinal symptoms in the elderly are compression fractures. When a patient breaks a bone, there is a considerable amount of pain which is aggravated by any movement at the fracture site. The spine is no exception. In the elderly, spinal fracture is less likely to be due to obvious trauma than from osteoporosis with or without injury. The vertebrae lose mineral content and become structurally weaker. The discs remain firm and rubbery and may bulge into the softened vertebral bodies. Patients who suffer from osteoporosis frequently develop aching pain from compression of the vertebral bodies which tends to be more pronounced in the thoracic region, where the normal kyphotic curve facilitates it. Increasing kyphotic deformity with loss of stature produces aching down the middle of the back that results from stretching of the ligaments. In addition, acute exacerbations of pain can occur because of collapse of vertebral bodies. All movements are markedly restricted because of pain, and complete rest is required to ease it.

In addition to common postmenopausal osteoporosis, numerous other conditions can cause weakening or destruction of the vertebral bodies and thus predispose to compression collapse. Myeloma is common in the elderly, as are metastases from primary tumors in the breast, prostate, thyroid, kidney, and other organs. In many of these conditions, patients frequently complain of a dull, boring, gnawing ache, especially at night. Superimposed on this might be a sudden exacerbation of symptoms when the bone fractures. Extensive disease may be present in the vertebrae and be asymptomatic until the fracture suddenly occurs. The patient then presents in the same way as any other patient with an acute compression fracture.

Management of these compression fractures is twofold: elucidation of the cause and treatment of the symptoms. Nothing is better for the acute distressing pain than bed rest. The patient should lie flat or be semireclining. He or she must not be propped up on pillows or be allowed to sit because this can only increase the tendency to further wedging. Active limb movement and deep breathing must be encouraged. As soon as the symptoms permit, the patient must be encouraged to begin standing and walking, gradually increasing these activities. Sitting should be discouraged for as long as possible. The majority of patients are out of bed within 1 to 2 weeks.

During the resting period the etiology of the condition can be investigated. For the patient previously known to suffer from osteoporosis or the elderly patient who sustains a compression fracture as a result of lifting a weight or bending excessively forward, there may be no need for further investigation. Should there be doubt of the diagnosis, then a complete blood count, a panel of serum chemistries, and urinalysis should be done. Unsuspected hyperparathyroidism or myeloma may be spotted and can be treated accordingly. If a metastatic lesion is suspected and the primary lesion is unknown, it is wise to have an orthopedist perform a needle biopsy. Judgment must be exercised, however, before taking such a step to be sure it will benefit the patient: If the diagnosis is made, will it materially alter the treatment or merely frighten the patient? Bracing should generally be avoided but is sometimes beneficial in those patients who suffer from repeated fractures.

Metastatic Growths and/or Chronic Infection

All of the conditions mentioned thus far have had symptoms aggravated either by change of position, movement, or posture, and relief is achieved in most instances by recumbency. Beware when the patient states that symptoms in the back or neck are most pronounced at bed rest and tend to be eased when the individual is up and about. This is frequently an indication of a disease process with gradual increasing destruction of bone. Such patients give no history of trauma, but there may be a history of malignancy or chronic lung disease, e.g., tuberculosis. Compression fractures related to disorders such as simple osteoporosis tend to get better with time. The clinician should be alerted when the patient complains of pain at night which tends to increase in severity with time, a symptoms suggestive of malignancy or possibly chronic infection. Varied neurological signs and symptoms may result from involvement of the spinal canal. A tumor may be within the spinal canal itself or in the vertebrae; or it may be invading directly from an adjacent viscus. Chronic infection such as tuberculosis can produce a similar picture. Aneurysms of the aorta and pancreatic tumors are notorious for causing unrelenting back pain of a dull, boring nature. Examination of the spine is usually quite normal.

Management

The reader should now be in a position to confidently undertake the management of the majority of patients presenting with vertebral symptoms. First, provisional diagnosis should be entertained; next, a decision should be made about appropriate investigations and a course of treatment formulated. Remember that you are treating patients and not x-rays. If you suspect that there are simple degenerative changes in the cervical spine, treat symptomatically, without taking x-rays. It is surprising how extensive degeneration can appear on an x-ray film even though the patient developed symptoms only 1 or 2 weeks previously. The x-ray interpretation "there are extensive degenerative changes in the bones of your neck" may serve only to frighten the patient. Each investigation must serve a specific purpose and not be merely an academic exercise.

SUMMARY

This lesson has been based on an experienced approach to the diagnosis and management of spine-related symptoms in the elderly. Although not invariably correct, it offers practical suggestions which avoid unnecessary investigation and expense in most cases. The vast majority of patients improve with a simple treatment regimen and are helped by explanation of the problem, reassurance, and understanding.

When caring for elderly patients, the physician should:

1. Know which conditions affecting the spine are particularly common in the elderly patient and how these may present clinically.
2. Have an orderly and rational plan for the assessment of patients who may have spinal problems, including appropriate use of diagnostic techniques and facilities.
3. Know the most appropriate and effective measures for management of the most common problems.

SUGGESTED READING

Brewerton, D. A. Rheumatic disorders. In: *Clinical Geriatrics*, 2nd ed., edited by I. Rossman. Lippincott, Philadelphia, 1979.

Brown, M. D. Diagnosis of pain syndromes of the spine. *Orthop. Clin. North Am.*, 6:233–248, 1975.

Brown, O. T., and Wigzell, F. W. The significance of span as a clinical measurement. In: *Current Achievements in Geriatrics*, edited by W. F. Anderson and B. Isaacs. Cassell, London, 1964.

Carter, A. B. The neurologic aspects of aging. In: *Clinical Geriatrics*, 2nd ed., edited by I. Rossman. Lippincott, Philadelphia, 1979.

Clarke, H. A., and Fleming, I. D. Disc disease and occult malignancies. *South. Med. J.*, 66:449, 1973.

Edeiken, J., dePalma, A. F., and Hoder, P. J. Paget's disease: osteitis deformans. *Clin. Orthop. Related Res.*, 45:141, 1966.

Exton-Smith, A. N. Bone aging and metabolic bone disease. In: *Textbook of Geriatric Medicine and Gerontology*, edited by J. C. Brocklehurst. Churchill Livingstone, London, 1973.

Fitzgerald, J. A. W., and Newman, P. H. Degenerative spondylolisthesis. *J. Bone Joint Surg.*, 58:184, 1976.

Garn, S. M. Bone loss and aging. In: *The Physiology and Pathology of Human Aging*, edited by R. Goldman and M. Rockstein. Academic Press, New York, 1975.

Jaffee, H. L. *Metabolic Degenerative and Inflammatory Diseases of Bone and Joints*. Lea & Febiger, Philadelphia, 1972.

Macnab, I. *Backache*. Williams & Wilkins, Baltimore, 1977.

Murray, R. O., and Jacobson, H. G. *The Radiology of Skeletal Disorders*, 2nd ed. Churchill Livingstone, London, 1977

Fundamentals of Geriatric Medicine, edited by
Ronald D. T. Cape, Rodney M. Coe, and Isadore
Rossman, Raven Press, New York © 1983.

Questions for Self-Assessment

DIRECTIONS: In questions 1–19, only *one* alternative is correct. Select the one
best answer and blacken the corresponding lettered box on the
answer sheet.

1. Dementia resulting from arteriosclerosis is *most* often due to:

    (A) Multiple infarcts
    (B) Reduced cerebral blood flow
    (C) Multiple small hemorrhages
    (D) Narrowing of the vertebral arteries
    (E) "Steal" of blood from the cerebral hemispheres to the brainstem

2. Of the following clinical states concurrent with organic brain syndrome,
   the one that is *most* likely to have the same cause is:

    (A) Obsessive compulsive neurosis
    (B) Hysterical personality disorder
    (C) Retarded depression
    (D) Visual hallucination
    (E) Involutional melancholia

3/4. An 80-year-old woman awoke one morning with pain at the back and sides
   of her neck radiating toward the left scapula. She did not have pain if she
   lay supine with one pillow only or if she were sitting, unless she rotated
   or flexed her neck. The neck pain was worse than the scapula discomfort.
   She had had similar but less severe episodes of neck pain during the past
   15 years. Usually symptoms were worst in the mornings, easing off during
   the day.

   Physical examination reveals an otherwise healthy woman. There is
   marked discomfort and restriction on rotation of the neck to the left and
   right, mild discomfort on flexion and extension, mild tenderness over the

lower part of the neck posteriorly. Movements and neurological examination of the upper limbs are within normal limits.

3. The *most* likely diagnosis is:

    (A) Metastatic disease
    (B) Collapsed vertebra
    (C) Cervical spondylosis
    (D) Ruptured disc
    (E) Subarachnoid hemorrhage

4. The *most* appropriate management is to:

    (A) Order roentgenograms of the cervical spine
    (B) Order complete blood count and urinalysis
    (C) Treat symptomatically
    (D) Order a bone scan
    (E) Refer the patient to an orthopedist

5. The *most* common cause of potentially reversible organic brain syndrome in elderly patients is:

    (A) Alcoholism
    (B) Subarachnoid hemorrhage
    (C) Senile dementia, Alzheimer type
    (D) Medications
    (E) Normal pressure hydrocephalus

6. In patients who have neurogenic bladder, involvement of the sacral cord is indicated by:

    (A) Uninhibited neurogenic incontinence
    (B) Detrusor instability
    (C) Overflow incontinence
    (D) A large atonic bladder
    (E) Confusion

7. The percentage of patients who die or suffer a permanent functional disability following their first stroke is:

    (A) 10%
    (B) 20%
    (C) 40%
    (D) 60%
    (E) 80%

8/9. A 69-year-old man developed the sudden onset of severe pain in the upper thoracic spine while walking. The pain persisted continuously for 6 days, and it was markedly aggravated by any movement. The pain did not radiate.

On physical examination, there is a small gibbus (prominence) at level T4–T5 with tenderness. All spinal movements are restricted by pain. The remainder of the physical examination and the neurological examination is within normal limits.

8. The *most* likely diagnosis is:

   (A) Ruptured disc
   (B) Rheumatoid arthritis
   (C) Sprained muscle
   (D) Collapse (fracture) of a vertebra
   (E) Intraspinal tumor

9. The *most* appropriate diagnostic study would be:

   (A) Roentgenogram of the thoracic spine
   (B) Bone scan
   (C) Myelogram
   (D) Excretory urogram
   (E) Aortogram

10. Of the following conditions, the one that has the *highest* potential for producing an organic brain syndrome is:

   (A) Arteriovenous malformation in the dominant parietal lobe
   (B) Meningioma in the occipital lobe
   (C) Pneumonia
   (D) Infarct of the basal ganglia
   (E) Basilar artery thrombosis

11. The *most* appropriate initial approach to a patient who has suspected pseudodementia is:

   (A) Evaluation for reversible organic etiology
   (B) A trial of major tranquilizers
   (C) A trial of minor tranquilizers
   (D) A trial of tricyclic antidepressants
   (E) Electroconvulsive therapy

12. Long-term therapy with aspirin has been shown the be effective in:

   (A) Reducing the incidence of stroke after a transient ischemic attack
   (B) Improving the clinical outcome after an acute stroke

    (C)   Preventing headache associated with cerebral hemorrhage

    (D)   Preventing lacunar infarction

    (E)   Improving cerebral blood flow in elderly patients

13.   Postponement of micturition is mediated by the:

    (A)   Sacral autonomic outflow

    (B)   Pons

    (C)   Musculature of the bladder

    (D)   Cerebral cortex

    (E)   Reticular formation

14.   Lacunar infarcts are caused by:

    (A)   Small hemorrhages in the deep gray nuclei

    (B)   Occlusion of small perforating vessels

    (C)   Emboli in the middle cerebral artery

    (D)   Thrombosis of the internal carotid artery

    (E)   Cerebral arterial spasm

15.   The *most* common cause of irreversible organic brain syndrome in elderly patients is:

    (A)   Atherosclerosis

    (B)   Syphilis

    (C)   Frontal lobe meningioma

    (D)   Depression

    (E)   Senile dementia, Alzheimer type

16.   The *most* common functional psychiatric disorder in elderly persons is:

    (A)   Hypochondriasis

    (B)   Anxiety

    (C)   Depression

    (D)   Paranoia

    (E)   Hysterical neurosis

17.   Annual statistics for the United States show that of all deaths due to falls, persons over 65 years of age account for approximately:

    (A)   30%

    (B)   50%

    (C)   60%

    (D)   70%

    (E)   80%

18/19.   Upon standing after a 10-hr transcontinental flight, a 67-year-old woman experienced acute pain in the low back, radiating down the posterior aspect of the left thigh and leg to the lateral aspect of the ankle. There was tingling over the dorsum of the foot extending into the big toe. On trying to walk, she had some weakness of dorsiflexion of her left ankle. The symptoms were totally relieved on recumbency; the pain was aggravated by bending, sitting, coughing, and sneezing. The limb symptoms were much more pronounced than the back symptoms.

Physical examination demonstrated tenderness in the lumbosacral region, marked limitation of flexion of the spine, sciatic pain produced by straight leg raising on the left side, weakness of dorsiflexion of the left ankle, hypoesthesia in the L5 dermatome (lateral aspect of the lower leg, across the dorsum of the foot to the big toe). The remainder of the examination was within normal limits.

18.   The *most* likely diagnosis is:

(A)   Collapsed vertebra
(B)   Acute prolapsed disc
(C)   Metastasis to the spine
(D)   Back strain
(E)   Aneurysm of the abdominal aorta

19.   The *most* appropriate management would be to:

(A)   Order a lumbosacral support
(B)   Order complete blood count and urinalysis
(C)   Refer the patient to a physical therapist
(D)   Refer the patient to an orthopedist or neurosurgeon
(E)   Order a bone scan

DIRECTIONS: In questions 20–34, *one or more* of the alternatives may be correct. You are to respond either *yes* (Y) or *no* (N) to *each* of the alternatives. For every alternative you think is correct, blacken the corresponding lettered box on the answer sheet in the column labeled "Y". For every alternative you think is incorrect, blacken the corresponding lettered box in the column labeled "N".

20.   True statements concerning paranoid ideations in elderly patients include:

(A)   Symptoms are frequently improved by environmental manipulation.
(B)   Sensory deficits (especially hearing) are frequent contributory factors.
(C)   Delusions usually involve family members or other persons emotionally close to the patient.

(D) It is useful for the physician to deny the validity of the paranoid ideation.

(E) Most patients have a history of psychiatric illness.

21. Drugs that affect continence include:

(A) Orphenadrine
(B) Chlorapromazine
(C) Diazepam
(D) Thioridazine
(E) Digitalis

22. Indications of an organic brain syndrome in elderly patients include:

(A) Cortical atrophy demonstrated on computed tomography (CT) scan of the head
(B) Impaired recent memory
(C) Hypothyroidism
(D) Seizure focus on electroencephalogram (EEG)
(E) History of syphilis

23. Falls by elderly persons frequently:

(A) Result in fractures of the wrist
(B) Result in fractures of the spine
(C) Occur in the absence of environmental hazards
(D) Cause temporary amnesia
(E) Are related to hyperextension of the neck

24. In patients who have involutional incontinence, there is associated:

(A) Dysuria
(B) Passive incontinence
(C) Episodes of "bladder infection"
(D) Autonomous neurogenic bladder
(E) Urethral stricture

25. In patients who have obstructive incontinence, there is:

(A) Constant incontinence
(B) Distention of the bladder
(C) Detrusor instability
(D) Overflow incontinence
(E) An absence of sacral cord reflexes

26. Cerebral emboli commonly arise from:

(A)   Plaques in the internal carotid artery
(B)   Plaques in the external carotid artery
(C)   The mitral valve of the heart
(D)   The distal end of a thrombus in the internal carotid artery
(E)   Congenital "berry" aneurysms

27.   True statements concerning depression include:

(A)   Depression in elderly patients may be precipitated by drugs.
(B)   Depression in elderly patients is frequently misdiagnosed as dementia.
(C)   Feelings of guilt are more common in elderly depressed persons than in young depressed persons.
(D)   Loss is a common precipitating event.
(E)   Feelings of anger are more common in elderly depressed persons than in young depressed persons.

28.   Cardiac dysrhythmias in elderly persons are often:

(A)   Asymptomatic
(B)   The cause of cerebral ischemia
(C)   Undetectable without the use of continuous 24-hr cardiac monitoring
(D)   Associated with organic heart disease
(E)   Of short duration

29.   Progression of a neurological deficit following a stroke can be due to:

(A)   Recurrent cerebral embolization
(B)   Cerebral edema
(C)   Distal propagation of a thrombus
(D)   Systemic hypotension

30.   Depression in elderly persons frequently presents with:

(A)   Agitation
(B)   Loss of weight
(C)   Withdrawal
(D)   Loss of memory
(E)   Hypochondriasis

31.   Logical extensions of organic brain syndrome in elderly patients include:

(A)   Frightening delusions
(B)   Stereotypy (redundant and illogical activity)
(C)   Nonfrightening auditory hallucinations
(D)   Provoked anger

(E)   Lability of affect

32.   True statements concerning orthostatic hypotension in elderly persons include:

(A)   It is a frequent cause of falling.
(B)   It is most likely to occur late in the day.
(C)   Incidence is increased in patients receiving antihypertensive medications.
(D)   Incidence is increased in patients receiving antidepressant medications.
(E)   Incidence is increased in patients with diabetic neuritis.

33.   Active incontinence refers to:

(A)   Failure to reach the toilet in time
(B)   Dysfunction of the sphincter muscle
(C)   Dysfunction of the detrusor muscle
(D)   Incontinence in the filling phase
(E)   Voluntary micturition at inappropriate times

34.   Changes in vision that occur with aging include:

(A)   Decreased ability to accommodate
(B)   Decreased ability to see at night
(C)   Decreased field of vision
(D)   Decreased tolerance to glare
(E)   Development of cataracts

Management

Fundamentals of Geriatric Medicine, edited by
Ronald D. T. Cape, Rodney M. Coe, and Isadore
Rossman, Raven Press, New York © 1983.

19

Overview

Isadore Rossman

Clinical management of the geriatric patient is in all respects more difficult than the management of younger patients, and there is less room for maneuvering or error. Only in recent years have we come to recognize some fundamentals of the therapeutic difficulties surrounding old age. The chapters in this section address appropriate concerns for management of some of the most common and most serious conditions that affect the elderly.

PHARMACOKINETICS

The importance of declines in lean body mass and renal competency in regard to dosage considerations in the elderly was disregarded for far too long. Major treatises in pharmacology had a striking absence of text concerned with age or aging. Although educators have taught us the validity and methodology of pediatric dosage, the equally valid concepts of geriatric dosage have only recently emerged on the therapeutic scene. Both the pediatric and geriatric dosage systems generally call for lower doses than those appropriate for the mature adult, but there the resemblance ends. Important pharmacokinetic differences are to be kept in mind, for an 8-year-old 80-pound child and an 80-year-old 80-pound woman are two quite different entities: The lean body mass, the volume of distribution, the plasma binding protein, and renal excretory capacity all undergo major alterations with aging. Even when allowances are made for all of these changes, the aged organism can still exhibit unpredictable adverse reactions which may be ascribed to age-related changes in end-organ sensitivity. Even the most cautious administration of certain sedatives or tranquilizers at the geriatric dosage level may produce such uncomfortable symptomatology as ataxia, dizziness, or confusion. There is a profusion of iatrogenic neuropsychiatric symptomatology in elderly patients that attests to their delicate balance.

INFECTIONS

Infections, increasingly lethal with aging, are everyday threats to old people. Diagnosed and undiagnosed bronchopneumonia is often the last event in a clinical sequence, supervening any other illness or disability. A common hazard is the pneumonia that quietly develops in what appears to be an ordinary viral respiratory illness—and is thus an avoidable cause of death. Because of declining immuno-competence, the elderly are the predisposed victims of pneumococcal and influenzal infections. To the extent that these infections are preventable, they become a special responsibility of the physician treating elderly patients.

In large part because of prostatic hypertrophy, elderly men are subject to urinary tract infections (UTIs). Because of the consequent necessary instrumentation and catheterization, these men are also often victims of serious gram-negative bacter-emias arising in the urinary tract.

Another important topic is asymptomatic bacteriuria. This is an overtreated con-dition almost unique to the older female and is best managed by a judicious and wary neglect. In most such women, repeated courses of treatment for the inevitable recurrences usually eventuate in the appearance of a resistant organism. Hence the well-intentioned physician's desire to clear the urine of infection may instead lead to hospitalization and protracted treatment of a serious UTI.

It has also become increasingly clear that some infections of old age have an environmental epidemiology. Discrimination increasingly has to be made between infections acquired in the community and those acquired in the long-term care facility. Just as we have come to recognize the serious nosocomial infections of the hospital setting, so may we also anticipate the likelihood of differences in the infecting organisms in environments such as the nursing home.

SLEEP DISORDERS

Sleep disorders, as all physicians with elderly patients well know, are an in-creasing source of complaint during old age. There are age-related changes in the central nervous system manifested by alterations in sleep patterns and the quality of sleep. Stage IV sleep, the sleep of innocent childhood, disappears before old age. Sleep often becomes lighter, fitful, and punctuated by episodes of wakefulness. It is very likely that there are two groups of oldsters who react differently to this experience. One group consists of persons who, for one reason or another, accept the sleep disorder and cope with it by various mechanisms that are self-generated. They may read for a while, turn on the radio, take an alcoholic drink, down some hot milk, and on the whole seem not to suffer too much. The physician is more likely to see those patients who appear in the office complaining bitterly of insomnia. Management of this second group of patients is fraught with the usual pharmaco-logical difficulties, and as yet there is no satisfactory drug or restorative for this manifestation of aging. The practical task for the physician may be to improve the elderly patient's sleep while assiduously avoiding the imminently hazardous line past which impairment and confusion begin to arise. The physician may also be asked to respond to the patient's relatives, who complain that he or she dozes all day and wanders all night. This inversion of normal sleep–wake relationships is likely to produce maximum distress in the family unit.

CONGESTIVE HEART FAILURE

Almost half the patient population of some of this country's first-rate facilities for the aged are on digitalis preparations. This points primarily to the formidable dimensions of congestive heart failure during old age. Congestive failure may be brought on by an illness (e.g., pneumonia), which may lead to digitalization and may eventuate in an unnecessary lifetime digitalization. Most physicians are inclined not to discontinue digitalis, though it has been safely done with a fair number of elderly patients in regular sinus rhythm. It is probable therefore that digitalization has been overutilized. However, the physician's greatest challenge comes from chronic congestive failure brought on by mostly irreversible myocardial events.

The introduction of vasodilator therapy with the success attendant on reduction of cardiac work is particularly important during old age. A formerly bleak picture has thus been greatly improved; edema, effusion, dyspnea, and angina may all respond notably. Here too the importance of adverse drug effects is stressed, for the delicate balance of all geriatric clinical management is nowhere more evident than in the cardiac patient.

PSYCHIATRIC DISORDERS

Mild states of depression in the elderly are often unrecognized, doubtless because they are thought to be natural parts of the aging process. The impact of more severe depression is illustrated by the fact that the highest suicide rate in any group is found in males over 65. Looming even larger in geropsychiatry is the most widespread of all mental disorders, the organic mental syndrome. Reversible and irreversible brain syndromes comprise the most important area of unfinished business anywhere in psychiatry. These disorders have widespread implications for management everywhere: in the chronic care facility, the hospital, and the community at large. Skilled management of such patients in the home setting may enable them to remain there rather than be institutionalized. In the acute care hospital, predisposed elderly patients seemingly develop the symptomatology almost without warning. It may be precipitated by pneumonia and fever on the medical service and by anesthesia and surgical trauma on the surgical side, and thus is an everyday challenge everywhere in the modern hospital. The details of management of this group of patients are therefore of importance to all who care for elderly patients.

CANCER

Annually, there are almost a quarter of a million deaths ascribed to cancer in individuals over 65, and silent or occult cancer is commonplace during old age.

Some of these cancers appear to evolve more slowly than in younger patients, although physicians caring for the elderly occasionally see highly aggressive malignancies. Hodgkin's disease may be more aggressive during old age, and cancers with poor prognosis (e.g., those of the stomach and pancreas) are unfortunately common in the elderly. The biology of tumor growth is of particular interest to the physician with elderly patients, with much yet to be learned. Thus the appearance of slowly growing carcinoma in a very old person may present more than the usual therapeutic options. The presence of other impairments or the actuarial probability of a short life span even in the absence of cancer can become major factors when weighing the various forms of management. Palliative treatment is often considered the best therapeutic choice. However, not enough is yet known about the hazards and rewards of cancer management in the elderly, e.g., with chemotherapeutic regimens. Thus the use of adjuvant chemotherapy with certain carcinomas of the elderly is yet to be worked out. We have much to learn about the transferability of findings from studies of young women to very elderly women, e.g., those over 80.

PAIN

Pain in elderly patients is well managed by the routine writing of pain prescriptions. As a group, geriatric patients are subject to all varieties of the pain experience: acute and lancinating, chronic and bone-breaking, and all combinations thereof. The pain syndromes run this gamut and present some paradoxes as compared to presentations in younger patients. Myocardial infarctions are more likely to be silent (15% or more), and the pain, when present, is far less likely to have the crushing and ominous intensity experienced by the middle-aged person. This alteration in the clinical aspects of myocardial pain has been commented on by numerous authors and is sometimes ascribed to a central diminution of the perception of pain.

On the other hand, it is mostly old people who have severe and really disabling herpes zoster. This is a common pain in old age, often not managed as successfully as it might be.

Arthritis and musculoskeletal conditions are almost ubiquitous in the elderly, and the management of the associated pain is often all that the physician can contribute. Cancer, the second most common cause of death in the age group 65 to 74, and the third most common in persons over 75, is a formidable challenge to anyone involved in the management of chronic pain.

CONCLUSION

The many pitfalls present in the clinical management of the elderly patient make geriatric medicine unique from that practiced with younger patients. The sleeping pill that is helpful to the middle-aged patient may generate pseudosenility in the older one. The standard digitalization program of the earlier years transferred into old age produces toxicity, with the early symptoms often overlooked or attributed to aging. A myocardial infarction may be painless; yet pain may be the only presenting complaint in a depression. Adverse drug and drug interaction effects are more common in the elderly, yet physicians cannot afford to be therapeutic nihilists; with respect to immunizations, prophylactic anticoagulation, and other courses, they must remain activists. The material in this section provides some of the essential information for management of serious conditions that commonly afflict the elderly.

Fundamentals of Geriatric Medicine, edited by
Ronald D. T. Cape, Rodney M. Coe, and Isadore
Rossman, Raven Press, New York © 1983.

20

Clinical Pharmacology of Aging

S. George Carruthers

The principles applied to prescribing medications for the elderly are no different from those employed in treating other age groups. Where possible, the following basic questions should be asked:

1. What is the basic diagnosis?
2. What are the defects in normal physiology?
3. What is the rational drug or nondrug therapy?
4. What can reasonably be expected from drugs?
5. How will improvement be assessed?
6. How long will treatment be pursued?
7. What is the appropriate dose of drug?
8. What are the potential problems?

The physician has a responsibility to identify each problem, to distinguish those conditions which can be helped by medication, and to follow the patient to ensure that the treatment has produced the desired effects and not adverse effects. Unfortunately, for a variety of reasons, medications are often used to treat the physical, psychological, social, and economic problems associated with aging, even when there is scientific evidence that drugs are the least appropriate way of managing some of these problems. Rather than having the quality of life improved, the elderly patient may actually suffer adverse effects of drug intervention which was initiated, presumably, with the best intentions. Overuse of medications in the elderly may result. Reasons for this include: ignorance of normal pathophysiology of aging, inaccurate interpretation of symptomatology, lack of appreciation of value and limitation of drugs, perceived physician-patient role models as giver and receiver of drugs, respectively, insufficient time or expertise to resolve certain problems without medications, insufficient understanding by the patient of why drugs are administered, and insufficient review and revision of therapy by the physician.

The elderly patient is therefore at risk of entering an "illness-medication spiral" (Fig. 1). Moreover, the aging person often lacks the resilience or homeostatic capacity of the younger patient to compensate for the adverse effects of drugs.

The numbers in Fig. 1 refer to the following possible events:

1. Because elderly patients tend to experience more illness as the result of declining body function or frank pathological change, they are likely to receive large numbers of medications.
2. The more medications a patient receives, the greater is the potential for interaction.
3. The more medications a patient receives, the greater is the risk of adverse reaction.
4. Drug interactions may produce adverse effects if the interaction leads to (a) impaired clearance of one or more drug(s), or (b) addition or synergism of the pharmacological effects of two or more drugs.
5. Drug interactions may exacerbate the original illness if the interaction leads to (a) increased clearance of one or more drug(s) or (b) less therapeutic effect if the pharmacological actions of the drugs are antagonistic.
6. Adverse reactions may be incorrectly interpreted. Instead of being associated with the medications, adverse effects are sometimes interpreted as "new illness," for which the physician may unwittingly prescribe further medication.

There are many common ailments in the elderly, e.g., constipation, aches and pains, dyspepsia, dyspnea, ankle edema, insomnia, anxiety, and depression. The aches and pains of "rheumatism" in the elderly patient may be treated with analgesics containing codeine or propoxyphene. For example, when constipation occurs, the patient receives a variety of laxative preparations. Confusion may lead to the use of major tranquilizers, which may aggravate drowsiness and cause postural hypotension or extrapyramidal problems. A male patient experiences severe grief at the loss of his spouse, for which a tricyclic antidepressant is prescribed. He develops a dry mouth and urinary retention for which he is referred to a urologist for possible prostatectomy.

It is important that this apparently dismal sequence of possibilities does not lead the physician to adopt a position of therapeutic nihilism except (a) when there is no good evidence of drug efficacy in a given clinical situation or (b) as a temporizing escape from the illness-medication spiral.

On the other hand, successful drug therapy in the elderly patient can be extremely rewarding for both the patient and the physician. There are, however, several simple

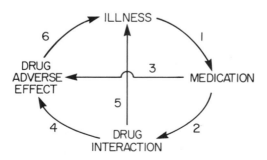

FIG. 1. Illness-medication spiral of problems to which the elderly are susceptible because of their multiple medical problems. See text for explanation of numbers.

guidelines which the physician should observe. Many simple common conditions may be more appropriately managed without drugs. Many conditions may be relatively brief and self-limiting. The ability of the elderly person to deal with the drug (pharmacokinetics) and the effect of the drug on the elderly patient (pharmacodynamics) may differ substantially from the manner in which the drug behaves in younger patients.

PATHOPHYSIOLOGY OF AGING

The physiology of aging was discussed in Chapters 4 through 9, but certain aspects are reviewed briefly here as they influence the manner in which the elderly patient responds to medications. These include: reduced total body weight, reduced skeletal muscle mass, reduced body water, increased body fat, reduced plasma protein concentrations, reduced cardiac output, reduced renal function, reduced hepatic oxidative function, altered responsiveness (of receptors, etc.), and common organic changes (e.g., vascular rigidity and prostatic hypertrophy).

Certain broad principles concerning drug use in the elderly can be developed directly from this information: (a) Older patients generally require smaller doses of drugs than younger patients. (b) The apparent volume of distribution of water-soluble drugs (e.g., digoxin) tends to be smaller. (c) The volume of distribution of fat-soluble drugs (e.g., diazepam) tends to be larger. (d) For highly protein-bound drugs, a given plasma concentration in an older patient is likely to be associated with a higher unbound or free drug concentration than the same total plasma concentration in a younger patient. (e) Drugs which are eliminated mainly by renal excretion leave the body more slowly in the elderly and hence may accumulate more insidiously. (f) Drugs which produce hypotension are more likely to cause faintness and syncope in older patients. (g) Elderly men are likely to be intolerant of powerful diuretics.

PHARMACOKINETICS IN THE ELDERLY

Absorption

Despite theoretical problems such as decreased gastric acidity, delayed gastric and intestinal motility, reduced gastrointestinal blood flow, and possible impairment of active transport mechanisms, there is little evidence that drugs are absorbed more slowly or less completely in the elderly than in younger patients. Indeed, preliminary studies suggest that the opposite may be true for drugs which undergo hepatic first-pass metabolism. As liver blood flow is reduced in the elderly, the first-pass hepatic clearance of drugs may be reduced if the extent of metabolism is limited by hepatic blood flow. Drugs which undergo significant first-pass metabolism include propranolol, morphine, meperidine, and propoxyphene. This particular possibility requires further extensive evaluation.

Distribution

Altered body composition leading to changes in distribution of both extremely fat-soluble and water-soluble drugs has already been mentioned. The volume of distribution (V_d) is an imaginary number which describes the apparent volume into which the drug has distributed by "mixing" in the body. If 100 mg of a drug is administered intravenously so that all is known to be in the body and produces a plasma concentration of 1 mg/L or 1 μg/ml, the volume of distribution is said to be 100 L. For a given dose of digoxin per kilogram of body weight, the plasma concentration will be lower in a muscular young athlete than in an elderly patient. This reflects the ability of digoxin to distribute in relatively large concentrations into skeletal muscle. The lower a patient's lean body weight, the less "space" there is for digoxin to distribute; consequently, plasma concentrations are higher. The converse is true for those drugs which tend to distribute predominantly into fat. Their plasma concentrations are likely to be higher in the lean young athlete than in the elderly patient whose total body fat content is higher.

When drug concentrations are measured in plasma, it is usual for the laboratory to report the total concentration, which includes both protein-bound and unbound (or free) drug. Only the unbound drug appears to be pharmacologically active, however. Alterations in protein binding are therefore of consequence only when a drug is extremely highly protein bound, e.g., > 90%. For example, if a drug were 98% protein-bound, hypoproteinemia might result in the fraction bound being reduced to 96%, i.e., twice the previous amount of unbound or active drug. Fortunately, there are compensatory mechanisms which preclude the need for major dosage alterations of drugs such as phenytoin (about 90% protein-bound). Some of the free drug is available for redistribution and clearance. However, when a serum phenytoin concentration is interpreted, it should be remembered that the usual 10% of unbound drug is increased by approximately 1% for every 0.1 g reduction of plasma albumin below 3 g/dl.

Warfarin is highly protein-bound (99.5%), which may explain in part the apparent sensitivity of older patients to this anticoagulant. Other possibilities are discussed later.

Metabolism

There are many metabolic pathways, but one of the most important is the mixed-function oxidase system. The classical yardstick of oxidative metabolism is antipyrine clearance. In many studies of elderly subjects, antipyrine half-life is prolonged 30 to 50% above the values in younger subjects. The half-life ($t_{1/2}$) of a drug influences the duration of its action as well as the time it takes for the drug to achieve a steady state in the body (i.e., when the amount of drug eliminated from the body each dosing interval is the same as that which is being administered, a period of approximately five half-lives). There are therefore two consequences of impaired hepatic metabolism: (a) a given plasma concentration will have a longer therapeutic or toxic effect; and (b) the drug will take longer to achieve the steady-state concentration, resulting in either delayed therapeutic benefit or an unexpectedly delayed onset of toxicity. Examples of drugs commonly used in the elderly which are metabolized in the liver include propranolol, lidocaine, phenytoin, phenothiazines, warfarin, and isoniazid.

It is probably better to think of clearance than elimination half-life, as clearance also recognizes the relevance of alterations in the volume of distribution. Clearance is expressed as a product of the elimination rate constant (k_{el} = $0.693/t_{1/2}$) and the volume of distribution (V_d). The half-life of diazepam in hours is approximately the same as the age of the patient expressed in years. However, the volume of distribution of diazepam increases with increasing age; therefore the clearance of diazepam is not much affected by age. Nevertheless, as mentioned earlier, the drug accumulates more slowly, and the effect of a given concentration is more persistent in the elderly.

Excretion

Age-dependent reduction in renal function appears to be a fairly consistent aspect of the aging process, e.g., creatinine excretion is 20 mg/kg/24 hr at age 20 and 8 mg/kg/24 hr at age 80. The presence of actual renal disease, of course, impairs renal function further. The serum creatinine level is not a good indication of renal function unless age, sex, and body weight are taken into consideration. A serum creatinine of 1.0 mg/dl in a 20-year-old male weighing 80 kg might reflect a creatinine clearance of about 120 ml/min, whereas the same serum creatinine level in an 80-year-old man weighing 50 kg would be compatible with a creatinine clearance of 40 ml/min, or only one-third that of the younger man. If renal function is stable and the patient is not acutely dehydrated or overhydrated, a reasonable prediction of creatinine clearance can be determined from knowledge of serum creatinine and the application of a nomogram such as that proposed by Kampmann and his colleagues (1).

DOSAGE ADJUSTMENT FACTOR

Knowledge of the fraction of a drug which is eliminated unchanged in urine and a patient's renal function enables determination of a "dosage adjustment factor" for that drug. A patient receiving digoxin (75% excreted unchanged) whose creatinine clearance is 50 ml/min would require a dosage adjustment factor of 2, i.e., the usual dosage interval must be prolonged by 2 or the usual dose divided by 2. As digoxin is usually administered on a once-daily basis, it is more appropriate to reduce the "usual" daily dose (if the patient had a creatinine clearance of 120 ml/min) rather than extend the dosing interval. In such deliberations, it is important that the dosage adjustment provides the patient with an acceptable dosage form and an acceptable dosage interval. A sophisticated calculation which determined the appropriate dose of digoxin to be 0.15 mg (usual tablets are 0.125 and 0.25 mg) at a dosing interval of 36 hr would be scientifically exact but practically absurd.

PHARMACODYNAMICS IN THE ELDERLY

Pharmacokinetic alterations in the absorption, distribution, metabolism, or excretion of certain drugs do not explain entirely the observations of increased "sensitivity" of older patients to certain drugs. True sensitivity appears to exist to these drugs; that is, for a given concentration of unbound drug, a greater or more sustained response is evoked. Some of the apparent sensitivity to warfarin appears to be impaired hepatic production of the clotting factors II, VII, and IX. Increased sensitivity to the analgesic meperidine may be the result of altered tissue binding of this drug. The number of beta-adrenoceptors appears to decrease in older patients.

"HAZARDOUS" DRUGS

Those drugs most likely to cause problems in the elderly can be defined in general terms. Any drug which has a narrow therapeutic margin between concentrations that produce therapeutic effects and those that produce toxicity is likely to cause problems. This statement clearly applies to all age groups.

Problems with drugs which possess a narrow therapeutic margin are compounded if the drug undergoes extensive renal elimination, e.g., digoxin, lithium, sulfonamides, cephalosporins, the aminoglycosides (gentamicin, streptomycin, kanamycin, tobramycin). Combination with a loop diuretic may aggravate these problems and, for example, increase the risk of aminoglycosides causing deafness.

Drugs which are more likely to upset homeostasis in the elderly include antihypertensives (dizziness and falls), diuretics (volume depletion), and anticholinergics (these include antiparkinsonian drugs, antihistamines, peptic ulcer remedies, tricyclic antidepressants, and disopyramide, which may aggravate prostatism and constipation).

Certain extrapyramidal effects of major tranquilizers appear to be more common in the elderly, e.g., parkinsonism and tardive dyskinesia. Impaired hepatic synthesis of clotting factors increases the activity of warfarin. The elderly myocardium is more likely to develop congestive cardiac failure following beta-blockade because of impaired muscle function and increased dependence on sympathetic tone.

The elderly brain becomes confused more readily under the influence of analgesics, psychotropic drugs, and drug-induced metabolic change. Drug-induced delays in gastric motility may readily precipitate severe constipation in the elderly patient.

OVER-THE-COUNTER PREPARATIONS

The complete drug history must include a record of over-the-counter (OTC) preparations consumed by the patient. Antacids, laxatives, decongestants, vitamins, cough mixtures, cold remedies, antihistamines, creams to remove "age spots," lotions for painful joints, solutions for bathing the eyes, drops for removing wax from the ears, and other patent medications of all sorts are consumed in vast amounts. Discouraged perhaps by how little our medications can do for their complaints, the elderly appear susceptible to the widely publicized claims of the manufacturers of OTC products. Their age may make them more willing to accept herbal and patent medications in the home, as most were adults before modern therapeutics were even conceived.

Laxatives are popular with the elderly. Chronic laxative use is a major medical problem, producing after many years an atonic, melanotic colon which is progressively resistant to most physiological and even pharmacological stimuli. Stronger cathartics, and ultimately combinations of agents with different properties, suppositories, and enemas become necessary to promote defecation. Mineral oil preparations may be associated with embarrassing incontinence of stool and may precipitate lipoid pneumonia. Antacids containing aluminum and calcium salts tend to constipate, whereas magnesium salts may cause diarrhea. Sodium bicarbonate may cause metabolic alkalosis in the presence of impaired renal function. Chronic salicylate use may cause occult gastrointestinal blood loss and chronic anemia, and occasionally causes massive gastrointestinal hemorrhage from peptic ulceration.

Pyridoxine (vitamin B_6) may impair the pharmacological action of levodopa. Iron preparations may interfere with tetracycline absorption. Antacids may reduce the gastrointestinal availability of digoxin and cimetidine. The combination of calcium salts taken for osteomalacia and vitamin D in excess may precipitate symptomatic hypercalcemia. Other problems include skin sensitization from topical preparations, excessive sedation from antihistamines, and drug rash from phenolphthalein (certain laxative preparations).

Unfortunately, patients may not even consider OTC preparations purchased at the corner drug store to be medications and may inadvertently give the inquiring physician an incomplete drug history unless the physician specifically inquires about their use.

SOCIAL DRUGS

Alcohol and tobacco remain the most widely used social drugs in our society. The medical problems associated with each are well known, but in addition they may influence the metabolism of other drugs. Smokers have increased metabolism of theophylline, and alcohol effects on drug metabolism are quite variable. The metabolism of some drugs is impaired if alcohol has recently been consumed, presumably by competition for enzyme activity. The metabolism of the same drugs may be enhanced by chronic alcohol use, presumably by oxidative enzyme induction. Cirrhosis may impair clotting factor synthesis and aggravate the hypoalbuminemia of old age.

PRACTICAL PROBLEMS

Compliance, the taking of medications as prescribed, is often poor in older patients. However, the elderly are not alone in this problem, and it is virtually impossible for a physician to predict the likelihood of compliance in a given patient. Most studies which have examined the problem of poor compliance concur that excessively complex regimens involving many drugs and dosage schedules increase the likelihood that medication orders will not be followed. Some studies also suggest that social isolation contributes to poor compliance.

It is common for legal packaging requirements to demand the use of childproof containers. The elderly patient may find it difficult to open these containers, especially if vision is impaired or if the patient suffers from muscular weakness or arthritis. Failing memory may make it difficult for the patient to recollect the times at which medicines are supposed to be taken. The patient may also have difficulty recalling whether the medication has been taken and so takes additional doses from time to time.

STRATEGIES TO IMPROVE MEDICATION USE IN THE ELDERLY

The preceding sections discussed the problems which arise in the drug treatment of elderly patients. We must now look at methods of improving the manner in which medications are used by the elderly. The physician, the patient, and friends or relatives of the patient may participate in this effort.

Emphasis has already been laid on the responsibility of the physician to define the disease state precisely, appreciate the natural prognosis of the condition, determine the benefit/risk of specific medications, determine the most appropriate drug, modify dose and dosing interval according to the patient's weight, hepatic, and renal function, and ensure that the dosage regimen is as simple as possible for ease of patient compliance. The physician should be reluctant to renew prescriptions without careful review of all current medications including OTC preparations. Each time a medication profile is reviewed, every effort should be made to discontinue those medications which are no longer indicated or which have not been effective in the condition for which they were prescribed. It is apparent that any medication causing a problem must be discontinued. Because of occasional difficulty in distinguishing adverse effects of drugs from unrelated ailments, the physician must develop a keen sense of suspicion that new problems may relate to drug therapy. In summary, the physician has a major responsibility to prescribe correctly and recognize adverse drug effects promptly when they occur. Labeling the medications according to indication is helpful when patients are taking many drugs, e.g., "Take one daily for fluid"; "Sleeping pill—take one at bedtime *only* if necessary"; "Antibiotic for chest—take every 6 hours until finished." In this way, not only the patient but interested and involved relatives or neighbors may identify more accurately the patient's medications. This will hopefully incur less risk of the patient taking a nighttime diuretic instead of an hypnotic!

It may be useful for the patient or a relative or friend to "dispense" the medications for a single day into a separate container or containers, so that the medications to be taken during the course of the day can be identified more readily. The patient can check the container around meal times, with a final check before retiring to ensure that the medications have been taken. This procedure has a virtue of solving several problems: the patient's difficulty in opening containers, removing the correct number of tablets, and recollecting if medications have been taken. The procedure offers a convenient form of supervision for the relative or friend as they visit with the patient during the course of the day. Such containers must, of course, be hygienic and convenient for the patient; they should not pose any risk to visiting children and so must be placed our of their reach. Composite blister-packing of medications according to the times at which they should be taken is an attractive but expensive and unrealistic concept at this time. A multicompartmental container (7 × 4 spaces) with transparent covers permits the storage and subsequent use of medications to a maximum of four daily dosage times over a 7-day period.

The measurement of drug concentrations in plasma can be a useful adjunct to therapy, especially if there are problems distinguishing between drug-related adverse effects and unrelated illness, e.g., vomiting by a patient receiving digoxin. Therapeutic drug monitoring may also serve a valuable role in the patient receiving a medication for prophylaxis of cardiac arrhythmia or seizure control. The dosage of the drug may be carefully tailored to the patient's needs, within the usual therapeutic concentration range, with less risk of the patient receiving inadequate therapy or suffering from toxic effects of the drug. Interactions between drugs may be identified more readily, and appropriate alterations in therapy may be made. Suspicion that the patient is not complying with therapy may be supported by the absence of drug in plasma or urine or the measurement of concentrations significantly lower than those recorded earlier when the patient took the medication under supervision. The ready availability of drug measurements must not, however, be abused, as the tests are often time-consuming and relatively expensive. The tests must always be interpreted in conjunction with a complete drug history and physical evaluation.

SUMMARY

The pharmacokinetics and pharmacodynamics of the elderly are reviewed, with particular reference to their relevance to drug administration and proper dosage. The factors involved in proper drug therapy for the elderly patient are considered, with the aim of increasing the benefits of the drug while reducing the risks.

When caring for elderly patients, the physician should:

1. Know what factors govern good prescribing practice.
2. Know what factors put elderly persons at particular risk of iatrogenic complications of drug therapy.
3. Know how the choice of drugs, dose, and dosing intervals can be adjusted to gain maximal benefit with minimal risk in the drug therapy of elderly persons.

REFERENCE

1. Hansen, J. M., Kampmann, J., and Laursen, H. Renal excretion of drugs in the elderly. *Lancet*, 1:1170, 1970.

SUGGESTED READING

Bochner, F., Carruthers, G., Kampmann, J., and Steiner, J. *Handbook of Clinical Pharmacology*. Little Brown, Boston, 1978.

Crooks, J., O'Malley, K., and Stevenson, I. H. Pharmacokinetics in the elderly. *Clin. Pharmacokinet.*, 1:280, 1976.

Davison, W. Drug hazards in the elderly. *Br. J. Hosp. Med.*, 6:83, 1971.

O'Malley, K., Judge, T. G., and Crooks, J. Geriatric clinical pharmacology and therapeutics in drug treatment. In: *Drug Treatment: Principles and Practice of Clinical Pharmacology and Therapeutics*, 2nd ed., edited by G. S. Avery, p. 158. Adis Press and Churchill Livingstone, Sydney, Australia, 1980.

Fundamentals of Geriatric Medicine, edited by
Ronald D. T. Cape, Rodney M. Coe, and Isadore
Rossman, Raven Press, New York © 1983.

21

Management of Infection in the Elderly

David W. Bentley

The main clinical syndromes that occur either more frequently or with increased severity in the elderly are included in this chapter. These infections may be difficult to diagnose because their onset is insidious and vague and/or the clinical manifestations may be remote from the actual site of infection. It is important, however, for physicians to detect these infections early because they can usually be cured (or at the very least improved), and other conditions that were adversely affected by the infection can thus also be improved, e.g., congestive heart failure, arrhythmias, anemia, confusion, incontinence, diabetes. Note that the recommended antimicrobial regimens and doses are for older persons with *normal* renal function. The physician must be aware that renal dysfunction occurs frequently in older persons despite minimal elevations in blood urea nitrogen (BUN) or serum creatinine. Appropriate dosage adjustments must be made for antimicrobials that are excreted primarily by the kidneys, especially aminoglycosides.

RESPIRATORY INFECTIONS

Upper respiratory infections (URIs) including the common cold, pharyngitis, and acute laryngitis affect older persons less frequently than younger persons but are important because they may be predisposing events for bacterial pneumonia. They are managed symptomatically. Acute sinusitis, which is usually complicated by bacterial infection, is treated with antimicrobials, e.g., ampicillin or dicloxacillin. Acute epiglottitis is a rapidly progressive cellulitis of the epiglottis and surrounding structures that can cause airway obstruction. Although usually rare, it may occur in adults, including older persons in whom *Haemophilus influenzae* type B is less frequent and pneumococci, staphylococci, and streptococci are more frequent.

Acute bronchitis is usually associated with a generalized respiratory infection due to common cold viruses (e.g., rhinovirus), with lower respiratory tract pathogens (e.g., influenza and parainfluenza viruses), or with adenovirus. The diagnosis is one of exclusion; treatment is symptomatic and directed primarily at controlling the cough. *Mycoplasma pneumoniae* as a cause may be diagnosed by appropriate laboratory methods and treated with erythromycin.

Chronic bronchitis with acute infectious exacerbations is frequently associated with emphysema and is a common problem for older persons. Antimicrobials (7- to 10-day course of ampicillin or amoxicillin, tetracycline, or erythromycin) are often directed against nontypable *H. influenzae* and *Diplococcus (Streptococcus) pneumoniae*, which are associated with exacerbations in approximately 50% of cases. Viruses account for fully 25% to 50% of cases. Prophylactic antimicrobials such as tetracycline or cotrimoxazole (trimethoprim-sulfamethoxazole) may be useful in highly selected patients who experience frequent exacerbations. Patients should receive yearly immunization with the current influenza vaccine and may benefit also from pneumococcal vaccine.

The largest group at risk for serious morbidity and mortality from *influenza virus infection* are the elderly. The classical syndrome of uncomplicated influenza (sudden onset, chills, fever, headache, cough, sore throat, myalgia, and malaise) is similar to that in younger persons. Morbidity and mortality are usually associated with lower respiratory tract complications (bronchitis or pneumonia, especially secondary to bacteria) which occur in up to 70% of persons 70 or older. For many years the U.S. Public Health Service's Advisory Committee on Immunization Practices has recommended annual revaccination of older persons, especially those 65 and over, plus those with chronic diseases, including poorly compensated congestive heart failure, compromised pulmonary function, chronic renal disease, or diabetes. The vaccines in current use are given by injection and contain inactivated materials representing antigens from the most recent types of circulating influenza viruses (usually A and B). It takes 2 to 3 weeks for influenza vaccine to achieve effectiveness, and the overall efficacy is about 65%.

When immunization is not feasible or when the vaccine is contraindicated (egg allergy) or not available, amantadine (100 mg p.o. q 12 hr) can prevent influenza A (but not B) viral infections. Amantadine can also shorten the period of symptomatology of influenza A infection. It should be started as soon as possible after onset of symptoms and continued for 24 to 48 hr after the disappearance of symptoms. Amantadine is primarily excreted by the kidney; toxicity (most commonly anticholinergic side effects plus central nervous system symptomatology) is more frequent in older persons if renal dysfunction is present.

Bacterial pneumonia is probably the most important infection of older persons because it occurs frequently and with increased morbidity and mortality. The initial presentation is often different from that seen in younger persons and includes an insidious or nonspecific deterioration in the patient's general condition, sudden deterioration or slow recovery from another primary disease, confusion, or a fall. Despite statements to the contrary, cough with purulent sputum is usually present in more than 50% of older persons; more than 75% have rectal temperatures greater than 100°F, including 33% with temperatures greater than 103°F. Rigors (shaking or teeth-chattering chills) are quite uncommon in the elderly, with a frequency of less than 10% even in patients with proved pneumococcal pneumonia. The physical examination also differs in that signs of consolidation may not be found, and rales at the lung bases mean little. The most frequent findings are nonspecific and apply equally to pulmonary embolus: tachycardia, tachypnea, and dullness to percussion. Seventy-five percent of older patients have a leukocytosis with white blood cell counts greater than 10,000/mm^3. Because of the problems noted, a chest roentgenogram (posterior-anterior and lateral views whenever possible) must be obtained when pneumonia is suspected. When using this reliable diagnostic tool, the physician should be aware that incomplete consolidation is the usual pattern, even with pneumococcal pneumonia, and resolution may be delayed as long as 14 weeks after its onset.

Laboratory diagnosis depends on demonstrating the etiological agent(s) in cultures of respiratory secretions, pleural fluid, or blood. An expectorated sputum adequate for microbiological study may be very difficult to obtain in the older person because of diminished cough reflex and dehydration. The gram stain of the sputum should be examined microscopically at $100\times$ power to determine the degree of oropharyngeal contamination prior to culture: Specimens containing fewer than 10 squamous epithelial cells per $10\times$ field are equivalent to specimens obtained by transtracheal aspiration. Those with 10 to 25 squamous epithelial cells are probably satisfactory, but specimens with more than 25 squamous epithelial cells per $10\times$ field should not be cultured. Nasopharyngeal aspiration is also frequently contaminated with organisms from the upper respiratory tract. Transtracheal aspiration is the most accurate technique for obtaining an appropriate specimen for culture. It is of great help in managing pneumonia in hospitalized older persons who have not responded to initial therapy. If satisfactory sputum or nasopharyngeal aspirates are not available and a transtracheal aspirate cannot be obtained, one or two blood samples for culture should be taken prior to starting the antimicrobial drugs. If pneumococcal pneumonia is suspected but the patient is already receiving treatment, examination of the urine for pneumococcal polysaccharide by counterimmunoelectrophoresis may be helpful.

Treatment

Early treatment with appropriate antimicrobials is necessary to decrease the high mortality of bacterial pneumonia in older persons. The initial choice of antimicrobials depends on the interpretation of the gram stain of the respiratory secretion (or pleural fluid), the patient's location, and whether the patient is receiving antimicrobials. If the gram stain demonstrates fewer than 25 squamous epithelial cells per $10\times$ microscopic field, drug regimens can be chosen according to the predominant bacteria noted. For patients with mild to moderate illness, either in the community or in institutions, procaine penicillin (600,000 units i.m. q 12 hr) is the drug of choice. This regimen can be used for both suspected mixed bacterial flora secondary to aspiration of oropharyngeal secretions or pneumococcal pneumonia. It has the advantage of low toxicity and little risk of suprainfection. For penicillin-allergic patients, clindamycin (300 mg i.m. q 8 hr) or cefazolin (250 mg i.m. q 8 hr) is an appropriate alternative. In patients with chronic bronchitis or chronic pulmonary disease, ampicillin (750 to 1,000 mg i.v. q 6 hr) may provide more effective coverage for possible *H. influenzae*. These initial regimens are satisfactory, even if gram-negative bacilli are part of the mixed flora.

Bactericidal combination regimens—e.g., cefazolin (1 g i.v. q 6 to 8 hr) and tobramycin (1.5 mg/kg i.v. q 8 hr)—should be started when gram-negative bacilli are the only bacteria noted or when (a) gram-negative bacilli are predominant, (b) the patient is seriously ill or has not responded within 72 to 96 hr to a "low-dose" regimen noted above, and (c) secretions cannot be obtained by transtracheal aspiration. The optimum duration of treatment has not been established but probably should be for approximately 3 days after the patient's clinical condition has returned to baseline for mixed bacterial flora, *D. pneumoniae* or *H. influenzae* and up to 7 to 10 days after returning to baseline when gram-negative bacilli or *Staphylococcus aureus* are involved. Chest physiotherapy, consisting of postural drainage, percussion, and vibration, may play an important role in the management of bacterial pneumonia by overcoming impaired clearance mechanisms such as decreased cough reflex and mucociliary function. Effective treatment of hypoxia is critical to avoid any adverse effects on the brain and myocardium.

Prevention

Specific measures to prevent bacterial pneumonia in older persons include: influenza vaccine (see previous discussion) and pneumococcal vaccine. The latter vaccine was licensed in January 1978 and contains purified polysaccharide from 14 of the 83 known pneumococcal types. Any older person for whom influenza vaccine is indicated should probably also receive pneumococcal vaccine. The dose is 0.5 ml subcutaneously. With the exception of local discomfort, very few reactions are noted, and antibody production is comparable to that in younger persons. The duration of protective antibody is at least 3 years and probably longer. Unlike influenza vaccines which are given annually, revaccination with pneumococcal vaccine is currently recommended at 3- to 5-year intervals. The cost of vaccination per year therefore is approximately the same for each vaccine. Although pneumococcal vaccine can be given at any time of year, it may be more convenient to give it in the fall along with influenza vaccination.

TUBERCULOSIS

The highest rates of tuberculosis in the United States occur among older persons. Active tuberculosis late in life is most commonly the result of reactivation of a dormant focus. More than 85% of new cases are pulmonary, but extrapulmonary disease is becoming more frequent in older persons, especially the miliary and genitourinary forms.

Tuberculosis is difficult to diagnose in the older person. The clinical findings in pulmonary tuberculosis of cough, sputum, and dyspnea are nonspecific and may be attributed to other medical problems. Miliary tuberculosis, especially the "cryptic" variety, occurs primarily in older persons with vague symptoms of weakness, anorexia, fatigue, weight loss, and intermittent fever. Genitourinary tuberculosis presents primarily with local signs and symptoms; fever is present in less than 10% of cases. The chest roentgenogram may demonstrate minimal findings in older persons despite active disease; nearly one-third with reactivation have findings in segments other than the usual apical-posterior region.

Pulmonary tuberculosis is diagnosed by examination of respiratory secretions for tubercle bacilli. Any findings suspicious of tuberculosis, including "stranding" or fibrosis on a chest roentgenogram, require sputum cultures. Sputum, spontaneous or induced, should be collected on three consecutive mornings prior to breakfast for examination by smear and culture. If sputum is not available, fasting morning gastric aspirates should be obtained before the patient moves or sits up and should be submitted for culture and fluorescein microscopy. Transtracheal aspirate or transbronchial biopsies obtained by fiberoptic bronchoscopy should be considered only when respiratory secretions and gastric aspirates are not helpful and the clinical suspicion of tuberculosis remains high.

Genitourinary tuberculosis should be suspected when persistent abnormal urinalyses are noted. Three consecutive first morning's urine specimens should be collected and submitted for culture. The most helpful diagnostic procedures for miliary tuberculosis are culture and histological examination of hepatic biopsy specimens. Bone marrow biopsy should be performed when hepatic biopsy is contraindicated or when anemia, leukopenia, or monocytosis are prominent findings. Older persons should be tested with PPD (5 tuberculin units), but this test may be negative in 10 to 20% of patients with proved active disease, especially miliary tuberculosis.

Successful treatment of pulmonary tuberculosis depends on early diagnosis, appropriate chemotherapy, and proper treatment of coexisting diseases. An effective regimen for uncomplicated (single lobe and no cavities) pulmonary tuberculosis is daily oral isoniazid (INH, 300 mg) and ethambutol (25 mg/kg for 2 to 3 months, then 15 mg/kg for the remainder of the course). The typical duration of 18 months poses a problem for many older persons who are unable to cooperate for this length of time. The newly recommended oral short-course chemotherapy regimen of INH and rifampin (600 mg) for 9 to 12 months may prove more acceptable. Streptomycin, though seldom employed, should be used with great care in the older person because of increased serum levels and vestibular toxicity secondary to unsuspected renal failure. The recommended dose for older persons is 0.5 g/day; serum levels should be followed even with mild renal failure. Older patients with fever, anorexia, and debility due to tuberculosis may benefit from steroids given concomitantly with effective antituberculous drugs.

Chemoprophylaxis (INH 300 mg/day for 12 months) is effective in decreasing bacterial populations in older persons with "healed" lesions and thereby reducing the risk of developing active disease. INH is also recommended for a number of conditions for which the risk of developing disease is greater than the risk of developing INH-associated hepatitis, which occurs in about 2 to 3% of persons over the age of 50. These conditions include recent PPD skin test conversion, household or intimate contact with an active case, or prior untreated clinical disease; they only rarely pertain to the older person. A fourth condition—chest roentgenogram compatible with old disease, no known prior clinical disease, plus other conditions (insulin-dependent diabetes, gastrectomy, impaired cell-mediated immunity secondary to steroids, immunosuppression or lymphoma-leukemia, or chronic diseases such as alcoholism, silicosis, or cancer)—is more pertinent to older persons, but the relative risks are not clearly defined.

Screening programs, based on chest roentgenograms and sputum cultures for tuberculosis, should be established in long-term care facilities where older persons frequently have active disease and/or a high prevalence of infection and are at risk of developing active disease.

URINARY TRACT INFECTIONS

Urinary tract infection (UTI) is the most frequent infection that afflicts older persons. Asymptomatic bacteriuria is the major clinical presentation, especially in women. Signs and symptoms of acute pyelonephritis in the absence of outflow obstruction or papillary necrosis associated with diabetes mellitus are seldom noted.

The diagnosis of UTI in older persons is therefore even more dependent on the careful collection of urine for culture. The reliability of a single midstream urine sample is dependent on the mental status and cooperation of the patient. When in doubt, a straight catheter with the smallest possible lumen and careful technique should be employed, especially in women. The frequent practice in long-term care facilities of attaching a "sterile" condom catheter collecting system to collect urine for culture in men is not recommended. As in younger patients, pyuria (counts of 5 to 10 white blood cells per high power field from a centrifuged urine specimen) is correlated with true bacteriuria in symptomatic UTIs. Traditionally, treatment of symptomatic UTIs requires collection of a urine specimen for culture and sensitivity tests, an appropriate antimicrobial agent given in adequate doses for 7 to 14 days, and follow-up cultures 1 week later. The choice of the antimicrobial agent depends on the patient's location. If at home where sensitive *Escherichia coli* accounts for 75 to 80% of infections, choose amoxicillin (250 mg q 6 to 8 hr) or cotrimoxazole (two tablets b.i.d.). If the patient is hospitalized or in a long-term care facility where resistant *E. coli*, *Proteus* species, or *Pseudomonas aeruginosa* are more frequent, it may be best to wait for identification and sensitivity test results. If this delay is not appropriate, begin treatment with oral carbenicillin or intramuscular injections of an aminoglycoside (e.g., tobramycin or gentamicin) and then be guided by sensitivity results.

Asymptomatic Bacteriuria

The majority of UTIs in older persons are uncomplicated. Avoid treating asymptomatic bacteriuria because: (a) most patients (especially women) are reinfected with different organisms within 4 to 12 weeks after stopping the initial treatment; and (b) there is no evidence that asymptomatic bacteriuria (in the absence of obstruction) is associated with renal impairment or hypertension.

Causes for acute or chronic urinary retention should be considered in any older patient with a UTI, especially if it is symptomatic. Such causes include fecal impaction, prostatic hypertrophy, atonic neuropathic bladder secondary to diabetes mellitus, and drug-associated causes, especially from antidepressants, antiparkinsonian drugs, and anticholinergics.

The frequently benign course of asymptomatic bacteriuria in older persons argues against vigorous urological work-ups, including intravenous pyelograms, which have excess morbidity especially in older persons. The genitourinary tract, both lower and upper, should be evaluated in women who have three or four recurrent symptomatic UTIs over several months with the same species, biotype, and resistant pattern as the original pathogen. Recurrent UTIs in men are frequently associated with abnormal genitourinary tracts; therefore men with one or two recurrent UTIs should be evaluated if chronic prostatitis can be ruled out or if it cannot be diagnosed (see below).

Chronic treatment with antimicrobials should mainly be reserved for recurrent symptomatic bacteriuria associated with serious morbidity (e.g., renal calculi, papillary necrosis) or the occasional patient whose symptoms are clearly associated with the bacteriuria. Chemoprophylaxis is indicated in older persons whenever bacteremia is associated with surgery or instrumentation of the genitourinary tract and underlying conditions of relatively high risk for developing infective endocarditis are present.

Acute bacterial prostatitis in older persons presents with fever, chills, low back pain, and symptoms of UTI, including urgency and dysuria. The prostate is warm, swollen, and tender on examination per rectum. Prostatic secretions can be expressed to demonstrate polymorphonuclear leukocytes and the infecting organism on gram stain; however, this may precipitate bacteremia and therefore should be avoided. Aerobic gram-negative bacilli are usually the etiological agents and can often be isolated from midstream urine cultures. Many antimicrobials diffuse well into the acutely inflamed prostate. Therefore systemic antimicrobial regimens that provide adequate blood levels are appropriate. During acute stages, urethral manipulation and indwelling catheters should be avoided.

Chronic bacterial prostatitis is the most common cause of recurring UTI in older men. It is very difficult to diagnose because there may be few or no symptoms related to infection. The main clues are perineal pain, low back pain, and difficulty urinating. Fever is low grade unless a septic local (pyelonephritis) or contiguous (vertebral osteomyelitis) process is present. Symptoms of UTI are periodic, and polymorphonuclear leukocytes in expressed prostatic secretions are not diagnostic. Diagnosis can be made only by quantitative localization techniques which evaluate simultaneous cultures of urethral urine (VB$_1$), midstream urine (VB$_2$), prostatic secretions expressed by massage (EPS), or by ejaculation and urine voided after massage (VB$_3$). Counts from EPS or ejaculate are 10 times larger than VB$_1$ or VB$_2$, or counts from VB$_3$ are 10 times larger than those from VB$_1$ or VB$_2$.

Chronic bacterial prostatitis is most commonly caused by aerobic gram-negative bacilli, especially *E. coli* (80%), but *Klebsiella* and *Enterobacter* species plus *Proteus mirabilis* and enterococcus may also be present. This entity is very difficult to cure because few antimicrobials adequately penetrate the noninflamed prostate. Cotrimoxazole (two tablets b.i.d. for 12 weeks) is presently the most effective therapy; approximately one-third of cases can be cured. If failure occurs, either treat the acute exacerbations of UTI or attempt chronic suppressive treatment with one-half dose per day. If enterococcus is present, treat with oral erythromycin (500 mg q 6 hr).

Acute symptomatic UTI associated with chronic indwelling catheters require prompt attention to avoid serious consequences, especially gram-negative bacteremia. Percuss the bladder to detect retained urine and look for leakage around the catheter, which indicates catheter dysfunction. If either is noted, remove the catheter promptly and carefully reinsert a new one to promote effective drainage. If a recent (within 2 to 4 weeks) urine culture is available, choose an appropriate antimicrobial to treat the UTI. If not available, select an aminoglycoside such as tobramycin or gentamicin (1.0 mg/kg/dose q 8 hr) that is effective against most gram-negative bacilli associated with catheter-related UTIs. The antimicrobial regimen should not be continued for the usual 10 to 14 days because infections cannot be eliminated so long as the indwelling catheter is in place and because colonization of the bladder with resistant organisms occurs frequently. Treat for 1 to 2 days after the patient's vital signs have returned to baseline values unless bacteremia is documented or strongly suspected. If this is the case, the regimen should be continued for 10 to 14 days. Asymptomatic bacteriuria associated with indwelling catheters in place more than 10 days should not be treated with either systemic antimicrobials or antibacterial bladder rinses.

HERPES ZOSTER

Herpes zoster is an important viral infection afflicting older persons. Zoster is caused by a herpes virus, the varicella-zoster virus, which produces a primary infection (chicken pox) in children and, after recovery, persists in the dorsal root ganglia without clinical manifestations until reactivation many decades later. Diagnosis of zoster in the older person is usually apparent once the unilateral eruption of vesicles appears. Disseminated zoster (i.e., 15 to 30 or more lesions distant from the primary dermatome) occurs frequently (15%) in the older patient. The distribution is generally sparse and is usually not associated with an underlying cause; there is no increase in morbidity or mortality with this type of dissemination. If the dissemination is generalized and profuse, the patient may develop signs of systemic involvement, especially of the pulmonary and central nervous systems. This picture is more commonly seen in patients receiving immunosuppressive therapy or in those with malignant disease, especially lymphomas. Laboratory assistance in the diagnosis of zoster infections is seldom required.

The most common cause of morbidity is postherpetic neuralgia (pain in the involved dermatome that persists for at least 2 months) that may be incapacitating for many months, and occurs with a frequency of 10 to 50% depending on whether older persons with zoster are seen in the community or admitted to a hospital. Analgesics, including oral narcotics, may be required to permit sleep or, in severe cases, normal daily activities. Systemic steroids given early in the course significantly reduce postherpetic neuralgia, and many authorities believe they should be used in all but the mildest of cases. A common regimen is prednisone (40 to 60 mg) each morning for the first week, 20 to 30 mg the second week, and 10 to 15 mg the third week, after which it is discontinued. The effect of steroids is not usually apparent until the second or third week of treatment. Therefore if pain dramatically decreases within several days of starting steroids, this response is most likely the natural course of the disease, and the steroids can be discontinued. Psychotropic drugs may be indicated to overcome depression. Vidarabine® (ara-A, adenine arabinoside) should be considered in older patients with generalized profuse eruption and visceral involvement. No specific treatment is required for uncomplicated zoster.

Prevention is not usually considered for the healthy elderly person with zoster because the illness is generally mild and self-limited. Although most older persons are not susceptible to varicella because of prior infection, contact with persons with varicella or zoster should be avoided if the older person is immunocompromised.

SUMMARY

The most common infectious diseases to afflict the elderly are respiratory and urinary tract infections, tuberculosis, and herpes zoster. Diagnosis may be difficult, as their onset may be insidious and the symptoms nonspecific. It is vital to arrive at a proper diagnosis and to treat the infection appropriately, however—not only to rid the patient of the offending organism but to avoid complicating other ongoing disorders. The treatments discussed herein are relevant only to patients with normal renal function. Patients whose kidneys are not functioning properly must have their doses and regimens adjusted according to need.

When caring for elderly patients, the physician should:

1. Know what infectious diseases are most likely to occur with great frequency or severity in elderly persons.
2. Know how the manifestations of infectious diseases may differ in elderly persons compared with younger persons.
3. Know what diagnostic techniques may be particularly helpful for evaluating the elderly person who may have an infectious disease.
4. Know how treatment regimens should be adjusted to the particular needs of elderly persons with infectious diseases.
5. Know what measures are appropriate in the prevention or prophylaxis of infectious diseases in elderly persons.

SUGGESTED READING

American Heart Association Committee on Prevention of Bacterial Endocarditis. Prevention of bacterial endocarditis. *Circulation*, 56:139A–143A, 1977.

Brocklehurst, J. C., Bee, P., Jones, D., and Palmer, M. K. Bacteriuria in geriatric hospital patients: its correlates and management. *Age Ageing*, 6:240–245, 1977.

Center for Disease Control. Guidelines for short-course tuberculosis chemotherapy. *Morbidity and Mortality Weekly Report*, 29:97–105, 1980.

Eaglestein, W. H., Katz, R., and Brown, J. A. The effects of early corticosteroid therapy on the skin eruption and pain of herpes zoster. *JAMA*, 211:1681–1683, 1970.

Gladstone, J. L., and Recco, R. Host factors and infectious diseases in the elderly. *Med. Clin. North Am.*, 60:1225–1240, 1976.

Hope-Simpson, R. E. Herpes zoster in the elderly. *Geriatrics*, 22:151–159, 1967.

Howells, C. H. L., Vasselinova-Jenkins, C. K., Evans, A. D., and James, J. Influenza vaccination and mortality from bronchopneumonia in the elderly. *Lancet*, 1:381–383, 1975.

Kasik, J. E., and Schuldt, S. Why tuberculosis is still a health problem in the aged. *Geriatrics*, 32:63–72, 1977.

Ledger, W. J. Infections in elderly women. *Clin. Obstet. Gynecol.*, 20:145–153, 1977.

Mandell, G. L., Douglas, R. G., Jr., and Bennett, J. E. *Principles and Practice of Infectious Diseases*, Vols. I and II. Wiley, New York, 1979.

Meares, E. M., and Stamey, T. Bacteriologic localization patterns in bacterial prostatitis and urethritis. *Invest. Urol.*, 5:492–518, 1968.

Phair, J. P. Aging and infection: a review. *J. Chronic Dis.*, 32:535–540, 1979.

Phair, J. P., Kauffman, C. A., Bjornson, A., Gallagher, A. L., and Hess, E. V. Host defenses in the aged: evaluation of components of the inflammatory and immune response. *J. Infect. Dis.*, 138:67–73, 1978.

Sourander, L. Urinary tract infection in the aged: an epidemiological study. *Ann. Intern. Med. Fenn.*, 55:7–55, 1966.

Sullivan, N. M., Sutter, V. L., Mims, M. M., Marsh, V. H., and Finegold, S. Y. Clinical aspects of bacteremia after manipulation of the genitourinary tract. *J. Infect. Dis.*, 127:49–55, 1973.

Fundamentals of Geriatric Medicine, edited by
Ronald D.T. Cape, Rodney M. Coe, and Isadore
Rossman, Raven Press, New York © 1983.

22

Management of Congestive Heart Failure in the Aged

Howard L. Moscovitz

Successful management of congestive heart failure requires an understanding of the altered physiological mechanisms at work, the possibility of extracardiac factors complicating the clinical picture, and the therapeutic modalities available. At the outset, it is of vital importance to determine if one is dealing with a surgically reversible factor (e.g., valve stenosis or insufficiency) or primarily ventricular muscle dysfunction. The imposing array of noninvasive techniques now available makes it feasible to study even the sickest patient at the bedside to determine the mechanisms operative in ventricular decompensation. The maximum age of potential surgical candidates is constantly rising.

Old age is often accompanied by alterations in drug absorption and disposition as well as increased receptor-site sensitivity to drugs. These factors may result in excessive drug accumulation, higher tissue and serum levels, and exaggerated drug effect and toxicity. Clearance of digoxin is accomplished largely by the kidney; as renal function declines with old age, the same dose of digoxin produces higher plasma concentrations in the elderly than in the young. The serum digoxin assay may be of limited value, as it is only an indirect reflection of digitalis tissue concentration. Quinidine is handled by both liver and renal clearance, and its plasma half-life is significantly prolonged in the elderly. This leads to higher steady-state quinidine levels at a given dose. The use of digoxin and quinidine simultaneously may quickly lead to digitoxicity due to rapid mobilization of tissue-bound stores of digoxin. The elimination half-life of lidocaine is prolonged in the aged, particularly in the presence of concomitant liver disease; thus central nervous system toxicity is frequent in the elderly on doses well tolerated by younger patients. Propranolol seems to achieve significantly higher plasma concentrations in aged subjects when compared to those in the young. At any given plasma concentration of coumadin, geriatric patients have a more prolonged prothrombin time than control patients of younger ages.

MYOCARDIAL INFARCTION

The clinical setting in which acute congestive heart failure most commonly takes place is acute myocardial infarction. Pump failure associated with acute infarction in the aged usually has an ominous prognosis, and when accompanied by shock the outlook is bleak. The heart's performance as a pump is quickly compromised when flow in a major coronary artery is interrupted. Cardiac contraction weakens within a few beats, and in a short time the ischemic area is visibly cyanotic, no longer effectively ejecting blood, and may bulge paradoxically with systole. The interval between the onset of ischemia and cell death is only a few hours, but during this initial interval of pump failure the cellular changes are potentially reversible and viability in the affected myocardium is retained. As this early pump failure is attributable to a lack of oxygen, interventions which either reduce the myocardial consumption of oxygen or enhance its delivery may improve the viability of the ischemic heart muscle. These measures include the use of an intra-aortic balloon pump, beta-blocking agents, coronary artery dilators, and certain controversial drugs, e.g., corticosteroids, hyaluronidase, and glucose-insulin-potassium solution.

Digitalis

Controversy surrounds the use of digitalis in the treatment of congestive failure associated with acute myocardial infarction. There have been indications that the ischemic myocardium is very sensitive to digitalis and that there is an increased incidence of digitalis intoxication in the setting of acute myocardial infarction. Because of its positive inotropic action, digitalis may increase myocardial oxygen demand and conceivably can result in expansion of the ischemic zone surrounding the myocardial infarction. However, when congestive failure is present, the reduction in ventricular size, wall tension, and tachycardia subsequent to digitalis therapy often results in a net reduction in myocardial oxygen requirement.

Digitalis may be potentially hazardous in a number of clinical situations and should be used with caution in elderly patients because of the following: (a) Digitalis may increase myocardial oxygen consumption in patients with acute myocardial infarction in the absence of cardiac enlargement or left ventricular failure. (b) It should be avoided when there are congestive symptoms in patients with mitral stenosis in regular sinus rhythm. (c) In hypertrophic cardiomyopathy, digitalis sometimes increases the left ventricular outflow obstruction by its positive inotropic action on the hypertrophic myocardium. (d) In some cases of atrial fibrillation secondary to the Wolfe-Parkinson-White syndrome, extremely rapid atrioventricular conduction may result from the decrease in refractory period secondary to digitalis therapy. (e) In the sick sinus syndrome patients may develop advanced digitalis-induced bradyarrhythmias.

One situation in which the indication for digitalis often is overlooked in the elderly is nocturnal angina. This clinical presentation is often due to occult, chronic left ventricular failure, and it responds better to digitalis and diuretics than to nitroglycerine. A decrease in left ventricular chamber size and wall tension results in reduced myocardial oxygen demand when digitalis is used in such patients. Paradoxically, ventricular ectopic activity, often considered to be a toxic manifestation of digitalis, may improve with the judicious use of digitalis. The addition of quinidine to the digitalized patient may mobilize tissue sources of digoxin and result in digitalis toxicity in the aged.

Vasodilators

More and more clinical studies have indicated a strikingly beneficial effect of vasodilators in myocardial infarction. In contrast to digitalis, drugs such as nitroprusside, hydralazine, and prazosin have no direct positive inotropic effects on the myocardium. Their principal hemodynamic action relates to a decrease in afterload by a reduction in peripheral vascular resistance and in some instances to a reduction in preload by an increase in venous capacitance. This effect results in normalization of the abnormally elevated left ventricular filling pressure and an increase in cardiac output. Other causes of acute heart failure (e.g. massive mitral or aortic insufficiency) are particularly responsive to vasodilator therapy by virtue of reduction in regurgitant volume and the enhancement of forward stroke output.

The medical management of chronic congestive failure consists of a reduction in the workload of the heart (rest, weight reduction, and control of hypertension), low salt diet, and the use of digitalis and diuretics. In cases of so-called refractory congestive heart failure that are resistant to all these therapeutic measures, vasodilators have come to the fore. They are useful not only in the acute clinical setting but also in the long-term management of clinical heart failure of varied causes. Cardiac output is reduced in many patients with chronic congestive heart failure, irrespective of etiology. In response to the reduction in cardiac output, there is an increase in peripheral vascular resistance which, when inappropriately elevated, causes a further reduction in cardiac output. Vasodilators interrupt this vicious cycle by reducing aortic impedance, permitting increased systolic ventricular emptying. The concomitant systemic venous dilation reduces ventricular preload, producing a salutary effect on both pulmonary congestion and myocardial oxygen demand.

Diuretics

Diuretics are the mainstay in the management of congestive heart failure. Modern diuretics are so potent in removing excess sodium and water that there is little need for a strict low sodium diet. In fact, vigorous diuretic therapy with a very low sodium intake without fluid restriction in the elderly may lead to serious hyponatremia secondary to the dilutional syndrome. This condition may be the result of failure of free water clearance by the congested kidney when the sodium load reaching the distal tubule is markedly reduced. This result is often overlooked in the zealous use of potassium supplements to prevent the more publicized hypokalemia, which may occur with the use of potent loop diuretics, e.g., furosemide. Potassium depletion results in potentiation of digitalis effect and may lead to digitalis toxicity in elderly patients; regular monitoring of electrolyte and digoxin levels are in order to detect this complication. Potassium supplements are best given in the chloride form to counteract the alkalosis often associated with hypokalemia.

As there is a modest increase in aldosterone levels in congestive heart failure, the use of aldosterone antagonists has an advantage over potassium supplements. In some patients the use of spironolactone or triamterene along with furosemide may be necessary, but here again electrolyte monitoring is necessary to prevent the occasional case of hyperkalemia which may occur with these diuretics, particularly in an elderly patient with borderline or actual renal insufficiency.

Overdiuresis of the aged cardiac patient exchanges the symptoms of peripheral or pulmonary edema for the syndrome of fatigue, low cardiac output, azotemia, and potentially dangerous electrolyte disturbances. At times the mechanical removal of pleural or peritoneal fluid avoids the problem of a rising level of blood urea nitrogen which accompanies the overenthusiastic use of potent diuretics in the elderly cardiac.

A school of thought has developed advocating that one should consider the use of hydralazine instead of digitalis in cases of congestive heart failure not satisfactorily controlled by diuretics alone. This may be especially true in the presence of regular sinus rhythm. Particularly in the elderly, the risk of the chronic use of digitalis for heart failure may outweigh its benefits because of the narrow therapeutic range of digitalis with consequent danger of toxicity. The effective dose of hydralazine, however, is difficult to predict in a given patient, and the incidence of side effects is high.

HYPOTENSION

Acute heart failure may present in the aged patient together with severe hypotension. In this clinical setting catecholamines were once widely used but were of little value in the elderly patient with cardiogenic shock. The use of dopamine, and more recently dobutamine—which has potent positive inotropic activity without the peripheral vascular, chronotropic, and arrhythmogenic effects of norepinephrine and isoproterenol—is of significant value in patients with heart failure and cardiogenic shock. Where previously the aged patient in cardiogenic shock had a miniscule chance of surviving, a substantial number of elderly patients have shown significant improvement with the use of dopamine and dobutamine.

The effectiveness of vasodilators in the management of low-output cardiac failure is due to their ability to reduce myocardial oxygen demand and simultaneously increase cardiac output and reduce pulmonary congestion. However, their usefulness in severe refractory congestive heart failure may be limited by concomitant hypotension. In such patients, a combination of a potent inotrope (dobutamine) and a vasodilator (nitroprusside) may result in better ventricular performance than either agent alone.

ACUTE PULMONARY EDEMA

Acute pulmonary edema is a common manifestation of heart failure in the aged. Although this condition is ascribed to acute left ventricular failure, the two ventricles should be considered as a delicate pair of scales which suddenly become unbalanced. By an incredibly refined mechanism, the two ventricles normally eject the same quantity of blood despite being separated by two widely different vascular systems, each of which is under complex neural and humoral control. At a heart rate of 100 beats per minute, if the ischemic left ventricle pumps only 1 ml of blood less per stroke than the right ventricle, within 2 to 3 min 400 to 600 ml of blood can accumulate in the lungs. When fluid flows outward from pulmonary capillaries into the lung, the interstitium increases to the same extent and the pulmonary lymphatics, which normally keep the lungs dry, are overwhelmed; massive pulmonary edema can then ensue. The pulmonary edema threshold is markedly reduced in elderly patients (a) who have low serum protein from chronic disease and therefore low colloid osmotic pressure, (b) who have been overloaded with volumes of crystalloid solutions, or (c) whose pulmonary capillary membranes are rendered more permeable by anoxia or sepsis.

The clinician faced with the therapeutic problem of acute pulmonary edema must restore the balance of the two ventricles (by improving left ventricular contractility perhaps with oxygen and digitalis) and by reducing the preload and afterload on the left ventricle (with the use of morphine, diuretics, and perhaps vasodilators).

HYPERTENSION

In the Framingham study the risk of developing heart failure was six times greater for hypertensive than normotensive patients. Emphasis has shifted to a consideration of ventricular afterload as a dominant factor in determining ventricular performance largely as a result of the fact that vasodilators alone can dramatically improve the symptoms of acute hypertensive heart failure. Blood pressure is the most easily measured component of afterload, but arterial compliance, peripheral resistance, stroke output, blood viscosity, and inertia are all involved in the determination of afterload.

The elderly hypertensive patient in heart failure presents several unique therapeutic problems. First, isolated systolic hypertension may well represent a completely different etiological and hemodynamic clinical situation, more closely related to a rigid aortic compression system than to an increase in peripheral resistance. Vigorous attempts at reducing systolic hypertension may only lead to vertigo or syncope due to orthostatic cerebrovascular insufficiency in the aged. Overdiuresis may stimulate the renin-angiotensin system, leading to an increase in outflow resistance and a lowered cardiac output. This may pose a serious problem for the patient in acute congestive failure whose cardiac output is critically low, leading to further diminution in intravascular volume. Sympathetic blockers (e.g., propranolol) may depress ventricular performance in the aged and exaggerate or precipitate congestive heart failure. Vasodilators at times induce a reflex tachycardia in the elderly hypertensive that limits their hypotensive effectiveness. No prospective double-blind trial has been carried out to assess the value of treatment in patients with isolated systolic hypertension. The increased mortality rate of elderly patients with systolic hypertension may be related more to the aortic disease it represents than to the systolic hypertension that merely reflects this loss of arterial compliance. Patients with deranged aortas die more quickly regardless of whether they have hypertension.

CONCLUSION

The ideal drug for augmenting the performance of the heart in congestive heart failure, acute or chronic, would have inotropic, vasodilator, and antiarrhythmic properties. It should have a low incidence of toxicity in therapeutic dosage (unlike digitalis) and be available in both parenteral and oral forms. Newer classes of drugs (e.g., captopril, amrinone, and the slow-channel calcium blockers) are currently being studied and give great promise in this direction.

Finally, the picture of cardiac surgery in the elderly patient with congestive heart failure appears to be brightening. The worst prognostic indicator in severe valve disease (e.g., aortic stenosis) is congestive heart failure. With the use of hypothermic cardioplegia, aged patients are surviving valve replacement and/or coronary bypass in larger numbers, even when their ventricular function is reduced to the point where they would previously have been rejected for surgery because of prohibitive mortality rates. Encouraging long-term survival, particularly in patients of advanced age with aortic stenosis, is now generally reported despite severe ventricular dysfunction. Significant aortic stenosis may be masked in elderly patients with depressed cardiac output when mean aortic valve gradients are less than 40 mm Hg. Every effort should be made to determine the actual orifice area in such patients before rejecting surgery as a viable alternative to severe and relentless heart failure.

When caring for elderly patients, the physician should:

1. Know about noninvasive diagnostic techniques that can be used at the bedside to clarify the situation.
2. Know how acute myocardial infarction can be managed so as to minimize the likelihood of congestive heart failure supervening, including the place of vasodilator drugs.
3. Know of the relationship between nocturnal angina and occult chronic left ventricular failure, and have some knowledge of appropriate management.
4. Know how the important role of diuretics in management of congestive heart failure in elderly patients can be safeguarded by appropriate attention to electrolyte and water balance.
5. Know the pathogenesis and management of acute pulmonary edema as a manifestation of congestive heart failure in elderly persons.
6. Know the importance of identifying surgically correctable lesions.

SUGGESTED READING

Amikam, S., Lemer, J. N., et al. Long-term survival of elderly patients after pacemaker implantation. *Am. Heart J.*, 9:445, 1976.

Burch, G. E. The special problems of heart disease in old people. *Geriatrics*, February:51, 1977.

Hollander, W. Role of hypertension in atherosclerosis and cardiovascular disease. *Am. J. Cardiol.*, 38:786, 1976.

Kannel, W. B. Implications of the recent decline in cardiovascular mortality. *Cardiovasc. Med.*, September, 1979.

Lloyd, B. L., and Smith, T. W. Contrasting rates of reversal of digoxin toxicity by digoxin specific IgG and Fab fragments. *Circulation*, 58:280, 1978.

Pomerance, A. Pathology of the heart with and without cardiac failure in the aged. *Br. Heart J.*, 27:697, 1965.

Quinlan, R., Cohn, L. H., and Collins, J. J., Jr. Determinants of survival following cardiac operations in elderly patients. *Chest*, 68:498, 1975.

Simon, A. B., and Zloto, A. E. Atrioventricular block: natural history after permanent ventricular pacing. *Am. J. Cardiol.*, 41:500, 1978.

Stephenson, L. W., MacVaugh, H., and Edmunds, L. H. Surgery using cardiopulmonary by-pass in the elderly. *Circulation*, 58:250, 1978.

Fundamentals of Geriatric Medicine, edited by
Ronald D. T. Cape, Rodney M. Coe, and Isadore
Rossman, Raven Press, New York © 1983.

23

General Approaches to Psychiatric Treatment of the Elderly

Alvin J. Levenson

The incidence and prevalence of late-life psychopathology exceed that in any other age range. Despite this, there is a significant quantitative and qualitative deficiency in mental health care delivery to the elderly. Quantitatively, 80 to 93% of the 2.5 to 5.5 million mentally ill aged in the United States are not having their needs met by existing resources. Qualitatively, a therapeutic nihilism underscores their treatment. The proponents of such nihilism espouse the view that because old age is "irreversible" late-life illnesses are likewise beyond significant assistance. As a consequence, psychopharmacological "control" and palliative measures often form the mainstay of treatment, with inadequate efforts directed to producing remissions in reversible states and to optimal rehabilitation. In fact, in skilled and caring hands, what is reversible in younger adult populations is likewise reversible in the aged. Suboptimal technique practiced in younger populations will generally find its way to the elderly, but with greater consequences.

As with younger adults, the treatment goal of late-life psychopathology should be optimal rehabilitation, defined as the removal of obstacles to the reattainment or reapproximation of the patient's premorbid baseline via optimal technique. Optimal geriatric mental health technique is defined as the application of mental health technique that is optimal for the general adult patient modified by age-related factors. The treatment modalities useful for younger age ranges are similarly useful for the geriatric patient. Further, the indications and contraindications for each do not differ.

It is not within the scope of this chapter to present a comprehensive view of geropsychiatric treatment, so an overview of various modalities and late-life modifications are offered. Psychiatric therapies can be divided broadly into organic and nonorganic types. Regardless, the goal of treatment is remission with a minimum amount of associated adverse reactions. The organic treatments involve primarily psychopharmacotherapy and electroconvulsive therapy (ECT).

PSYCHOPHARMACOTHERAPY

Four drug groups are available for the treatment of psychopathology: major tranquilizers, minor tranquilizers, antidepressants, and mood/affect stabilizing agents. The more commonly prescribed members of each group are listed in Table 1.

TABLE 1. *Commonly prescribed psychotropic agents*

Drug	Relative equipotency
MAJOR TRANQUILIZERS	
Phenothiazines	
Aliphatic subgroup	
Chlorpromazine (Thorazine®, CPZ)	1
Piperidine subgroup	
Thioridazine (Mellaril®)	1
Mesoridazine (Serentil®)	2/3
Piperazine subgroup	
Acetophenazine (Tindal®)	1/5
Prochlorperazine (Compazine®)	1/6
Perphenazine (Trilafon®)	1/10
Trifluoperazine (Stelazine®)	1/20
Fluphenazine (Prolixin®)	1/50
Thioxanthenes	
Thiothixene (Navane®)	1/25
Chlorprothixene (Taractan®)	1
Butyrophenone	
Haloperidol (Haldol®)	1/50
Dibenzoxazepine	
Loxapine succinate (Loxitane®)	1/10
Dihydroindolone	
Molindone (Moban®)	1/10
MINOR TRANQUILIZERS[a]	
Benzodiazepines	
Diazepam (Valium®)	
Oxazepam (Serax®)	
Lorazepam (Ativan®)	
Chlordiazepoxide (Librium®)	
Diphenylmethane antihistaminics[a]	
Hydroxyzine (Vistaril®)	
TRICYCLIC ANTIDEPRESSANTS[a]	
Amitriptyline (Elavil®)	
Noritriptyline (Aventyl®)	
Protriptyline (Vivactyl®)	
Imipramine (Tofranil®)	
Desmethylimipramine (Pertofrane®)	
Doxepin (Sinequan®)	
MOOD/AFFECTIVE ACTIVE AGENTS[a]	
Lithium carbonate	

[a]Refer to standard sources for dosage ranges. Relative equipotencies are not well established.

Principles of Use of Psychoactive Drugs

Clinical Aspects

The health care provider must have a working knowledge of the psychopharmacologically responsive psychiatric syndromes, as well as a structured means of assessing the patient with respect to them. Furthermore, he or she must be able to differentiate between functional and nonfunctional states. As mentioned previously, the initial clinical approach when nonfunctional psychopathology is suspected is to evaluate thoroughly for an organic etiology and then to reverse the illness where possible. There is a tendency to assume that late-life psychopathology is irreversibly organic and to perform little more than palliative procedures. Although irreversible organic states are more frequent in old than young populations, much of the irreversibility may be ascribed to failure to treat what was once reversible or to mistakes in assessment. A functional state in elderly adults is the same as in the young. Where an organic state is suspected, it is unwise to prescribe psychotropic medications. They may not only worsen an abnormality (e.g., by lowering the seizure threshold where an epileptic focus may be present or by aggravating a cardiac conduction defect-induced cerebral hypoperfusion state) but may also cloud an existing clinical picture. Once an organic etiology is ruled out or cannot be delineated, psychotropic medications may be prescribed for specific indications and in the absence of contraindications.

The prepsychopharmacological physiological evaluation must include the history (including H.P.I., MROSS, patient's medical history, family history), physical examination, and appropriate laboratory data. This information forms the basis for developing relative and absolute contraindications to the prescription of a particular class of psychotropic agents. Although psychopharmacological agents may be extremely efficacious for a psychiatric state, they are not innocuous. Therefore appropriate clearances must be obtained prior to their prescription and appropriate intraprescription monitoring implemented during the course of treatment.

Drug Effects

The clinician must be aware of psychoactive and physiological differences in the various groups of psychotropic drugs, the principal one being therapeutic efficacy. Attempts to prove intraclass differences in clinical effectiveness have been fruitless. All of the more commonly prescribed intraclass components have been found equally efficacious, irrespective of age. Selection of a component agent therefore must be based on other considerations, e.g., physician prescribing experience, previous patient response (both desired and undesired), and the physiological propensities of the intraclass component member. Previously existing physiological dysfunction, so common in the elderly, predisposes them to untoward, drug-related reactions (Chapter 20). Consequently, differences in pharmacological effect of the various component agents are of paramount importance when selecting a psychotropic agent for the geriatric patient. In general, these effects are of two major types: pharmacodynamic and idiosyncratic. Pharmacodynamic effects involve the action of the pharmacoactive agent at receptor sites. The most common nontarget receptor sites are cholinergic (acetylcholine) and adrenergic (dopamine and norepinephrine), and the most common action at the receptor site is blockade. Actions at these sites yield the anticholinergic, soporific, and adrenolytic effects noted commonly with major tranquilizers and tricyclic antidepressants and the antidopaminergic effects peculiar to major tranquilizers alone, albeit with intra- and interclass varying potentials. For example, with respect to interclass differences, tricyclic antidepressants as a class have more anticholinergic potential than major tranquilizers. Within the major tranquilizers class (intraclass), antidopaminergic potential varies from one agent to another. The butyrophenone haloperidol (Haldol®) possesses the highest antidopaminergic potential of any major tranquilizer, and the phenothiazine thioridazine (Mellaril®) possesses the lowest. All other major tranquilizers can be arranged in varying order or potential between these extremes. Anticholinergic effect tends to be in inverse relation to antidopaminergic potential; hence the most anticholinergic major tranquilizer is thioridazine, and the least is haloperidol. Soporific potential tends to be proportional to anticholinergic potential within major tranquilizers and tricyclic antidepressants alike.

Idiosyncratic properties represent effects peculiar to certain agents which cannot be attributed directly to pharmacodynamics as described above. These are seen usually with major tranquilizers and include such effects as seizure-lowering potential (more common with chlorpromazine), pancytopenic effects (more common with fluphenazine), and the production of a retinitis pigmentosa-like syndrome (seen only with thioridazine in doses above 800 mg per day).

Pharmacokinetics and Pharmocodynamics

Pharmacokinetics includes such factors as the effects of smoking, antacids, and route of administration on rate of absorption and peak blood level attainment, as well as factors affecting rates of catabolism and blood levels of free, active agents. Pharmacodynamics involves protein binding, skeletal muscle mass, and rate of elimination (discussed in Chapter 20). Another factor, however, is the effect of concomitant medication administration on blood levels (drug-drug interactions). This is a key issue in the elderly because of widespread polypharmacy. The combination of major tranquilizers and tricyclic antidepressants is of greatest concern because of widespread use and the fact that the former increases the plasma concentration of the latter by a factor of approximately three. This requires a two-thirds reduction in tricyclic antidepressant dosage when administered with major tranquilizers to avoid dose-related side effects, in addition to any adjustments for age.

Psychiatric Aspects

The clinician must possess a working knowledge of the biogenesis of psychiatric states with presumed biochemical etiologies (e.g., schizophrenia, delusions, hallucinations, retarded depression, hypomania/mania). In addition, he or she must appreciate the postulated loci and mechanisms of action of the various psychotropic drug groups, especially as they relate to biological etiology. For example, it is important to understand that tricyclic antidepressants elevate central nervous system (CNS) levels of biogenic amines, notably norepinephrine, dopamine, and 5-hydroxytryptamine (serotonin). CNS levels of biogenic amines are postulated to be elevated in schizophrenia (dopamine, norepinephrine, and serotonin). Consequently, administration of a tricyclic antidepressant medication to a patient with one of the above catecholamine-elevated psychiatric states will risk a worsening of that state. However, if the schizophrenia, mania, and/or delusion(s) were first treated to remission with major tranquilizers (the psychotropic drug class of choice for these states) and the patient continued on the agent, tricyclics could then be added in the appropriate dosage, assuming there is an indication and that no contraindications exist.

Drug Regimens

The clinician must coalesce the foregoing concepts and data into a pragmatic format, i.e., principles of use which may then be applied to *any* psychotropic drug class. Components of this format include the indications (Table 2), relative and absolute contraindications, and selection of a component agent (discussed previously). In addition, the format should contain the design of a dosage regimen, as well as the factors affecting dosage and the dosage regimen (e.g., age, stature, relative bioequivalence, and disease state). A dosage regimen is a structured, physiologically and age-appropriate plan designed to attain and maintain remission with the lowest incidence of side effects possible. It includes starting dosage; incremental increase in dosage en route to remission; plateau dosage (lowest dosage required to produce remission); incremental decrease dosage en route to the maintenance

TABLE 2. *Functional and irreversible nonfunctional psychiatric indications for psychotropic drug groups*

Group	Indications
Major tranquilizers	Any syndrome which includes incipient or manifest schizophrenia, incipient or manifest delusions, or hallucinations
	Severe anxiety (agitation) or severe anxious depression (agitated depression)
	Agitation of acute mania while awaiting the therapeutic effects of lithium carbonate
	Lability of affect
	Stereotypy
	Pathological resistance
Minor tranquilizers	Mild to moderate anxiety or mild to moderate anxious depression
Tricyclic antidepressants	Retarded depression without incipient or manifest schizophrenia, incipient or manifest delusions, or hallucinations
Lithium carbonate	Acute mania or hypomania without incipient or manifest schizophrenia, incipient or manifest delusions, or hallucinations

dosage level[1]; and the maintenance dosage itself (lowest dosage required to maintain remission). The factors affecting dosage and the dosage regimen are of great importance in treating the geriatric patient. Individuals over approximately 50 years of age and of frail stature should receive one-fourth to one-third the usual starting and incremental increase dosages.

The issue of relative equipotencies pertains primarily to the major tranquilizers and has two components. The first concerns intramuscular versus oral administration. At the same dosage, intramuscularly administered major tranquilizers are approximately three times more potent than those given per os; e.g., chlorpromazine 25 mg i.m. is equipotent to 75 mg p.o. The second component concerns the relative equipotency differences among major tranquilizers (Table 1). Relative equipotencies have not been devised well for the other classes of psychotropic agents, and so the clinician must depend on recommended standard and acceptable dosage ranges for these drugs. Psychiatric states affect starting and incremental increase dosages as well as the length of time the patient is kept at the plateau and maintenance dosages. For more detailed information, the reader is referred to standard comprehensive texts.

Adverse Reactions

It is important to know side effects and those agents which are more commonly associated with untoward reactions. Side effects are a major problem among the aged. For various reasons cited earlier, the incidence of medication-related illness is considerably higher in the elderly than younger populations. Most unnecessary side effects in the geriatric age group are caused by failure to adjust dosage to the age of the patient. Standard adult dosages increase the concentration of free, active agents available to act on target and other receptor sites, thereby increasing the risk of physiological dysfunction.

Cogniactive Agents

Although not usually included under psychotropic agents, the cogniactive agents have come into wide use and deserve some comment. These can be grouped into at least three subclasses: cerebral vasodilators (e.g., papaverine, cyclandelate), neuronal metabolic stimulators (e.g., ergot alkaloids, methylphenidate, anabolic steroids), and replacement compounds (e.g., lecithin, deanol). It should be clear that the primary indication for these agents is for the pure cognitive intellectual and memory deficits of the irreversible organic brain syndromes (primary and secondary neuronal degenerative states). While the extent of their efficacy is not completely clear, agents such as Hydergine are widely used in many areas of the world.

---

[1]Unless there is significant cause, major and minor tranquilizers and tricyclic antidepressants should not be abruptly withdrawn. A withdrawal reaction may result, including seizures (minor tranquilizers).

When evaluating their inadequate effects, one must consider several facts. In regard to the primary and secondary states, dead neurons cannot be revived. With specific respect to the secondary (vascular) state, the cerebral arterial vasculature is already maximally dilated under hypoxic conditions. Further, agents alleged to be cerebral vasodilators are in fact peripheral vasodilators and may even shunt blood away from an infarcted area. Unquestionably, the clinician must await further information on clinical trials of these agents and on the etiologies of irreversible organic brain syndrome.

ELECTROCONVULSIVE THERAPY

The indications and contraindications for the use of electroconvulsive therapy (ECT) in the elderly are believed to be the same as for younger adults. The major indication is the retarded depression (depressed mood, affect, and/or thought content in the presence of psychomotor retardation); additional ones including acute undifferentiated schizophrenia and acute catatonic stuporous schizophrenia. Consensus holds that a trial of psychotropic medications should precede ECT where possible. The major absolute contraindications to ECT are the presence of a space-occupying mass and status after myocardial infarction. The key relative contraindications include serum electrolyte imbalance (particularly Na^+/K^+) and a significantly fragile or diseased skeletal structure.

It is most important to take great precautions when administering ECT to the aged patient. First, cardiorespiratory instability may necessitate the use of lower doses of anesthetic, succinylcholine, and atropine. Second, a more comprehensive pre-ECT evaluation is required. In addition to the history and physical examination, this must include a complete blood count with differential, BUN, creatinine, electrolytes, uric acid, chest x-ray, electrocardiogram, electroencephalogram, computed tomography scan of the head, skull series, as well as radiographs of the cervical, thoracic, and lumbosacral spine. Additional laboratory determinations should be ordered as indicated. Prior to ECT, patients must have had nothing by mouth for at least the preceding 12 hr, have voided prior to the treatment, and been carefully checked to be certain there are no loose objects in their mouths, including dentures.

The nonorganic therapies include psychotherapy and other intervention designed to reattain or reapproximate the patient's premorbid baseline.

PSYCHOTHERAPY

There are two main types of psychotherapy: investigative and supportive. Investigative psychotherapy seeks to penetrate protective psychological defenses en route to an unconscious conflict, to elevate the unconscious conflict to conscious attention, and to then work through the conflict at the conscious level in an attempt to resolve it. Its only true application is for the neuroses. Neuroses are syndromes manifested by signs and symptoms of inappropriately deployed mechanisms which protect the individual from the anxiety evoked by conscious recognition of the conflict and/or an unpleasant thought or memory. Neuroses are rare during late life, although they do occur. Presumably then, investigative psychotherapy could be employed. However, several factors mitigate against its use in most elderly. It is long term (years), requires frequent visits, is expensive, is anxiety-provoking, and strips protective defenses, leaving the individual with few emotional alternatives.

Supportive psychotherapy seeks to support and strengthen (rather than penetrate) existing defenses which are adaptive (promote coping and psychological comfort) and to make more adaptive or delete those which do not serve the individual well. It is used for all psychiatric diagnostic entities either alone or in combination with other forms of treatment, e.g., pharmacotherapy. This is the most commonly utilized form of psychotherapy in the elderly, as it is frequently time-limited, requires infrequent visitation, is supportive, and in skilled hands is rarely anxiety-provoking. Although investigative and supportive psychotherapy are usually applied in the individual therapy session, they can be employed in a couple, family, or group format.

Psychiatric Referrals

Often nonpsychiatrist clinicians choose not to treat psychiatric illness. As a result, the major initial service they can and should render is psychiatric referral. Failure to arrange for such services may be partly responsible for the significant number of elderly patients with untreated psychiatric illness.

One obstacle to referral is the absence of a structured and rapidly administered clinical approach for rendering such decisions. The Rapid Psychiatric Assessment (RPA) permits such an approach. It can be administered in approximately 5 to 30 min, depending on the patient and clinician's practice with the instrument. The reader is referred to its listing in the "Suggested Reading" at the conclusion of this chapter.

SUMMARY

The elderly patient can and does suffer psychiatric illnesses. This chapter suggests appropriate goals for the treatment of these individuals. The major indications and contraindications for drug therapy, ECT, and psychotherapy are outlined. Psychiatric referral is urged if the clinician does not want to treat a patient with psychiatric problems.

When caring for elderly patients, the physician should:

1. Know the extent to which health care delivery systems in the United States fail to meet the needs of elderly patients with psychiatric illnesses.
2. Know the major goals and priorities in rendering psychiatric care to the elderly patient.
3. Know the principal modalities of psychiatric treatment for elderly persons.
4. Know some of the most important principles to be followed in use of psychopharmacological agents in elderly patients.

SUGGESTED READING

Busse, E. W., and Blazer, D., editors. *Handbook of Geropsychiatry.* Van Nostrand Reinhold, New York, 1980.

Butler, R. N. *Why Survive? Being Old in America.* Harper & Row, New York, 1975.

Dewald, P. A. *Psychotherapy: A Dynamic Approach.* Basic Books, New York, 1964.

Freedman, A. M., Kaplan, H. I., and Sadock, B. J. *Modern Synopsis of Comprehensive Textbook of Psychiatry.* Williams & Wilkins, Baltimore, 1972.

Hollister, L. E. *Clinical Use of Psychotherapeutic Drugs.* Charles C Thomas, Springfield, IL, 1973.

Klein, D. F., and Davis, J. M. *Diagnosis and Drug Treatment of Psychiatric Disorders.* Williams & Wilkins, Baltimore, 1969.

Levenson, A. J. *Basic Psychopharmacology for Health Professionals.* Springer, New York, 1980.

Levenson, A. J., and Tollett, S. M. Rapid psychiatric assessment of the geriatric patient for immediate psychiatric referral. *Geriatrics,* 35:113–120, 1980.

Verwoerdt, A. *Clinical Geropsychiatry.* Williams & Wilkins, Baltimore, 1976.

Fundamentals of Geriatric Medicine, edited by
Ronald D. T. Cape, Rodney M. Coe, and Isadore
Rossman, Raven Press, New York © 1983.

24

Sleep Disorders in the Aged

Charles W. Pollak

About 30% of women and 14 to 16% of men aged 60 years or more complained of insomnia in a survey of more than one million people by the American Cancer Society. Sleep disturbances, though common in the older population, have unfortunately not been well understood. Too often treatment has consisted of the prescription of a sleeping pill.

Our knowledge concerning sleep disorders has expanded dramatically over the past several years. Clinical and laboratory assessments in the newly organized Sleep Disorders Centers have made it possible to detect underlying diseases, including certain ones that may be completely occult in the elderly. Treatment plans are now often more complex than a prescription but more likely to be effective and safe. As greater knowledge and resources become available to physicians, it can be predicted that the expectations of the public will also rise. The elderly, disproportionately affected by sleep disturbances, especially require effective detection and treatment of the disorders discussed in this chapter.

SLEEP AS AN AGE-RELATED PROCESS

Most persons view normal sleep as a simple state of inactivity and mental oblivion. In reality, sleep is a complex process consisting of several distinct states—rapid eye movement (REM) sleep and several forms of non-REM sleep—which are temporally organized into cycles of approximately 90 min. duration. These cycles, in turn, are modulated by a circadian (approximately 24 hr) cycle of sleep and waking.

The sleep-wake process is continually modified during the course of normal development and senescence. The newborn sleeps about 16 hr per day, half of this in REM sleep. As maturation of the central nervous system proceeds, a circadian pattern of sleep and wakefulness develops. Non-REM sleep stages become associated with high-amplitude, slow electroencephalographic (EEG) activity, and both total sleep time and REM sleep decrease in duration. The familiar "8 hr" of sleep is achieved during the early teen years, at a time when daytime alertness is sustained at a high level. Later in life, a slow decrease of total sleep time to approximately 6 hr appears to take place.

The physician should recognize, however, that figures for total sleep time are often unreliable. Subjective estimates of sleep, always problematical, are especially so in the elderly. Even polygraphic sleep recordings fail to provide accurate data if only the nighttime portion of the 24-hr day is included. The recorded amount of sleep may be incomplete if daytime naps are not recorded, or misleading if a reasonable level of daytime alertness cannot be maintained. Sleep in the elderly is often fragmented by awakenings and is less stable because of frequent sleep stage changes. There is some evidence that the waking period is also fragmented by periods of drowsiness or sleep. Thus the overall circadian sleep-wake cycle loses some of its strength (amplitude).

Other effects associated with aging include decreased amplitude of the large, slow, delta-shaped EEG waves that are characteristic of non-REM sleep stages 3 and 4. As a result, these "deep" sleep stages may become completely undetectable. There may also be attenuation of the rhythmic EEG configurations called spindles that are normally associated with non-REM sleep stages 2 and 3. It is possible that the fragmentation and instability of sleep in the elderly is correlated with the reduction of such normal EEG phenomena. It also seems possible that sleep that has lost its former EEG features is more susceptible to interruption by external or internal signals (noise, pain), but this has not been investigated in the elderly.

THE INSOMNIAS

The recognized causes of insomnia and other categories of sleep disorders have recently been listed and described (1). In this chapter, we are primarily concerned with the way to approach the older patient with a sleep disorder. Rather than mention every possible sleep disorder, I describe only the most significant ones.

History

The first step in the successful evaluation of the insomnia patient is a complete medical history, complete physical examination, basic laboratory examinations, and, if indicated, psychiatric evaluation. It is essential to extract a clear, concise, chief *complaint*. The complaint may be difficulty initiating sleep (DIS), difficulty maintaining sleep (DMS), or both (DIMS).

DMS may refer to unwanted awakenings during the night, premature awakening in the morning, or poor "quality" of sleep. Some patients have no such complaint; instead, they feel tired during the daytime and infer that sleep must be insufficient or abnormal in some way. This is not necessarily true, however, as daytime symptoms may originate from illnesses or psychogenic mechanisms. Similarly, patients who have become dependent on sleeping pills may experience little or no difficulty sleeping so long as they take their pills but complain of severe insomnia whenever they attempt to discontinue the drugs. The patient's inference that an underlying, chronic insomnia has been suppressed by the sleeping pills may be unwarranted, as chronic use of hypnotics usually leads to drug tolerance and withdrawal symptoms that include insomnia.

The onset of the sleep disturbance may be vague, but often there is a clear precipitating event, as in the following case:

> A 66-year-old woman with insomnia was able to recall the exact date of its onset 40 years earlier. She had been married and was pregnant by her husband when another married man began to "pursue" her. Being rich, influential, and persistent in his efforts, she eventually agreed to marry him. After obtaining a divorce and undergoing an abortion, she arrived in a foreign city where she was to marry her lover. He failed to appear that day, however, and she was unable to sleep all night. The next day, he again failed to appear. It soon became obvious that she had been abandoned. She rapidly turned to sleeping pills, "to put me out", and has never again been able to sleep unless she took large doses of hypnotics or alcohol.

We next wish to know the *course* and *previous treatment* of the sleep difficulty. In the patient just described, the hypnotic drugs and alcohol were utilized continuously for all the years since the original trauma. Actual difficulty sleeping was experienced only occasionally, when she tried to reduce dosages. The initiating insomnia had clearly been severe and psychogenic in nature, but the current problem seemed to be related mostly to the "treatment" itself—the use of hypnotics and alcohol. This was borne out when these substances were gradually withdrawn, without any adverse effects on sleep.

It is useful to obtain from the patient a detailed *description of a typical 24-hr day*. The description should start at bedtime: At what time, and how regular and what preparations, including drugs or alcohol, precede going to bed? How long after lights out does it generally take to fall asleep? Once sleep has been initiated, is it experienced as a solid period or as a broken, interrupted one? Is medication taken if an awakening occurs during the night? At what time does the patient awaken? Is the awakening spontaneous or induced by an alarm? What are the patient's work hours (if any) and daytime activities? The dynamics of the patient's sleep-wake behavior are best portrayed by means of a graphical log. The log used at the Sleep-Wake Disorders Center of Montefiore Hospital is shown in Fig. 1. By making entries each morning, the patient builds up a 2-week profile of the daily interval spent in bed, the interval spent sleeping, and the relationship of these intervals to each other. Numerical data (e.g., sleep latency and total sleep time as well as their 2-week means) are also collected. Keeping this log requires no more than a few minutes of the patient's time each morning. It is useful both for diagnosis and to assess the response to treatment efforts.

Treatment

In most cases, the sleep pattern is at least moderately irregular, and one of the first steps in treatment should be to impose a regular schedule: a regular bedtime, a regular time for arising (by alarm), and no opportunity for sleep at other times. The amount of time to be assigned to the patient for sleep should be estimated from the average of the 14 nightly sleep times recorded in the log. This average, which

SLEEP–WAKE DISORDERS CENTER
Montefiore Hospital and Medical Center

YOUR NAME

Please Complete Both Sides

EACH MORNING DO THE FOLLOWING:

1. Write in today's day and date.
2. With an arrow pointing down, mark the time that you STARTED TO TRY to go to sleep last night.
3. With a plain line, mark the time you THINK YOU FELL asleep last night.
4. With plain lines, mark whenever you woke up and fell back asleep during the night.
5. With another plain line, mark the time you woke up this morning.
6. With an arrow pointing up, mark the time you got out of bed this morning.
7. If you took any naps, mark them the same way.
8. Answer all 8 questions.

E X A M P L E S

DAY	DATE	MID-NIGHT	1 AM	2 AM	3 AM	4 AM	5 AM	6 AM	7 AM	8 AM	9 AM	10 AM	11 AM	12 AM	1 PM	2 PM	3 PM	4 PM	5 PM	6 PM	7 PM	8 PM	9 PM	10 PM	11 PM	MID-NIGHT
MON.	5/7/79				SLEEP									NAP												
TUES.	5/8/79			SLEEP		SLEEP								NAP												

Questions (answered each morning):

1. How long did it take you to fall asleep last night? (Mark minutes or hours.)
2. Did you take any sleeping pills or alcohol at bedtime? (Mark "yes," or "no.")
3. How many times did you wake up? (0, 1, 2, etc.)
4. How much sleep did you get last night? (Mark minutes or hours.)
5. By what time did you HAVE to be up this morning? (If none, leave blank.)
6. How did you awaken? (Mark "M." for "myself," "A" for "alarm," or "D" for "disturbed.")
7. How did you feel immediately after getting up? (Mark number from the scale on back.)
8. Were you awake and alert all day yesterday? (Mark "yes," or "no.")

	M	Tu	W
1	2 hrs.	45 M	
2	Yes	Yes	
3	1	0	
4	4½ hrs.	8½ hrs.	
5	8 AM	8 AM	
6	M	D	
7	3	2	
8	Yes	No	

is likely to be in the range of 5 to 7.5 hr, may surprise the patient, who believes she or he sleeps less. The patient may therefore resist efforts to limit the time in bed to that actually estimated as being utilized for sleep. We generally assign 0.5 to 1 hr more than the log average as the opportunity for sleep. We have found that the imposition of a rational, rigid sleep schedule early in treatment is of great value. Patients who succeed in adhering to the schedule often improve symptomatically. Some fail to follow the recommended schedule, however, and the reasons for that failure are almost certain to be relevant to understanding the origin of the patient's symptoms. For example, the most common deviation from a recommended schedule is spending more than the recommmended number of hours in bed; usually, the patient retires too early, reasoning that the likelihood of obtaining an adequate amount of sleep will thereby be increased. To the contrary, the amount of time required to fall asleep (sleep latency) is often increased by this strategy. The mechanism underlying "onset insomnia" may thereby be clarified.

Polysomnography, a diagnostic technique available only in sleep disorders centers, should be considered when the diagnosis remains unclear after the approach just outlined has been tried or if there is reason to suspect a sleep-related physiological abnormality. An example is sleep apnea (described later). Polysomnography is usually performed for two or more consecutive nights and may be used to obtain quantitative sleep data for comparison with the patient's subjective impressions, as reported in a questionnaire shortly after awakening in the laboratory the following morning.

Subjective Insomnia with Limited Findings

Sleep laboratory evaluation in the insomniac patient occasionally reveals that sleep is normal for age or less abnormal than the complaints suggest. The causes vary. Patients whose sleep subjectively improves in the laboratory may have been adversely conditioned to their usual sleep environment.

> A 71-year-old woman complained of inability to sleep without "sedation." She had been widowed for 3 years and now lived alone in the central city. Her children lived in other cities. She had no occupation but had long been active in clubs, charities, and cultural affairs. Although her circle of friends had contracted since her husband's death, she was able to socialize a few times a week, always making certain to return home before dark because of the risk of being mugged. As a result, she spent most of the day in her apartment, including 11 hr in bed reading, watching television, but mostly trying to sleep. She estimated that she slept an average of 6 hr per day and had no difficulty maintaining alert wakefulness when she was up.

We pointed out to her that her efforts to sleep more than 6 hr per day were likely to continue to fail, as the sleep she was obtaining appeared to be physiologically

FIG. 1. Two-week sleep log used by the Sleep-Wake Disorders Center, Montefiore Hospital and Medical Center. (Note: Forms may be obtained from Metrodesign Associates, 684 Allen Street, Syracuse, NY 13210.)

sufficient. She was advised to reduce the time in bed, especially the time spent in efforts to sleep. Such efforts are unpleasant and may contribute to insomnia by adversely conditioning the patient to associate the usual sleep conditions (dark, quiet, repose) with the inability to fall asleep. At first she rejected this advice because she could not see a way to use the additional waking hours that would become available. The implication—which she did not deny—was that she tried to use sleep to rid herself of empty time. In this case, therefore, we confronted a generic problem of the aged, disguised as a sleep disorder. What was lacking was a useful daytime occupation, not sleep. This case also brings out the subjective aspect of "insomnia": the physician must ascertain both how a patient sleeps and how he or she *expects* to sleep.

One should remember that the majority of insomniac patients do have demonstrable abnormalities of sleep but that the subjective sleep disturbance is often greater than the objective one. The reasons for this discrepancy are not known. It is sometimes useful to obtain polysomnograms as an objective basis for reassuring the patient. Patients who claim that they "never" sleep or sleep only a few minutes a night can almost always be shown to sleep for several hours in the laboratory. Such patients may also be assured that the lack of sleep will not "kill" them as they sometimes fear.

Use of Hypnotics

Hypnotic drugs eventually lose their effectiveness during chronic use: None has been shown to be effective for more than 1 month of nightly use. This means that long-term treatment of insomnia with barbiturates (e.g., Seconal®, Nembutal®, Tuinal®), benzodiazepines (e.g., Dalmane®), or other drugs (Placidyl®, Doriden®, Noctec®, alcohol) has no place at this time. One implication of tolerance is that such drugs may be withdrawn gradually without adversely affecting sleep. Rapid withdrawal, on the other hand, may precipitate severe insomnia, and withdrawals of barbiturates or alcohol may also cause an increase and intensification of REM sleep ("REM rebound") accompanied by unpleasant dreams. For this reason, patients' own efforts to stop the use of hypnotic drugs often fail. Indeed, patients may misinterpret the insomnia of drug withdrawal as the resurgence of the insomnia that originally led to the use of sleeping pills or alcohol. It therefore seems useless to the patient to persist in the effort to withdraw. New efforts will probably be made, however, and a pattern of recurrent insomnia due to partial, drug-alcohol withdrawal is established. Even in regular use, short-acting sedatives (e.g., barbiturates and alcohol) may lead to partial drug withdrawal symptoms such as REM sleep nightmares and unwanted awakenings during the latter part of the sleep period when the drugs taken at bedtime have been partially metabolized. Long-acting hypnotics such as flurazepam, on the other hand, are prone to accumulate to toxic levels in elderly patients with impaired drug-clearing mechanisms. Serious impairment of performance and judgment may result.

To summarize, the long-term use of hypnotics is ineffective because of tolerance and may itself cause sleep disturbances through intentional but incomplete or unintentional withdrawals. We therefore withdraw hypnotic drugs as an early step in the management of insomnia, along with the imposition of a regular sleep-wake schedule. Drug withdrawal is especially desirable in the elderly patient with irregular or impaired drug absorption and handling.

Once the patient has been convinced of its desirability and the likelihood of any adverse effects on sleep, hypnotic drug withdrawal can usually be accomplished on an outpatient basis without major problems, especially if the physician remains in frequent contact with the patient. Patients require constant reassurance about transient sleep disturbances and nightmares. Long-acting hypnotics may be acting mostly as tranquilizers, and the possibility of instituting regular daytime doses of a tranquilizer should be considered in appropriate patients. Standard withdrawal schedules for barbiturates and other hypnotics may be followed: We have found that a halving of the dose every 4 to 6 days and total elimination within 2 to 3 weeks is usually well tolerated. Patients should be forewarned, however, that some discomfort may be experienced. The most frequent symptoms in our experience are anxiety and difficulty falling asleep. As bedtime approaches, the patient becomes increasingly apprehensive about the likelihood of falling asleep. This anticipatory anxiety itself may delay sleep onset, thereby confirming the patient's expectations and setting up the conditions for a new round of insomnia the following night. This unfortunate situation can probably be attributed to the personality of the patient more often than anything else, although the possibilities that the drug(s) has been withdrawn too rapidly or that the patient is not being encouraged and reassured often enough by a physician must be considered. It should also be kept in mind that all "sleeping pills" are sedatives, often with tranquilizing properties that persist well into the waking period. Apprehensive patients may therefore do better if a tranquilizer is prescribed in small but regular doses (e.g., diazepam, 2 mg t.i.d.) until withdrawal has been completed. The question of continued use of the tranquilizer should then be decided in terms of the patient's overall emotional status. Withdrawal of REM suppressant hypnotics (e.g., barbiturates) may cause an increased amount and intensity of REM sleep (REM rebound), accompanied by vivid, disturbing dreams. The patient may be reassured that the effect is transitory. If anxiety, insomnia, or nightmares seem excessive, the dose of the hypnotic may be held at the same level for several nights before withdrawal is resumed.

Insomnia Associated with Depression

Elderly patients who complain of difficulty maintaining sleep, with or without difficulty falling asleep, should be carefully assessed for evidence of *depression*. Sleep complaints are common in patients with major depression, representing one of the more unpleasant of the "vegetative" features that include disturbances of appetite, weight, bowel habits, and libido. Classically, the depressed patient complains of "early morning awakenings," but close questioning and sleep logs reveal that sleep is repeatedly and increasingly interrupted as the night progresses. DIS is also common but usually less severe. Polygraphic recordings of sleep have demonstrated that the first REM sleep period of the night occurs abnormally early and the rapid eye movements are more abundant. These sleep pattern abnormalities are among the earliest events in the development of each depressive episode; their response to antidepressant drug therapy is predictive of the way in which the affective disturbance will respond to treatment. It may therefore be of value to perform a polysomnographic examination in some depressed insomniacs. It is worth reminding the reader that depressed affect is a common psychiatric symptom which does not imply that a patient will respond to antidepressant drugs. Psychiatric consultation is often worthwhile, as adequate antidepressant drug therapy in selected depressives may eliminate even severe degrees of insomnia along with the other symptoms of the illness.

Sleep Apnea

Breathing abnormalities are common during sleep, including the sleep of the elderly, and may account for the complaint of DMS. Most often, ventilation decreases in volume (hypopnea) or ceases (apnea) in a discrete, episodic fashion. Occasionally, ventilation and arterial oxygen saturation decrease during sleep to an abnormal but limited degree, without marked fluctuations ("sleep hypoventilation").

An apneic episode is initiated during sleep or during a transition into sleep, lasts about 30 (20 to 50) sec, and is terminated by arousal. Cycles of sleep onset apnea arousal may be repeated hundreds of times a night, resulting in a profound disruption of the sleep stage pattern. As a result, patients may complain of disabling daytime sleepiness while remaining totally unaware of the abnormal events during sleep from which it arose. Indeed, sleep apnea may be totally asymptomatic. In such cases the diagnosis of sleep apnea will be made only if the physician is alert to the possibility and arranges for polysomnography. Fortunately, patients or their spouses are often aware of untoward events during sleep. Sleep apneics may be aware of awakening frequently, for example, if the awakenings last a few minutes or longer and may then present themselves to a physician with the complaint of DMS. The spouse may observe stoppages of breathing or a variety of abnormal behaviors during sleep. Sleep apneics sometimes experience breathlessness just as they awaken from an apneic episode, resembling paroxysmal nocturnal dyspnea in patients with congestive heart failure.

One of the most common symptoms of sleep apnea is loud snoring. Snoring may be a serious annoyance in its own right, especially to spouses whose sleep is fragile, but its larger significance lies in the fact that snoring usually originates from partial obstruction of the pharynx during sleep. Indeed, apneic events during sleep usually include an obstructive phase that follows the initial cessation of breathing associated with sleep onset ("mixed" apnea). The upper airway obstruction is terminated by arousal, and patients occasionally experience a choking feeling as they wake up. This form of sleep apnea is strongly age-related: Peak prevalence is at around age 50. Apneas of both the obstructive and nonobstructive types are well known to occur in the elderly, perhaps especially those with chronic obstructive lung disease.

Sleep apneics are especially sensitive to the respiratory depressant effects of barbiturates, opiates, and general anesthetic agents. The possibility that such drugs pose special risks in elderly patients with decreased drug-handling mechanisms, and especially those with some degree of chronic lung disease, is currently being investigated. Meanwhile, sedative drugs should be withheld from elderly patients with symptoms suggestive of sleep apnea, especially at bedtime. It also seems prudent to emphasize frequent vital sign checks during sleep in hospitalized elderly patients, especially after surgery utilizing general anesthesia. Cardiovascular complications may also develop directly in severe cases; various arrhythmias, systemic and pulmonary hypertension, cor pulmonale, polycythemia, and occasional sudden death have all been reported.

Polysomnography is the only currently available method of accurately diagnosing and grading the severity of sleep apnea. Treatment varies with type and severity of sleep apnea and should be selected in consultation with a Sleep Disorders Center or someone experienced in the field. The possibilities include the use of low-flow oxygen during sleep, mechanical ventilation, diaphragmatic pacing, respiratory stimulants such as medroxyprogesterone, weight loss, permanent tracheostomy, or simply expectant watchfulness.

Other Causes of DIMS

Many other causes of DIMS in the elderly can be uncovered by a thorough history and physical examination. Painful arthritides, gastroesophageal reflux, nocturnal angina, or certain symptoms of congestive heart failure (paroxysmal nocturnal dyspnea, orthopnea, nocturia) may be apparent to the patient himself as the cause of insomnia. Parkinson's disease and other neurological disorders may be associated with absent sleep spindles and a refractory insomnia.

Elderly patients who report being awakened repeatedly by frightening or morbid dreams should be asked if they have ever been deeply traumatized, as in a prisoner of war or concentration camp; unfortunately, there is no satisfactory treatment in such cases of "REM interruption insomnia."

An occasional patient with DMS may report frequent, sometimes violent movements of the extremities during sleep. The spouse may have been kicked, and the patient may experience soreness of the legs in the morning. This condition has been termed "nocturnal myoclonus," but the movements are actually rather slow, nonmyoclonic flexions of one or both lower extremities. Polysomnography reveals the movements to be strokingly periodic, and we therefore prefer to call the condition *periodic movements in sleep* (PMS). The individual movements are sometimes associated with brief arousals, but PMS is usually an incidental, asymptomatic polysomnographic finding which we have recorded in patients with a wide variety of sleep disorders. The affected patients are somewhat older than other sleep disorders patients.

A disorder termed *restless legs syndrome* is closely related to PMS and is often associated with DIS. The patient experiences intense unease in the legs and an impulse to move them. When he does so by stretching, walking, or even jumping, the feeling can be dispelled but returns as soon as he makes a new attempt to fall asleep. During sleep, PMS can be demonstrated in practically all cases. An effective treatment has never been demonstrated for PMS or restless legs syndrome, although improvement has been reported with clonazepam.

Aging or some concurrent process is associated with alterations of the sleep pattern, including the fragmentation of sleep by multiple nocturnal awakenings. Such awakenings are not necessarily associated with alterations of daytime alertness, mood, or performance. Patients who are otherwise healthy and not thought to have other causes of DMS and who complain of unwanted awakenings should be reassured and enjoined from using hypnotics or extending the time spent in bed trying to sleep.

It has frequently been observed that some elderly people doze frequently during the day. Detailed studies of this phenomenon have not yet been made. In particular, it is not known to what degree the dozing may be facultative, i.e., the result of limitations of those physical, intellectual, and emotional activities that help wakefulness to be sustained and/or if age-related deterioration takes place in the central nervous mechanism for the maintenance of alert wakefulness. We have observed particularly severe impairment of wakefulness, along with DMS, in some patients with Parkinson's disease. It seems possible that the circadian sleep-wake cycle as a regulated physiological process breaks down with age or certain diseases.

Disorders of the Circadian Sleep-Wake Cycle

DIS is uncommon as an isolated symptom (i.e., not associated with DMS) in the elderly. The restless legs syndrome has already been mentioned as a possible cause of DIS. Another cause is a delay of the phase of the sleep-wake cycle. By "phase" we mean the clock time at which some event of the sleep-wake cycle (e.g., sleep onset or morning awakening) takes place. The phase of the sleep-wake cycle may become delayed for any of several reasons, including shiftwork (evening or night shift), jet lag (rapid travel westward), a bout of insomnia that includes DIS, or personal preference. Once the phase of sleep has been delayed, it may be difficult for the patient to restore it to the original time by retiring and arising early. As a result, the patient may lie awake for hours after retiring.

Sleeping pills and alcohol are usually ineffective. Ruminations often fill the hours before sleep onset and may give rise to psychological explanations of the insomnia. Characteristically, sleep is relatively normal if it is allowed to end spontaneously in the late morning or early afternoon. The successful management of this problem therefore depends on modifications of the way sleep is scheduled.

Patients who have not experienced repeated or prolonged bouts of DIS in the past and have recently become phase-shifted should respond if hypnotics are gradually withdrawn, a regular sleep-wake schedule is imposed, and the sleep phase is then advanced by a small amount each day, until the desired phase is reached.

Patients with a long history of DIS, by contrast, are likely to have an intrinsic limitation of the capacity for phase advancement (delayed sleep phase syndrome).

The phase of sleep in such patients can be advanced only indirectly, by *delaying* the sleep period in much the same way that some digital clocks can only be reset "forward." As a practical example, if the sleep period spans 4:00 a.m. to 10:00 a.m. and it is desired to advance the phase to 12:00 a.m. to 6:00 a.m., the schedule should be delayed 3 hr per day for seven consecutive days (day 1: 7:00 a.m. to 1:00 p.m.; day 2: 10:00 a.m. to 4:00 p.m.; day 3: 1:00 p.m. to 7:00 p.m.;....; day 7: 12:00 p.m. to 6:00 a.m.).

Elderly men and women who are physically inactive and understimulated by their environment often nap during the day. The nighttime sleep pattern may thereby be altered, leading to further daytime napping, and so on. The nocturnal wakefulness may cause disruption of the household or inconvenience to the nursing staff. Often hypnotic drugs are prescribed. By disturbing the sleep pattern or causing confusion or paradoxical excitement, however, drugs may add to the problem and perpetuate it. It may be an oversimplification to indict schedule irregularities alone, especially when an organic brain syndrome is present, but efforts should always be made to provide physical and mental stimulation during the day to help consolidate nighttime sleep.

SLEEPINESS IN THE ELDERLY

Sleepiness in the elderly patient has a wide variety of possible causes that include endocrine and metabolic disorders (hypoglycemia, hypothyroidism, apathetic hyperthyroidism, uremia, liver failure, hypercapnia), neurological disorders (raised intracranial pressure of any cause, hydrocephalus, heart trauma, diencephalic tumors, chronic meningitis) and others. The possibility of drug overdose or accumulation as well as drug interactions with alcohol or other drugs should be carefully investigated. Of patients who complain of *chronic* excessive daytime sleepiness (EDS), 80% are eventually diagnosed by our Sleep Disorders Center as having either *sleep apnea* or *narcolepsy*.

Sleep apnea and related hypoventilation syndromes have already been mentioned as causes of insomnia, but they are more often a cause of EDS. This complaint is especially prominent and disabling among middle-aged men who are often obese and hypertensive and are found by polysomnography to have predominantly mixed apneas (hypersomnia-sleep apnea syndrome; HSA). HSA is progressive and may lead to serious complications, including cardiac arrhythmias and progressive pulmonary hypertension. The most reliable and effective treatment is permanent tracheostomy. EDS may be fully cleared up by this means.

Narcolepsy is a neurological disorder that affects more than 100,000 men and women in the United States. EDS is the most obvious and disabling feature of the disorder, but a phenomenon termed cataplexy—sudden weakness precipitated by laughter, anger, or other emotions—is the most specific feature. This weakness is believed to be caused by the inappropriate triggering of an inhibitory mechanism that is normally active during REM sleep. This mechanism may also be triggered by the act of falling asleep or waking up (sleep paralysis). Another normal feature of REM sleep that occurs in an unusual context in narcolepsy is dreaming, which may appear as vivid hallucinations (usually visual) as the narcoleptic is falling asleep (hypnogogic hallucinations). Strong efforts by the sleepy patient to stay awake may result in lapses of attention and performance due to brief, unnoticed episodes of sleep, and he may perform activities such as driving in a continuous but inconsistent manner (automatic behavior). Partial complex seizures may be mimicked.

The symptoms of narcolepsy make their first appearance during the late teens or early twenties and only rarely after the mid-thirties. EDS of later onset should therefore be attributed to other causes. The disorder runs a nonprogressive, lifelong course. Despite its usual onset during the second to third decades, patients may reach an advanced age without a correct diagnosis or effective plan of management. The diagnosis can be objectively confirmed by means of polysomnographic recordings that demonstrate abnormally rapid transitions (15 min) from wakefulness to REM sleep. The treatment of EDS due to narcolepsy requires the use of an analeptic drug. In our experience, pemoline (Cylert®) is the best tolerated one, with only weak sympathomimetic effects.

SUMMARY

A large number of the elderly population in the United States complain of insomnia. The sleep cycle changes as a person ages, and the physician must take these physiological changes into account when treating the "insomniac." However, the insomnia must also be explored from a psychological viewpoint as well: The problem may not be an actual lack of sleep but a perceived lack of sleep. Appropriate strategies for diagnosis and treatment are outlined.

When caring for elderly patients, the physician should:

1. Know the normal age-related changes in the sleep-wake process.
2. Understand that sleep is a complex process with physiological and psychological dimensions.
3. Know how to evaluate and recognize the sleep disorders most common among the elderly.
4. Understand the role of hypnotic drugs in the treatment of sleep disorders.

REFERENCE

1. Association of Sleep Disorders Centers. Diagnostic classification of sleep and arousal disorders: first edition. *Sleep*, 2:1–137, 1979.

SUGGESTED READING

Coleman, R. M., Pollak, C. P., and Weitzman, E. D. Periodic movements in sleep (nocturnal myoclonus): relation to sleep disorders. *Ann. Neurol.*, 8:416, 1980.

Guilleminault, C., and Dement, W. C., editors. *Sleep Apnea Syndromes*. Alan R. Liss, Inc., New York, 1978.

Guilleminault, C., Dement, W. C., and Passouant, P., editors. *Narcolepsy.* Spectrum Publications, New York, 1976.

Kripke, D., Simons, R., Garfinkel, L., and Hammond, E. C. Short and long sleep and sleeping pills. *Arch. Gen. Psychiatry*, 36:103–116, 1979.

Sleeping Pills, Insomnia and Medical Practice. Report of a study by the Institute of Medicine. National Academy of Sciences, Washington, DC, 1979.

Weitzman, E. D. Sleep and aging. In: *Neurology of Aging*, edited by R. Katzman and R. Terry. Davis, Philadelphia *(in press)*.

Fundamentals of Geriatric Medicine, edited by
Ronald D.T. Cape, Rodney M. Coe, and Isadore
Rossman, Raven Press, New York © 1983.

25

Management of Cancer in the Elderly

W. Bradford Patterson

Cancer is predominantly a disease of aging, and so physicians need to be particularly alert to the diagnosis in older patients. Right lower quadrant pain in an 80-year-old means cancer of the right colon until proved otherwise. This is in sharp contrast to the same pain in an 18-year-old, for whom appendicitis is far more likely the correct diagnosis. Moreover, physicians must be aware of the increased occurrence of almost all types of cancer in the older patient. They watch the old farmer or sailor for skin cancer caused by prolonged actinic exposure. They know that a patient with peptic ulcer operated on long ago may have an increased risk of gastric cancer. They suspect that a woman with Plummer-Vinson syndrome may develop gastric cancer when she reaches her sixties. They know that the patient from whom a colonic polyp or a colonic cancer has been removed is at increased risk of subsequent cancer in the same organ. Periodic rectal examinations and tests for occult blood in the stool (Hemoccult™) are strongly indicated in the older population.

Certain factors simplify the management of cancer in the aged, whereas others make it more difficult. For example, most elderly women with stage I breast cancer accept a simple mastectomy with axillary dissection, an operation which can be done with minimal anesthesia and very little risk, whereas the typical 25-year-old woman with a similar lesion requires careful consideration of the different treatment options, lengthy discussion, and often specialized multidisciplinary care. Scars following the excision of skin cancers in the elderly heal with hardly a trace because the elastic tissue is gone, whereas scars from the same cancer and same excision in a young person may need the most skillful plastic surgery to avoid a poor result. Also, compared to younger patients, the elderly may accept the threat to their life with equanimity, so long as they are not frightened by what the death event itself may hold. Conversely, for younger people, the threat of death often poses an enormous problem.

Although cancer in the aged is sometimes easier to manage, operations and other treatment modalities present increased risks, and extra precautions are mandatory. Major abdominal or chest surgery in the elderly whose lungs and blood vessels have been impaired by a life of heavy smoking and heavy eating is much more difficult. Likewise, patients with narrowed cerebral vessels pose major risks during the postoperative period. The geriatric patient may find medication compliance difficult because of arthritis or impaired mentation, and fragile health may prohibit aggressive tumor-directed therapy of any kind.

Thus cancer in the aged presents specific diagnostic and treatment options for the physician to resolve and often requires special management techniques.

OBJECTIVES OF THERAPEUTIC MANAGEMENT

In the geriatric patient, the first objective may not always be to initiate a direct attack on the primary cancer itself. In many patients the mandate may be to:

1. Relieve symptoms.
2. Prevent catastrophic complications such as pathological fractures.
3. Determine the appropriate therapeutic setting for a particular patient, e.g., hospital, nursing home, extended care facility, home care.
4. Institute good supportive care when life is ending.

These criteria make evident many differences in cancer management according to the patient's age. In the elderly, breast cancer may deserve only the simplest local therapy, which often is a simple mastectomy with removal of palpable axillary nodes. When disseminated disease is in evidence, hormones can be tried cautiously, knowing that stilbestrol may provide lasting symptomatic relief so long as fluid retention is controlled. The problems with metastatic breast cancer which must be avoided include hypercalcemia, malnutrition, and pathological fractures of long bones, particularly the femur. If pain in the hip or thigh leads to bone scans and x-rays which show a lytic lesion in the femur, prophylactic insertion of a nail and radiotherapy are almost mandatory.

With colon cancer, a different set of treatment modifications are considered. One classic problem is the elderly patient with a nearly obstructing cancer in the left or descending colon who already has palpable hepatic metastases. Surgeons sometimes do a colostomy as a precautionary measure if resection and anastomosis are impossible, yet this is not always good management. A colostomy in a geriatric patient is a great burden and may be avoided by a careful diet which permits continued bowel elimination. This more conservative treatment requires a low-residue diet, a nonabsorbable sulfa drug by mouth to reduce the bacterial content (and thus the bulk) in the stool, plus regular magnesium citrate to assure a soft, moist stool. Patients can often be coaxed along on this regimen for months, passing occasional soft stools through a nearly obstructed sigmoid colon until they succumb from hepatic failure.

Cancer of the lower esophagus and gastric cardia poses other problems in the geriatric patient. Radiotherapy can be remarkably effective to forestall complete obstruction of the esophagus. Feeding tubes, bouginage with minimal anesthesia, or Celestin tubes may provide a sufficient lumen so that saliva and nutriment can be swallowed (7).

Electrocoagulation of cancer is a tissue-conserving technique which may be particularly useful in the geriatric patient. Crile and Turnbull (3) have used this technique in low-lying rectal lesions to avoid an abdominoperineal resection with colostomy. The wound created by the electrosurgical instrument heals painlessly by second intention, and the scarring is minimal. Some of the same advantages can be obtained with cryosurgery.

SPECIAL PROBLEMS PECULIAR TO THE AGED

Tolerance to Surgery

It has been stated that if the kidneys, lungs, and blood vessels are all right old patients tolerate anything that young patients can. Unfortunately, because of lung and heart damage due to smoking and because of sclerotic blood vessels, in many old patients tolerance to operative procedures requiring anesthesia is greatly reduced. As a result, anesthesia must be minimized, and local anesthesia is often preferred. Preoperative medication should be reduced. Similarly, the use of postoperative narcotics which cause increased periods of somnolence and which promote atelectasis must be reduced. The older patient is susceptible to postoperative hypoxemia. Endotracheal tubes must be kept in place longer to ensure that patients are fully awake and breathing on their own.

Major organs (e.g., lungs and liver) have less reserve in geriatric patients. Thus hepatic or pulmonary resections for cancer should almost always be limited to the subsegments or lobes whose removal is absolutely necessary to encompass a cancer. Also wounds heal more slowly in older patients. Often this can be attributed to a poor diet preoperatively, which leads to low serum albumin levels and depleted stores of vitamin C (Chapter 31).

Radiotherapy

It was once thought that x-ray therapy was easily tolerated in a patient too fragile for a major operation. Today it is recognized that a full course of 5,000 to 6,000 rads is markedly stressful, and no easy assumptions can be made about its use in elderly patients who may have deficiencies in cerebration, muscle strength, nutrition, or motivation. Maintaining nutrition and hemoglobin levels is critical. When conventional voltage radiotherapy was used, the tolerance of atrophic aging skin was a problem. Now, however, megavoltage radiotherapy spares the skin and expends its energy beneath it.

Radiotherapy in geriatric patients is commonly used to relieve symptoms and "buy time." Bone pain from skeletal metastases, like symptomatic inoperable cancers of the lung and esophagus, can often be palliated effectively with doses in the range of 3,000 to 3,500 rads. Radiotherapy for a cancer of the prostate which is diagnosed when a transurethral resection is done for urinary retention yields a control rate similar to that obtained by radical prostatectomy (6).

Chemotherapy

Chemotherapy presents a real therapeutic dilemma. In patients over 70, modern aggressive chemotherapy is poorly tolerated if carried to maximum dosages. Severe bone marrow reactions occur, nutrition often cannot be maintained, and an unacceptable rate of side effects is common. Some oncologists have tried to avoid this by reducing the dosage, but such a tactic will also reduce the percentage and duration of remissions obtained by full-dose chemotherapy. Consequently, aggressive chemotherapy is generally restricted to situations where such treatment appears to be the only means of combating intolerable symptoms such as pain or other distress.

SPECIAL CANCERS

Prostate

Prostatic cancer in the geriatric patient should be treated only if it is symptomatic. Aggressive treatment of localized, asymptomatic prostatic cancer by radical prostatectomy has not shown any benefit. In disseminated prostatic cancer, the use of estrogens is associated with an increased death rate from cardiac complications, and this balances out the slight decrease in prostatic cancer deaths. Thus prophylactic treatment has little justification in the elderly patient, either for very early or very late disease. Transurethral resection is excellent as palliation for the elderly man with prostatic cancer who cannot void. At this stage, operation can be legitimately combined with orchidectomy and/or estrogens to gain additional time free of symptoms. Radiotherapy and chemotherapy both provide additional palliation.

Colorectal

Colon resections with anastomosis are well tolerated in the elderly. Lesions of the right, transverse, descending or sigmoid colon should almost always be resected, as they lead to anemia, bleeding, and obstruction if operation is deferred because of age. Stage for stage, the cure rate is actually better than for younger persons. This, of course, does not apply if the patient has diffuse metastases and if pulmonary or hepatic decompensation is already occurring.

Abdominoperineal resections for cancer of the rectum have high morbidity and mortality rates in patients over 75. Therefore conservative methods for small distal rectal cancers should be considered in place of abdominoperineal resection. These include electrocoagulation and the Papillon technique, which uses high doses of contact radiotherapy applied through a special sigmoidoscope (5). For large rectal lesions of questionable operability, preoperative radiotherapy is often of great usefulness. In my opinion, it should almost always precede an attempted resection. In some instances the subsequent operation is made easier, and in a few patients complete disappearance of the lesion means that operation can be omitted. Although no improvement in cure rate is proved, perineal recurrences, very difficult to manage, are significantly reduced.

Skin

Some basal cell carcinomas are so indolent that immediate treatment is not essential. It is usually safe to follow a small basal cell cancer at intervals of 2 to 3 months before deciding to remove it. Fortunately, surgery of the skin in older patients is well tolerated, and results are excellent. Radiotherapy can also be used in such areas as around the eye, where skin coverage may be difficult to obtain. In general, one should remove suspicious, enlarged regional lymph nodes, but prophylactic regional node dissection is warranted only for the strongest indications. One might recommend an axillary dissection in conjunction with primary excision of an ulcerating melanoma on the upper arm.

Benign skin lesions in the elderly are ubiquitous. Most of these are seborrheic keratoses. These are slightly elevated, tan to brown, soft to scaly, and have no penetration into the deeper layers of the skin. Because they are benign and superficial, they should not be widely excised; they respond well to monopolar electrodesiccation, which is really done for cosmetic and not therapeutic reasons.

Stomach

Fortunately, cancer of the stomach is diminishing in incidence and is a much less common problem than in earlier years. When cancer is identified in the stomach, exploration is indicated unless advanced metastatic disease is already present, often in the liver. With the best surgical operative techniques, resection and re-establishment of continuity in the gastrointestinal tract is always worth the risk. Neither radiotherapy nor chemotherapy are good alternatives, although either may be used occasionally in an attempt to relieve pain. When an inoperable cancer obstructs the distal end of the stomach, the wise surgeon will not simply do a gastrojejunostomy but will divide the stomach proximally and exclude the antrum prior to the gastrojejunostomy. This provides better emptying of the gastric pouch.

RESECTION OF METASTASES

It has become recognized during recent years that the outlook for survival after resection of selected metastatic lesions in the lung is as good or better than the record for resection of primary lung cancer (4). Thus there are instances when a pulmonary resection for a solitary metastatic focus of cancer in a geriatric patient is justified. Factors to be considered include anticipated longevity without the cancer (i.e., whether the patient is otherwise robust and has a low operative risk) and the patient's wishes. The same philosophy governs resection of hepatic metastases; however, because the outcomes are less favorable, candidates for resection are few.

Resection of metastatic, symptomatic lesions in other parts of the body should not be avoided simply because of age. We have seen solitary metastases of melanoma, soft tissue sarcoma, and lymphoma in the small or large intestine. When these cause obstruction or bleeding, resection is generally indicated and often leads to months or years of satisfactory palliation. The same aggressive approach applies to enlarged metastatic regional lymph nodes, in that node dissections are done with light anesthesia, do not involve any of the body cavities, and have low morbidity rates. It is not necessary to leave a geriatric patient with markedly enlarged nodes in the neck or axilla if these are removable and an operation can thus promise great psychological and physical comfort.

ADVANCED CANCER

In the geriatric patient, fear of death is less an issue than is the fear of dying. Terminal patients need reassurance that the final event will not be accompanied by strangling, exsanguination, or terrible pain. Once reassured that a combination of medication and the natural biological processes can make the event reasonably peaceful, the elderly patient usually is able to accept advanced cancer with equanimity.

The good clinician treats avoidable symptoms and recognizes that certain symptoms (e.g., weakness and sadness) are unavoidable. Modern care of terminal patients makes it possible to provide relief of pain in most situations without the obtundation which leads to confusion and coma (1,2). The most important keys to pain medication in patients with advanced cancer are surprisingly simple:

1. Believe the patient. Do not assume he or she has "supratentorial" pain. Increase the strength and amount of analgesics as needed.
2. Remember that tolerance can develop to codeine, morphine, and other narcotics. Occasionally, dosage may have to be escalated to quite high levels (e.g., 60 mg morphine every 3 hr).
3. Give these medicines by the clock, not p.r.n., in order to stay ahead of the pain.
4. Provide oral pain-relieving drugs at the bedside, and let patients who are able determine their own schedule and amount.

The expert care to be found in the modern hospital palliative care unit or hospice has provided great assistance for aged patients who are dying. Perhaps the greatest solace is the sympathetic attendance from members of the health care team, including nurses, social workers, volunteers, and helpers, and the frequent visits from family. This is in sharp contrast to the dying cancer patient of earlier years, who most of all sensed abandonment and the loss of familiar contacts.

SUMMARY

In the aged, physicians should be on the lookout for signs of cancer, a disease common to this age group. Whereas certain factors tend to simplify treatment of cancer in the elderly, others present added risks.

Major objectives of the physician treating a cancer patient should be the relief of symptoms, preventing catastrophic complications, determining the proper therapeutic setting, and providing supportive care during the patient's final days.

Cancers particularly common in the elderly are discussed with regard to special problems in treatment of this age group. The appropriate settings in which to use chemotherapy, radiotherapy, and/or surgery are outlined.

When caring for elderly patients, the physician should:

1. Know the conditions of early life which predispose individuals to the development of cancer in late life.
2. Know how issues in diagnosis and treatment differ between elderly patients and young patients.
3. Know how operative techniques can be adjusted to the tolerance of elderly patients for anesthesia.
4. Know the salient clinical features of the most characteristic tumors of elderly patients.
5. Know the principles of effective and humane management of the patient with advanced cancer, including the management of pain.

REFERENCES

1. Bonica, J. J., and Ventrafridda, V., editors. *Advances in Pain Research and Therapy*, Vol. 2. Raven Press, New York, 1979.
2. Brocklehurst, J. C. *Textbook of Geriatric Medicine and Gerontology*, Chap. 16. Churchill-Livingstone, New York, 1978.
3. Crile, G., Jr., and Turnbull, R. B., Jr. The role of electrocoagulation in the treatment of carcinoma of the rectum. *Surg. Gynecol. Obstet.*, 135:391–395, 1972.
4. Mountain, C. F. The basis for surgical resection of pulmonary metastases. *Int. J. Radiat. Oncol. Biol. Phys.*, 1:749–953, 1976.
5. Papillon, J. Endocavity irradiation in the curative treatment of early rectal cancer. *Dis. Colon Rectum*, 17:172–180, 1974.
6. Ray, C. R., Cassady, J. R., and Bagshaw, M. A. Definitive radiation therapy in carcinoma of the prostate: a report on 15 years of experience. *Radiology*, 106:407–418, 1973.
7. Takita, H. Endoesophageal intubation for advanced esophageal carcinoma. *NY State J. Med.*, Nov. 1:2526–2529, 1977.

Fundamentals of Geriatric Medicine, edited by
Ronald D. T. Cape, Rodney M. Coe, and Isadore
Rossman, Raven Press, New York © 1983.

26

Management of Pain

Edith R. Kepes

Acute pain, the response to a nociceptive event, is an early signal of a disease process; it serves a useful purpose and usually responds to medication and treatment. When pain persists for a prolonged period, it is no longer a symptom but becomes the disease itself. The reaction to continuing pain is often accompanied by behavioral changes, depression, and anxiety; the magnitude of these, in turn, is related to ethnic, cultural, and socioeconomic factors as well as the secondary gain which results from chronic pain behavior.

There is still a great void in our knowledge about the mechanism and pathophysiology of chronic pain syndromes. Because of their complexity, a number of hospitals have developed pain centers staffed by specialists in psychiatry, orthopedics, neurology, surgery, oncology, anesthesiology, nursing, rehabilitation medicine, and sociology. Chronic pain patients who come to such pain centers have usually already received multiple modalities of therapy, undergone one or more surgical procedures, and become habituated to narcotic and other drugs. Most have all the symptoms of reactive depression, e.g., sleep disturbance, loss of appetite, and lack of interest in social and recreational activities. For many, pain becomes their central focus, dominating their lives.

Most patients have extensive treatment records and hospital discharge summaries, and have had x-ray studies, electromyographic studies, etc. At our Pain Treatment Center (P.T.C.), a screening questionnaire is used to evaluate the patient's attitude toward work, family, and society, as well as his self-esteem. In addition to a careful neurological examination, all patients are seen by a psychiatrist whose special interest is the psychological response to chronic pain. If additional information is needed, psychological testing is used. We use the Minnesota Multiphasic Personality Inventory (MMPI), which is computerized and obviates the need for consultation with a psychologist. In some cases, the use of differential spinal or epidural block reveals whether a patient is a placebo reactor or one who has somatic, sympathetic central, or psychogenic pain.

THERAPY OF DISORDERS PRODUCING INTRACTABLE PAIN

Low Back Pain

Low back pain is one of the most common disabling disorders, affecting patients of all ages. The etiology may be congenital or acquired, due to injury or age. Age-associated changes in the spine, including deterioration of intervertebral discs, arthritis, and osteoporosis, make low back pain relatively common in the elderly. Metastatic tumors and Paget's disease are causes to remember, and in elderly, debilitated patients coccygeal pain is common.

There is no single uniformly successful treatment of backache and sciatica, and many modalities have been tried. The majority of patients recover with such conservative measures as bed rest, massage, heat, traction, and exercise, or with point injections, acupuncture, or transcutaneous electrical nerve stimulation. Those who do not respond to the above measures have several further options.

Epidural steroid injection. The author has found epidural steroid injections most successful for the acute exacerbation of chronic low back pain in patients who have had no previous laminectomies and are not addicted to drugs. The efficacy of this injection is thought to result from bathing the inflamed and compressed nerve roots with a local anesthetic that contains a corticosteroid, thus reducing the swelling and inflammation responsible for the pain.

Facet block. The medial branch of the posterior ramus of the spinal nerve gives off small nerve filaments to the facet joint. The medial descending branch then continues caudally, giving off muscular and cutaneous branches and sending five branches to the medial side of the superior facet below. Injection of the lumbar facets with a local anesthetic alone or with Depo-Medrol® gives long-term relief in some cases.

Facet rhizolysis. If pain relief is obtained with facet blocks, the nerve can be destroyed utilizing radiofrequency coagulation. In carefully selected patients, a significant percentage of incapacitating chronic back pain can be rapidly relieved.

Discectomy. The most frequently used surgical procedure since 1930 is the removal of the herniated disc through laminectomy. Reported results vary from 30 to 85% major improvement. Only 35% of the patients return to work following surgery for industrial back injuries.

Stimulation technique. Transcutaneous electrical nerve stimulator (TENS), dorsal column stimulation, and epidural stimulation may be useful (see below). The benefits of all these methods can be significantly improved if they are combined with back exercises which strengthen abdominal and back muscles, and diminish the lumbar lordosis. Obese individuals should be encouraged to lose weight. Drug-habituated patients should be detoxified and narcotics substituted with nonsteroidal anti-inflammatory drugs, salicylates, and antidepressant medication. Patients should be encouraged to resume moderate social and work activities. Relaxation exercises can be taught with the aid of biofeedback. Selected elderly patients may benefit from group psychotherapy.

Headaches

Overall, complaints of headache appear to be less common in the elderly than in younger individuals. Migraine headaches, particularly those of recent onset, are relatively rare and warn of possible subsequent development of transient ischemic attacks or stroke. If the usual treatment methods are unsuccessful, selected elderly persons may be helped with biofeedback.

REFLEX SYMPATHETIC DYSTROPHIES

In general, all conditions classified under the reflex sympathetic dystrophies (RSD) have in common a triad of symptoms: pain, vasomotor disturbances, and trophic changes. The etiology is vast, as seen in Table 1.

In the elderly, RSD is most commonly seen after myocardial infarction, hemiplegia, herpes zoster, Colles' fracture, and thrombophlebitis. Despite various etiologies, the underlying physiopathological mechanisms are very similar. Probably local tissue damage initiates a reflex disorder which in some way involves the sympathetic nervous system. Interruption of the sympathetic fibers either modifies, improves, or cures the disorder.

Clinical Features

The diagnosis can be made from the history of recent or remote trauma, infection, or disease. Persistent pain of a burning, aching, throbbing character, not related to specific dermatomes, is typical. In the beginning, the skin feels warm, red, and dry; later it becomes moist, cyanotic, and cold. The edema spreads, joints become increasingly stiff, a muscular wasting sets in, the hair is coarse, and nails are brittle. The x-rays may show patchy osteoporosis. Measurement of skin temperature gives a good indication of sympathetic tone. Hyperactivity of the sympathetic system results in decreased skin temperature. Electrical skin resistance is also altered in the affected extremity and can be measured by a portable dermometer.

TABLE 1. *Reflex sympathetic dystrophies*

Major reflex dystrophies	Minor reflex dystrophies	
	Posttraumatic	Diseases
Causalgia	Sudeck's atrophy	After myocardial infarction
Phantom limb pain	Traumatic arthritis	After hemiplegia
Central pain	Posttraumatic spreading neuralgia	Vasospastic arterial disease
	Posttraumatic osteoporosis	After herpes
	Posttraumatic pain syndrome	Thrombophlebitis
	Posttraumatic edema	After frostbite
	Posttraumatic angiospasm	After trombotic painful edema
	Shoulder-hand syndrome	

Pathogenesis

Many theories have been suggested to explain the pathogenesis of reflex sympathetic dystrophy. None is able to explain all the features of causalgia. Afferent sympathetic fibers, both from the intestine and the blood vessels, are pain-conducting neurons. Distention and contraction of the intestine and changes in caliber of blood vessels stimulate these nerves. Also, chemical substances released from damaged tissue are implicated in autonomic fiber stimulation. The most acceptable theory is that continuous afferent impulses alter the internuncial neuron activity in the spinal cord. The abnormal activity of the internuncial pool may spread widely and implicate anterior and lateral horn cells, resulting in excessive skeletal and smooth muscle activity. As the condition progresses, the disturbance may ascend up to the higher centers and to the cortex. This explains the importance of early treatment and lack of response to treatment in longstanding cases.

Treatment

The following management strategies are available:

1. Local treatment: removal of causative lesion, if any.
2. Analgesic blocks.
   a. Local infiltration: In early cases, infiltration of a local anesthetic into the site of the lesion may be effective.
   b. Sympathetic blocks: Sympathetic blocks are of both diagnostic and therapeutic value. Most of these disorders involve either upper or lower extremity; blocking the stellate ganglion and lumbar sympathetic chain are the methods of choice in most cases. Usually a series of blocks is necessary. The response varies from patient to patient, and in general the earlier the therapy is instituted the better. In selected cases, if the response is transitory after repeated blocks, sympathectomy can be done.
3. Regional intravenous injection of sympatholytics (e.g., reserpine and guanethidine) has been used with good results.[1]
4. Physical therapy.
5. Psychotherapy.
6. Transcutaneous electrical nerve stimulation. It appears that sympathetic tone can be altered in some cases with the use of TENS.
7. Surgery: thoracic or lumbar sympathectomy.

PHANTOM LIMB PAIN

The majority of amputees are elderly, and within this group phantom limb pain is a commonly encountered condition. Immediately following amputation of a limb,

---

[1] In the author's experience, the safety and duration of sympathetic block with intravenous regional guanethidine has been found superior to conventional nerve blocks. Unfortunately, only oral guanethidine is approved at present in the United States.

there is always awareness of the absent part. For most amputees, this discomfort gradually fades. In 5 to 10% of patients, a disagreeable sensation, variously described as cramping, shooting, burning, or crushing, persists.

Although many theories have been advanced, the etiology of phantom limb pain is obscure. A recent conceptual model proposes that a portion of the brainstem reticular formation exerts a tonic inhibitory effect on transmission at all levels of the somatic projection system. The loss of sensory input after amputation would decrease the tonic inhibition and increase the probability of self-sustaining neural activity. Modulation of the sensory input by anesthetic blocks or intense stimulation by electrical stimulation would abolish the self-sustaining activity and produce pain relief. In addition, psychotherapeutic methods, biofeedback, relaxation, mood elevators, and antidepressants may be helpful.

A careful psychiatric assessment is of immense value. The ability of individuals to cope with stress varies greatly, and other aspects are involved, e.g., personality, reaction to the lost limb, economic and family background. Some patients with a low pain threshold can be encouraged with training to be more tolerant and to accept their disability more stoically.

Phantom limb pain is a most distressing condition because knowledge of its cause is incomplete and treatment is unsatisfactory and unreliable in the majority of individuals. A survey of treatment methods used in the United States was carried out recently (1), revealing that of 68 treatment methods 50 were in current use. Only a few were even moderately successful when subjected to the criterion of low failure rates after 1 year. Nonsurgical treatment methods were far more successful than surgical ones. The authors suggested that phantom limb pain is a single symptom class caused by many different disorders.

HERPES ZOSTER AND POSTHERPETIC NEURALGIA

Herpes zoster (H.Z.; shingles) is an infectious disease caused by the varicella zoster virus. Shingles increases in incidence with age and strikes 1 to 2% of the elderly each year. The pain of the acute stage subsides after 3 weeks to 6 months in over 80%, but the rest develop the postherpetic syndrome. The symptoms of postherpetic neuralgia can be explained by damage to afferent fibers, with the most injury to the large fast-conduction fibers. When the inhibitory influence of the faster larger fibers is lacking, burning pains of long duration mediated via the small fibers result. The pains of H.Z. are of three types: burning pain with cutaneous hyperesthesia; sharp, shooting, intermittent pain; and a continual background ache. Recent evidence suggests that this intractable pain can be prevented by a series of sympathetic nerve blocks during the acute stage or within the first month of the presenting symptoms. In the author's experience, this method brings impressive pain relief, the lesions heal rapidly, and neuralgia is prevented.

Once postherpetic neuralgia has developed, a variety of treatments have been suggested (e.g., nerve blocks, neurectomy, subarachnoid neurolytic agents, cordotomy, and TENS), all with disappointing results. The most rewarding treatment is supportive therapy with tricyclic antidepressants, anticonvulsives, and pheno-thiazines. Drugs must be carefully administered in the elderly (Chapter 20), as side effects and intolerance are frequent. Amitriptyline 10 to 75 mg at bedtime with fluphenazine 1 to 3 mg during the day usually produces results after 2 weeks. Fluphenazine should be discontinued if signs of parkinsonism or tardive dyskinesia are present. Impressive results have been achieved with carbamazepine 600 to 800 mg/day or diphenylhydantoin 300 to 400 mg/day together with 50 to 100 mg nortriptyline in divided doses, depending on the age and physical status of the patient. Patients should be admitted for the initial treatment, as side effects, although self-limiting, are frequent during the first 2 weeks of therapy. They consist of drowsiness, diplopia, tremor, and gastrointestinal symptoms, e.g., nausea and an-orexia.

CANCER PAIN

Patients referred to a Pain Treatment Center have usually exhausted all benefits that can be derived from surgery, radiation, and chemotherapy. These individuals may have pain caused by the treatment of the disease, e.g., postsurgical pain, peripheral neuropathy due to chemotherapy, direct involvement of nerve plexuses due to spread of the malignancy, or radiation fibrosis.

In addition, such patients with cancer pain, knowing that their disease is incurable, develop feelings of hopelessness, depression, anger, and anxiety. Some patients become so discouraged and desperate as to contemplate suicide. Management has to be directed toward both pain and its psychological effects. Patients who are cured and suffer pain due to "the treatment" should be managed as other chronic benign pain patients. For those individuals whose life expectancy is shortened, pain man-agement should be directed toward modulation of the symptoms in order to maintain alertness and social interaction.

Depending on the location of pain, one or more of the following procedures may be applied:

1. Nerve blocks.
    a. Peripheral nerve block with phenol or absolute alcohol causes neurolysis which may give pain relief for up to 6 months. This is suitable if pain is limited to one to three dermatomes.
    b. Celiac plexus block with alcohol is indicated for visceral pain, especially pain due to cancer of the pancreas.
    c. Subarachnoid phenol and alcohol is especially useful for pain of the thoracic and upper lumbar segments.
    d. Chemical hypophysectomy. This method of relieving intractable pain in inoperable cancer was introduced in 1963. It appears to be of value in two classes of patients with inoperable cancer: those with cancers known to be hormone-dependent (e.g., carcinoma of the breast) and those suffering from continuous severe pain. Through a transnasal, transsphenoidal ap-proach with the aid of an image intensifier, alcohol is injected into the

pituitary fossa, which destroys the gland in whole or in part. Complications include rhinorrhea, diabetes insipidus, and visual defects.
2. Neurosurgical procedures, including rhizotomy, percutaneous chordotomy, and thalamotomy.
3. Drug treatment.

ANALGESICS AND RELATED DRUGS FOR CHRONIC PAIN

Many patients become habituated to depressant and addictive drugs. In our experience, the most frequently misused drugs are the barbiturates, diazepam, oxycodone, pentazocine, and propoxyphene. Detoxification is important, and if necessary hospitalization in one of the pain centers is recommended. The nonnarcotic analgesic derivatives of salicylic acid, paminophenol pyrasolone, indole, and many other nonsteroidal anti-inflammatory drugs are useful, especially for pain of musculoskeletal origin. In our experience, the most effective drugs are acetylsalicylic acid, lidomethacin, ibuprofem, naprosyn, and sulindac. A newly available and very potent analgesic in this group is zomepirac. Unfortunately, not every patient can tolerate these drugs because of gastrointestinal disturbances and bleeding tendencies. Acetaminophen, which is free of these side effects, is much less effective.

Today, it is generally accepted that anxiety and depression intensify pain arising from nociceptive sources and may even give rise to pain in the absence of painful inputs. Psychotropic agents have been used successfully during the last 10 years to reduce anxiety, provide nighttime sedation, elevate mood, and potentiate analgesia. Among the tricyclic antidepressant drugs, we have found amotriptyline and doxepin useful. They can be taken at night if insomnia is present. Imipramine is used if the former drugs cause too much sedation. Side effects (e.g., dry mouth, blurred vision, urinary retention, constipation, glaucoma, parkinsonism, and such cardiovascular changes as tachycardia and blood pressure changes) must be carefully monitored, especially in the elderly patient. The doses used for reactive depression due to pain are small, e.g., amitriptyline 10 mg at night, which can be gradually increased. Seldom is more than 30 mg amitriptyline tolerated by the elderly without side effects. Antidepressants can be combined with antianxiety drugs and tranquilizers with caution.

Among the phenothiazine derivatives, we have found the following drugs useful: fluphenazine especially for herpes zoster, chlorpromazine if nausea is a problem. Methotrimeprazine is excellent for use at night to potentiate analgesia and sedation. Side effects are similar and even more frequent than with the tricyclic antidepressants. There may be serious complications (e.g., dystonia and tardive diskinesia) if these drugs are used for long periods.

In central thalamic pain and in some neuralgias, anticonvulsant drugs are often effective. Phenytoin sodium, carbamazepine, and valproic acid are examples of drugs we have used successfully. Minor tranquilizers (e.g., meprobamate, chlordiazepoxide, diazepam, hydroxyzine) are not used. They not only cause habituation and withdrawal symptoms (e.g., convulsion) but most have no antipsychotic properties.

Mild and strong narcotic analgesics are used only in patients who have a limited life expectancy or whose pain is due to cancer. Narcotics are singularly capable of modifying both the perception of and reaction to pain as well as inducing a sense of calm indifference to psychological stresses frequently experienced by the patient with cancer. This sense of well-being and euphoria is most desirable in the dying patient. Narcotics act centrally to relieve pain, which is an important property when treating patients with widely disseminated cancer. When milder simple nonnarcotic analgesics have been found wanting, we use narcotic drugs. Among the milder narcotic analgesics, propoxyphene, codeine, oxycodone, pentazocine, and meperidine have been tried and used. If tolerated by the patient, these can be administered at the maximum dose before changing to a more potent analgesic. If these drugs are ineffective, more-potent analgesics are indicated, e.g., morphine, hydromorphone, levorphanol, and methadone. These drugs must be taken regularly throughout the 24 hr, as changing blood levels of the drug with breakthrough of pain causes anxiety, depression, and more pain.

When all these methods have failed to produce adequate pain relief, we have found that an intravenous drip of morphine for 24 to 48 hr is useful to titrate the patient for narcotic requirement. After calculation of the 24-hour requirement, the patient is given oral methadone. This is more readily absorbed from the gastrointestinal tract than morphine and has the longest duration of action.

In addition, antidepressant, antianxiety medication is indicated. Nausea is often a problem, and antiemetics such as prochlorperazine or cyclizine are useful. If the narcotic analgesics cause too much sedation during the day, stimulants such as amphetamine and dextroamphetamine are indicated. Constipation is often a problem with large doses of narcotics, and attention should be paid to this if fecal impaction is to be avoided.

If undesirable side effects are to be eluded, the principles of drug treatment in the aged must be strictly followed (Chapter 20). Absorption, transport, distribution, metabolism, and excretion are all decreased during old age. The biological half-life of drugs is therefore increased. Smaller doses at less frequent intervals must be used if undesirable side effects are to be avoided. Family members should be informed of toxic effects and instructed to stop medication and consult the physician if such effects are observed.

STIMULATION OF PERIPHERAL NERVES, SPINAL CORD, AND BRAIN FOR PAIN RELIEF

Pain relief by stimulation of various parts of the nervous system is generally as successful as destructive procedures, with considerably less risk. Current techniques include transcutaneous stimulation of peripheral nerves, spinal cord and brain.

1. *TENS.* Stimulators are small, portable, battery-powered devices available from a number of manufacturers. In general, they supply a variable square wave

or spike pulse, with controllable pulse width, frequency, and voltage. A large selection of electrodes is available. There are few contraindications, but patients with cardiac pacemakers should not be given this device. Electrodes are applied over major nerve trunks supplying the painful area. After several days of education, the patients are allowed to use the device. A 1- to 2-month trial period is advisable before purchasing the device in order to establish if a placebo response is present. TENS may be effective by a combination of large-fiber stimulation with its gating effect on small pain fiber input and the stimulation of endorphin secretion in the midbrain. Chronic pain which responds most often to TENS is that due to peripheral nerve trauma, low back and chronic neck problems, phantom limb pain, and postherpetic neuralgia or reflex sympathetic dystrophy. Pain from diabetic neuropathies, central nervous system injuries, or psychogenic origin does not appear to improve to a degree beyond the accepted placebo response.

2. *Peripheral nerve stimulators.* These are embedded electrodes. After an initial period of enthusiastic use, they have now come to be reserved for patients with pain caused by peripheral nerve injuries. In other pain syndromes, the beneficial result was short-lived.

3. *Spinal cord stimulation.* This involves laminectomy and implantation of electrodes over the posterior column. This operation is now seldom performed and has been replaced by stimulation of the spinal cord or cauda equina by electrodes which can be threaded through an epidural needle into the epidural space.

4. *Brain stimulation.* Electrodes have been introduced into various target points, e.g., sensory nuclei of the contralateral thalamus, posterior capsule sensory cortex, and midline posterior thalamic area, the site of the opiate receptors. Brain stimulation is used for thalamic syndrome, anesthesia dolorosa, and dysesthesia following cordotomy and rhizotomy.

BIOFEEDBACK

Elderly patients are less responsive to biofeedback than their younger counterparts. Biofeedback is an educational method in which ordinarily unavailable information in an individual's own bodily processes is presented continuously to the individual, enabling the patient to make adjustments that would have been impossible or difficult without access to the information. Examples of the functions which can be trained are muscle tension, skin temperature, and blood pressure. The most commonly used methods are:

1. *Electromyographic (EMG) feedback.* In procedures using EMG feedback, electrodes are placed on the patient's skin overlying the muscle or muscle group to be trained. The electrical activity is converted into a sound the subject can hear through a speaker or headphones. The sound, clicking, or tone varies directly with the amount of electrical activity emanating from the muscle. For example, a greater number of clicks or a higher-pitched tone indicates more muscle tension.

EMG feedback is useful in tension headaches. The data from the published reports indicate a reduction in the headache activity coincident with the acquired ability to relax the frontalis muscles and the surrounding muscles of the forehead. The most successful subjects have been those who practice relaxation regularly at home.

2. *Temperature feedback.* A heat-sensitive electrode is taped to the part of the body where temperature change is desired. In visual feedback, the temperature registers on a dial. The needle indicator moves to the left when the temperature drops and to the right when it rises. In audio feedback, the pitch of a tone goes down as the temperature rises and goes up as the temperature falls. Raynaud's disease has been treated by teaching the patient to warm his extremities. Some investigators have reported that they have been able to train migraine patients to warm their hands and thus to decrease or eliminate the occurrence of migraine headache episodes.

FUTURE GOALS AND DIRECTIONS

It is clear that improvements in the care of the elderly with pain will require considerable effort in both research and education. More research is needed on the neurological, biochemical, and psychological mechanisms of pain. There is a need for new drugs which produce pain relief qualitatively similar to that of morphine, are effective when administered by mouth, have no sedative or psychotomimetic effects, cause little or no respiratory or circulatory depression, and are nonaddictive with little or no development of tolerance. It is hoped, because of the recent interest in the opiate receptors and endorphins, that there will be a search for peptides that can function as oral analgesics. There is an urgent need to critically evaluate the results of old and new treatment modalities for pain. These evaluations must be disseminated among health professionals involved in the management of the elderly patient with pain. Every nurse and doctor should understand that pain is a psycho-biological phenomenon modulated by the patient's mood, interpretation of the pain, and many other factors.

SUMMARY

This chapter identifies conditions associated with severe pain that are particularly common in the elderly patient. The clinical features of some of the pain syndromes are useful to the physician for making the diagnosis and choosing the proper form of therapy. A number of these therapies are outlined.

When caring for elderly patients, the physician should:

1. Know what conditions involving severe, acute, or chronic pain are particularly common in elderly persons.
2. Know how the clinical features of certain common pain syndromes may aid in their differential diagnosis.
3. Know what medical or surgical therapeutic measures not involving drugs may be helpful in the management of pain syndromes.

4. Know the indications for and dangers of drugs in the management of pain in elderly patients.
5. Know how drugs can be used effectively in the management of pain in terminally ill patients.

REFERENCE

1. Sherman, R. A., Sherman, C. Y., and Gall, N. G. A survey of current phantom limbs: pain treatment in the United States. *Pain*, 8:85–99, 1980.

SUGGESTED READING

Marcus, N., and Levin, G. Clinical application of biofeedback. *Hosp. Community Psychiatry*, 28:21–25, 1977.

Melzack, R. Phantom limb pain: implications for treatment of pathological pain. *Anesthesiology*, 35:409–419, 1971.

Melzack, R. *The Puzzle of Pain*. Basic/Harper Torchback, New York, 1973.

Moricca, G. *Progress in Anesthesiology. Proceedings of the Fourth World Congress Anesthesiology*, p. 266. Excerpta Medica, Amsterdam, 1968.

National Institutes of Health. Pain in the elderly: patterns change with age. *JAMA*, 241:2491–2492, 1979.

Shealy, C. N. Transcutaneous electrical stimulation for control of pain. *Clin. Neurosurg.*, 21:269–277, 1974.

Sternback, R. A. *Pain Patients: Traits and Treatment*. Academic Press, New York, 1974.

Swerdlow, M., editor. *Relief of Intractable Pain*, 2nd ed. Excerpta Medica, Amsterdam, 1978.

Winnie, A. P., Hartman, J. T., Meyers, H. L., Ramamurthy, S., and Barangan, V. Pain clinic. II. Intradural and extradural corticosteroids for sciatica. *Anesth. Analg.*, 51:990–999, 1972.

Fundamentals of Geriatric Medicine, edited by
Ronald D. T. Cape, Rodney M. Coe, and Isadore
Rossman, Raven Press, New York © 1983.

Questions for Self-Assessment

DIRECTIONS: In questions 1–17, only *one* alternative is correct. Select the one
best answer and blacken the corresponding lettered box on the
answer sheet.

1. Narcotic analgesics are drugs of choice for elderly patients who have:

    (A)   Causalgia
    (B)   Phantom limb pain
    (C)   Herpes zoster
    (D)   Trigeminal neuralgia
    (E)   None of the above

2. In a 68-year-old woman with excessive daytime sleepiness since age 23, the
    most likely cause is:

    (A)   Hypothyroidism
    (B)   Narcolepsy
    (C)   Sleep apnea
    (D)   Depression
    (E)   Chronic insomnia

3/5. An 80-year-old woman with no evident defects in her cardiopulmonary re-
    serve and no other serious chronic illnesses has a 3-cm hard mass with skin
    dimpling in the outer quadrant of her pendulous right breast. In the right
    axilla, one 2.5-cm lymph node is palpable. An invasive intraductal carcinoma
    is diagnosed by needle biopsy of the breast. The liver is not palpable and
    LFTs are within normal limits.

3. The staging procedures should include roentgenogram of the chest and:

    (A)   Complete blood count (CBC)
    (B)   CBC and bone scan

(C)   CBC, bone scan, and liver scan
(D)   CBC, bone scan, liver scan, and brain scan

4.   Assuming no metastases have been demonstrated, the *most* appropriate management at this time would be:

(A)   Total (simple) mastectomy plus conservative axillary dissection
(B)   Removal of the mass plus radiation therapy
(C)   Therapy with diethylstilbestrol
(D)   Radical mastectomy and postoperative radiation therapy
(E)   Observation but no immediate treatment

5.   Three years later metastases have developed. The *least* likely complication from the metastases is:

(A)   A fractured hip
(B)   Constipation
(C)   Intestinal obstruction
(D)   Jaundice
(E)   Chest pain

6.   The *most* important therapeutic goal of psychiatric treatment of the elderly patient is:

(A)   Getting the patient to adjust to circumstances that are beyond his or her control
(B)   Improving their socialization
(C)   Helping the family to adjust to the patient's condition
(D)   Reapproximation or reattainment of premorbid baseline status
(E)   Getting the patient into a safe, secure nursing home situation

7.   Diuretics control nocturnal angina in elderly patients by:

(A)   Increasing coronary flow
(B)   Correcting occult congestive heart failure
(C)   Controlling the rate of atrial fibrillation
(D)   Producing an antihypertensive effect
(E)   Producing vasodilatation

8.   Successful treatment of phantom limb pain is usually accomplished by:

(A)   Transcutaneous electrical nerve stimulation (TENS)
(B)   Biofeedback
(C)   Nerve blocks
(D)   Excision of neuroma
(E)   None of the above

9. Of the following, the finding that is *least* common in elderly patients who have bacterial pneumonia is:

   (A) Cough with purulent sputum
   (B) Fever
   (C) Leukocytosis
   (D) Tachycardia and tachypnea
   (E) Signs of consolidation

10. The *best* established therapeutic indication for administration of major tranquilizers is:

    (A) Acute schizophrenia, schizoaffective manic subtype
    (B) Acute mania
    (C) Insomnia
    (D) Provoked anger
    (E) Agitation associated with alcohol withdrawal

11. The *best* established therapeutic indication for administration of tricyclic antidepressants is:

    (A) Acute schizophrenia, schizoaffective manic subtype
    (B) Mental retardation
    (C) Reserpine-induced depression
    (D) Hypothyroid stupor
    (E) Retarded depression

12. A 75-year-old man who had a coronary artery bypass graft 2 years ago has rectal bleeding. There is a 2-cm irregular tumor on the anterior rectal wall 4 cm in from the sphincter. Biopsy demonstrates adenocarcinoma. The remainder of the examination is within normal limits, except for moderate obesity and absent dorsalis pedis pulses. The *most* appropriate management is:

    (A) Symptomatic treatment (analgesics and iron supplements)
    (B) Local treatment of the carcinoma (electrocoagulation or contact radiation therapy)
    (C) Abdominoperineal resection
    (D) Chemotherapy using 5-fluorouracil intravenously, once weekly
    (E) Radiation therapy

13. The condition or finding that is *most* likely to obscure the clinical diagnosis of aortic stenosis in an elderly patient who has ventricular dysfunction is:

    (A) Low cardiac output leading to a low aortic ejection gradient

(B)   A loud systolic ejection murmur
(C)   Pleural effusion
(D)   A murmur at the mitral valve area
(E)   Poor compliance of the stiffened ascending aorta

14.   Treatment with digitalis is hazardous for an elderly patient who has congestive heart failure if:

(A)   Atrial fibrillation is present
(B)   The patient is receiving quinidine concomitantly
(C)   The heart is enlarged past the anterior axillary line
(D)   There is a history of myocardial infarction
(E)   Hypertension is likely to occur

15.   In elderly patients, prevention of the development of postherpetic neuralgia has been *most* often achieved by:

(A)   Treatment with analgesics
(B)   Transcutaneous electrical nerve stimulation (TENS)
(C)   Sympathetic blocks
(D)   Administration of antidepressants
(E)   Administration of amantadine

16.   For a 5-mg dose of haloperidol administered intramuscularly, the equipotent dose of chlorpromazine administered orally is:

(A)   5 mg
(B)   50 mg
(C)   100 mg
(D)   250 mg
(E)   750 mg

17.   Of all elderly persons in the United States who are mentally ill, the percentage whose mental health needs are presently being met is approximately:

(A)   5%
(B)   20%
(C)   30%
(D)   50%
(E)   75%

DIRECTIONS: In questions 18–36, *one or more* of the alternatives may be correct. You are to respond either *yes* (Y) or *no* (N) to *each* of the alternatives. For every alternative you think is correct, blacken the corresponding lettered box on the answer sheet in the column labeled "Y". For every alternative you think is incorrect, blacken the corresponding lettered box in the column labeled "N".

18. Studies that should be part of a prepsychopharmacological evaluation include:

   (A) Complete blood count with differential
   (B) Glucose tolerance test
   (C) Serum triglyceride level
   (D) Liver function test
   (E) Evaluation of renal function

19. The use of hypnotic drugs in the elderly may be risky because:

   (A) Occult sleep apnea may be increased
   (B) Drug dependency may develop
   (C) Nocturnal myoclonus may be increased
   (D) Drugs with long half-lives may accumulate
   (E) Drug interactions are more likely

20. Drugs that are useful for the treatment of refractory congestive heart failure in elderly patients include:

   (A) Dopamine
   (B) Methyldopa
   (C) Dobutamine
   (D) Propranolol hydrochloride
   (E) Amrinone

21. True statements concerning the use of pneumococcal vaccines for elderly persons include:

   (A) The principal immunization component is a polysaccharide antigen.
   (B) The duration of protection is at least 3 years.
   (C) Pneumococcal and influenza vaccines should not be administered concurrently.
   (D) Elderly persons receiving pneumococcal vaccine should probably also receive influenza vaccine.

22. True statements concerning the relationship of specific drug effects to the age of the patient include:

   (A) Isoniazid hepatotoxicity is more common in patients who are more than 35 years of age than in younger patients.
   (B) In an elderly patient with hypothermia who has a history of psychiatric illness, hypothermia (35.2°C) is more likely a side effect of phenothiazines than of antidepressant drugs.

(C)   Elderly patients are particularly susceptible to postural hypotension with "fainting" or falls when given propranolol for treatment of hypertension.

(D)   In an elderly patient under treatment with levodopa for parkinsonism, writhing movements of the right ankle with inversion of the ankle are an indication for a higher dose of levodopa.

(E)   To achieve anticoagulation in an elderly patient with a serum albumin level of 2.7 g/dl will require a greater dose of warfarin than in a young adult with an albumin level of 4.0 g/dl.

23.   Problems associated with the use of laxatives include:

(A)   Hypokalemic metabolic alkalosis
(B)   A "fixed" skin eruption
(C)   Aspiration pneumonia
(D)   Crampy abdominal pain
(E)   Fecal incontinence

24.   A 74-year-old, otherwise healthy woman was unable to fall asleep whenever she omitted her usual dose of nightly secobarbital 200 mg. This implies that:

(A)   Her insomnia requires continuous drug therapy.
(B)   Drug tolerance may have developed.
(C)   Withdrawal from secobarbital would be unlikely to succeed.
(D)   More gradual, supervised withdrawal might produce fewer symptoms.
(E)   Sleep will be normal once secobarbital has been completely withdrawn.

25.   True statements concerning adverse drug effects in elderly patients include:

(A)   Deterioration in renal function is generally compensated for by improved drug clearance by the liver.
(B)   Adverse drug effects commonly result from the increased number of medications received for numerous concomitant ailments.
(C)   Although elderly patients usually weigh less than younger patients, they are often resistant to drug therapy and require larger daily doses of most drugs.
(D)   The volume of distribution of water-soluble drugs (e.g., digoxin) is likely to be reduced in elderly patients.
(E)   Phenytoin toxocity (unsteadiness, nystagmus) may occur at serum concentrations within the usual therapeutic range as less of the drug is protein-bound in hypoalbuminemic patients.

26.   The following are characteristic of the insomnia associated with major depression:

(A)   Difficulty maintaining sleep
(B)   Early onset of REM sleep

(C) Increased eye movements during REM sleep
(D) Repeated awakening during the night
(E) Difficulty initiating sleep

27. Pain restricted to dermatomes is seen in:

(A) Neuralgia
(B) Shoulder-hand syndrome
(C) Phantom limb pain
(D) Thrombophlebitis
(E) Neuritis

28. True statements concerning tuberculosis in elderly patients include:

(A) In the United States the prevalence of active disease is greatest among the elderly.
(B) Clinical findings are usually specific.
(C) Roentgenograms of the chest commonly show lesions outside the usual apical-posterior region.
(D) The PPD-S skin test is a reliable diagnostic tool.
(E) The risk of INH-associated hepatitis is lower in older patients than in younger patients.

29. Radiation therapy is appropriately used for palliation of:

(A) Malignant obstruction of the esophagus
(B) Symptomatic solitary skeletal metastases
(C) Carcinoma of the prostate with local invasion
(D) Diffuse intra-abdominal metastases
(E) Hepatic metastases with jaundice

30. True statements concerning the management of cardiac arrhythmia in elderly patients include:

(A) The rate of clearance of lidocaine is related to the patient's hepatic function.
(B) Disopyramide exerts sufficient anticholinergic activity to precipitate acute urinary retention.
(C) In the majority of elderly patients, the isolated finding of 4/min unifocal premature ventricular contractions (PVCs) warrants antiarrhythmic drug therapy.
(D) First-degree heart block in association with nausea and vomiting in a patient whose serum digoxin concentration is 2.5 ng/ml 12 hr after the last dose of digoxin is highly suspicious of digoxin toxicity.
(E) Patients whose creatinine clearance is 25 ml/min should have one-half the usual digoxin dose.

31. Drugs that are used for vasodilation in patients who have advanced congestive heart failure include:

    (A) Hydralazine
    (B) Nitroprusside
    (C) Furosemide
    (D) Prazosin
    (E) Digoxin

32. True statements concerning urinary tract infections (UTIs) in elderly patients include:

    (A) Asymptomatic bacteriuria is the most common type.
    (B) Asymptomatic bacteriuria as an isolated finding requires treatment.
    (C) Pyuria (5 to 10 leukocytes/high power field from a centrifuged specimen of urine) indicates a high likelihood of true bacteriuria in patients with symptoms of UTIs.
    (D) Expressed prostatic secretions containing polymorphonuclear leukocytes are diagnostic for chronic bacterial prostatitis.
    (E) In patients who have acute symptomatic UTIs associated with a continued indwelling catheter, initial treatment should be limited to the usual 10- to 14-day course.

33. A short delay from sleep onset to first REM sleep is associated with:

    (A) REM interruption insomnia
    (B) Major depression
    (C) Narcolepsy
    (D) Hypersomnia-sleep apnea syndrome
    (E) Normal aging

34. Addictive drugs include:

    (A) Barbiturates
    (B) Diazepam
    (C) Pentazocine
    (D) Tricyclic antidepressants
    (E) Propoxyphene

35. True statements concerning treatment with aminoglycosides in elderly patients include:

    (A) Age-related changes in renal function modify the serum levels of aminoglycosides.
    (B) There is evidence that the combination of an aminoglycoside and a

loop diuretic (e.g., furosemide or ethacrynic acid) is more likely to precipitate deafness than either drug given alone.

(C) Age-related changes in hepatic function modify the serum levels of aminoglycosides.

(D) Peritoneal lavage with aminoglycoside solutions is a safe procedure as these drugs are poorly absorbed from the peritoneum.

(E) If aminoglycosides are to be prescribed for prolonged periods, formal hearing and renal function tests are essential.

36. In elderly persons:

(A) Influenza vaccine must be given at least 2 weeks prior to contact in order to be effective.

(B) Influenza vaccine has an overall efficacy of approximately 85%.

(C) The only contraindication to influenza vaccine is allergy to eggs.

(D) Infection with type B influenza virus is prevented by prior administration of amantadine hydrochloride.

(E) Influenza infection that is treated with amantadine hydrochloride should have the therapy continued for 1 week following the disappearance of symptoms.

Controversies in
Geriatric Medicine

Fundamentals of Geriatric Medicine, edited by
Ronald D. T. Cape, Rodney M. Coe, and Isadore
Rossman, Raven Press, New York © 1983.

27

Overview

Richard W. Besdine

Controversy in clinical medicine generally exists when definitive data are not available concerning optimum management and different opinions are espoused by the proponents of various positions. At one extreme opinions are based on anecdote, and at the other extreme truly conflicting data generate differing views. Between these extremes is a spectrum of opinion and suggestive data which produce fruitful controversy and grounds for further investigation, culminating in definitive studies that identify the ideal clinical approach. Historical examples abound, e.g., discovery of the etiology and treatment of tuberculosis or typhoid fever or more recently the accelerated elucidation of Legionnaires' disease.

Until recently, medical controversy concerning care of the elderly was rare, largely because health care of older individuals was not identified as having a data base separate from that for younger people. Controversy in geriatric medicine was largely the statement of strong anecdotal views by different individuals or groups arguing from a predetermined perspective on the elderly. However, controversy in geriatrics has now taken an exciting new form. Traditional medical myths about elderly patients are being refuted by new data from reliable clinical studies, making controversy of this sort transient. Much of the controversy addressed by the chapters in this section falls into this transient category, in which medical controversy evolves from polemic to research to sound practice (2).

One manifestation of elderly patient neglect is the shortage of clinically relevant research on which to base geriatric health care. Therefore it is gratifying and reassuring to note the sharp increase in age-related academic activity in American medicine. Curriculum and faculty development in gerontology and geriatric medicine are at least agenda items if not high priorities at a majority of medical schools (3). Implicit in efforts to improve clinical care of the elderly through education is a clinical research mandate to expand boundaries of knowledge about health and disease during old age. In no other field is there such ripe opportunity to improve health care through direct clinical research, with both the well elderly (to derive expanded standards of normative age-related differences) and the sick elderly (to learn more about disease and treatment differences in old age) (4). The ultimate goal is a synthesis of information from studies of normal aging and disease in the eldery, yielding a data base that allows quantification of and differentiation between age effect and disease effect in each functionally impaired old person. As each organ system and functional unit is better understood, old controversies will dissolve and new ones will crystallize for the solution of geriatric problems.

CLINICAL ETHICAL ISSUES IN GERIATRIC MEDICINE

In addition to the major specific categories covered in this section, there is another kind of controversy in geriatric medicine that is less amenable to research clarification. Ethical questions abound and intrude daily into the practices of physicians treating elderly patients, and yet efforts to help identify and clarify the impact of ethical issues in care of aged individuals are just beginning (1). When is the quality of life so reduced by intense or prolonged suffering caused by the treatment that the treatment itself should be withheld? When is life so painful or intolerable that treatment should be withheld solely to allow relief through death? Should there be different standards for intervention with the cognitively impaired elderly? Do elderly individuals with cognitive loss have a basic right to diagnostic evaluation of their losses? Should nursing home residents have different treatment standards, considering the negative societal view of nursing home living? When these and other ethical questions complicate treatment issues in elderly patients and the physician is not aware of the ethical component, frustration and endless fruitless consultation often further confuse the basic unidentified dilemma.

The most essential aspect of successful management of clinical ethical problems in elderly patients is early detection. From the first encounter with a complicated, ill, elderly patient, the physician must identify ethical components and consider them concurrently with the technical biomedical aspects of diagnosis and treatment. Failure to identify and evaluate the ethical aspects of an illness guarantees that clinical decisions will be fragmented, based on an incomplete data set, and inadequate over the long term. For example, the initial decision to insert a nasogastric feeding tube, when based solely on the patient's inability to obtain nutrition and hydration per os, neglects the inevitable dilemmas and complications engendered by continuing the feedings. If quality of life is poor or nonexistent, it is much easier to withhold treatment originally than to discontinue measures once begun. Ventilatory support of a patient with respiratory failure raises the same issues but is additionally complicated by the expensive technology of the respiratory intensive care unit. Again, withholding endotracheal intubation or tracheostomy is far easier than discontinuing either based on the delayed recognition that the life being preserved is an agonizing, continuing burden to the patient and family.

Once ethical components of a clinical problem are identified, an even greater chore looms for the clinician. How does one determine when treatment of a treatable condition should be withheld? The supervening principle governing the decision to withhold treatment is based on life quality, suffering, and pain. If life quality is terrible or likely to become so even if treatment is successful, then one must consider withholding that treatment, allowing death to relieve present agonies and prevent future ones. Certain guidelines can and should be established governing decision-making when such problems arise: (a) Treatment should never be withheld solely because of a patient's age. (b) When conscious and competent, the patient must be the primary decision maker if treatment is to be withheld; however, when deciding whether to initiate heroic or extreme treatment, the physician, in collaboration with the patient, family, and other relevant persons, has primary responsibility for the decision. (c) Withholding treatment should be considered only when a reasonably certain diagnosis and prognosis can be made. (d) If the proposed treatment produces extreme suffering and reduced life quality, likely worse than the progression of the disease itself, then treatment may best be avoided. (e) In the temporary absence of requisite information necessary for deciding to withhold treatment, the treatment should be vigorously initiated.

Employing these general guidelines, useful individual clinical clues for deciding to withhold treatment of a potentially treatable disease must be vigorously pursued from all available sources, including the patient, family, friends, and previous caregivers. Each patient problem must be evaluated individually by the entire health care team, providing clear information to patient and family, allowing them meaningful participation. Any further categorical rules about withholding or initiating treatment would be restrictive to the decision makers, who have the profound responsibility of life and death.

SUMMARY

The investigative mandate generated by controversy in care of the elderly is clear. Only when gerontological and geriatric medical studies have enlarged the data base of geriatrics will we be able to draw on an adequate scientific foundation to allow optimum care of ill elderly. Until then clinicians must be receptive to any data in controversial but inadequately studied areas which might suggest opportunities for improved care.

REFERENCES

1. Beauchamp, T. L., and Childress, J. *Principles of Biomedical Ethics*. Oxford University Press, New York, 1979.
2. Besdine, R. W. Geriatric medicine: an overview. *Annu. Rev. Gerontol. Geriatrics*, 1:135–153, 1980.
3. Institute of Medicine. *Aging in Medical Education*. National Academy of Sciences, Washington, DC, 1978.
4. Rowe, J. W. Clinical research on aging: strategies and directions. *N. Engl. J. Med.*, 297:1332–1336, 1977.

Fundamentals of Geriatric Medicine, edited by
Ronald D. T. Cape, Rodney M. Coe, and Isadore
Rossman, Raven Press, New York © 1983.

28

Hypertension in the Elderly

William B. Kannel, Fred Brand, and Daniel McGee

Epidemiological investigations at Framingham and elsewhere have yielded data which emphasize the importance of hypertension as a contributor to cardiovascular morbidity and mortality (19,34,36,40). Because cardiovascular disease (CVD) is a prominent cause of death and disability in the aged, a detailed examination of the role of blood pressure in the development of CVD in the elderly is warranted.

The clinical significance of hypertension in the elderly is in doubt (16), and some clinicians question if vigorous treatment of hypertension in the elderly is worthwhile or safe. Some even appear to consider the rise in pressure observed with aging as an inevitable and normal physiological occurrence necessary to maintain perfusion of vital organs to compensate for progressive sclerosis of the arterial system.

METHODS

In the Framingham Study a cohort of 5,209 men and women aged 30 to 62 years at the start of the study has been followed biennially for a period of 20 years. Each biennial examination included blood pressure determinations and a cardiovascular examination to determine which members of the cohort had developed CVD. The criteria for CVD and the methods employed for the investigation of its possible precursors have been published elsewhere in detail (40). The cardiovascular sequelae of hypertension which were examined include coronary heart disease, cardiac failure, atherothrombotic brain infarction, and occlusive peripheral arterial disease. All cases of CVD evolving in the cohort are included in the present report. This includes patients who were not hospitalized, cases which were suddenly fatal, cases of unrecognized disease, and cases not under medical care. Follow-up has been reasonably complete, with 85% of subjects taking each clinical examination and only 2% lost to follow-up for death.

Each new case of CVD was verified by a second physician examiner, and the final diagnostic decision was made by a panel of investigators applying uniform criteria (40). Blood pressures were determined with the patients seated with their arm on a desk using a cuff large enough to encircle the most obese arm. A mercury sphygmomanometer was employed. Three blood pressure readings were obtained on each biennial examination, two by a physician and one by a nurse.

The contribution of hypertension and blood pressure to the occurrence of cardiovascular sequelae was determined by estimating univariate and multivariate coefficients for the regression of incidence of CVD on blood pressure (40,44).

RESULTS

During the first 20 years of follow-up there were enough persons in the age range 65 to 74 to provide 3,876 person-years of experience for men and 5,924 person-years for women. During this period at risk, there developed 108 cardiovascular events in men and 128 in women. Among this age group there were 160 deaths in men and 133 in women.

PREVALENCE

The Framingham Study defines definite hypertension as systolic blood pressures above 160 mm Hg or diastolic pressures over 95 mm Hg (40). By this definition, about 22% of men and 34% of women between 65 and 74 years of age were hypertensive (Table 1).

Examination of age trends in blood pressure indicate that systolic blood pressure rises almost linearly with age, whereas diastolic blood pressure rises until the mid-fifties in men and the early sixties in women, and then begins to decline (9). This is consistent with a decrease in arterial capacitance and progressive loss of elasticity of the arterial system. Because of the differing age trends for the two components of blood pressure, the prevalence of isolated systolic hypertension increases with age to a high level in the elderly. Using the commonly accepted definitions of systolic hypertension (i.e., systolic pressure over 160 mm Hg and diastolic pressure concurrently below 95 mm Hg), 30% of women and 18% of men have this condition (Fig. 1), commonly attributed to an inelastic vasculature. Data from peripheral pulse wave recordings using the depth of the dicrotic notch to reflect the elastic recoil of the vasculature is consistent with this notion. Flattened or absent dicrotic notches were noted with a prevalence of 1.3% between age 45 and 54, increasing to a prevalence of 10.8% between ages 65 and 74 (6).

TABLE 1. *Average prevalence of hypertension in Framingham cohort over 20 years of follow-up, age 65–74*

Blood pressure status	% Prevalence	
	Men	Women
Normotensive	39.5	24.8
Borderline	38.7	40.8
Hypertensive	21.8	34.4

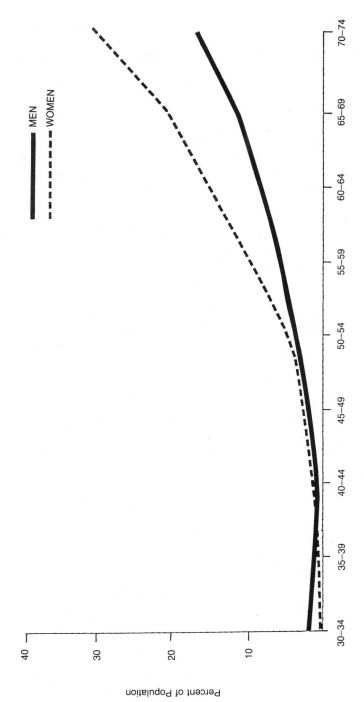

FIG. 1. Prevalence of isolated systolic hypertension (%): Framingham study, 20-year follow-up.

This rigidity of the vasculature did not appear to inhibit the lability of the pressure, as the degree of lability, determined from standard deviations of three pressures, actually increased with age. Also, contrary to expectation, the lability increased with the level of the pressure. Lability was not characteristic of elderly persons from one examination to another (10).

CARDIOVASCULAR SEQUELAE

Hypertension is a recognized prominent contributor to overall mortality, for which it generally doubles the risk, and to cardiovascular mortality, for which risk in the hypertensive is tripled compared to that in normotensive persons (20). This takes on added significance in the elderly because the absolute risk is greater than in the younger hypertensive.

Attributable risk, which takes into account the high prevalence of hypertension and the high relative risk, is as great in the elderly as in the young. This is also apparent in computation of coefficients for the regression of CVD on blood pressure (Table 2).

The impact of hypertension is greatest for stroke and least for occlusive peripheral arterial disease, comparing the risk ratios of the elderly hypertensive subject with normotensives the same age within each sex. In terms of *absolute* incidence, coronary heart disease is still the most common sequela in the hypertensive elderly, as it is in the young (Table 3).

There is no evidence that elderly women tolerate hypertension better than elderly men. Relative risks are just as large for women, and the attributable risk for women is actually greater over age 65 than for men (Tables 2 and 3). Regarding stroke and cardiac failure, even the absolute risks are no better in women than men.

It is not safe to await evidence of target organ involvement in the elderly hypertensive before instituting treatment. About a third of the cardiovascular sequelae which occurred in the hypertensive elderly appeared before such evidence could be ascertained on biennial examinations (Table 4).

The risk of developing CVD is higher when there is evidence of organ involvement. The occurrence of left ventricular hypertrophy (LVH) on the electrocardi-

TABLE 2. *Risk of CVD according to age in hypertensives: Framingham study, 20-year follow-up*

Age	Incidence per 1000		Risk ratio[a]		Regression coefficient		Attributable risk	
	Men	Women	Men	Women	Men	Women	Men	Women
45–54	23.6	9.7	2.7	3.6	.521	.654	16.4	17.4
55–64	43.9	23.7	2.8	3.9	.544	.668	17.9	26.5
65–74	51.0	35.6	3.0	4.1	.575	.654	18.8	26.9
All ages	35.7	20.6	2.8	3.5	.537	.643		

[a]Risk ratio = rate in HBPs/rate in normotensives.

TABLE 3. *Risk of specified cardiovascular events according to hypertensive status: Framingham study, 20-year follow-up, age 65–74*

Blood pressure status	Coronary disease[a]		Stroke		Peripheral arterial disease		Cardiac failure	
	Men	Women	Men	Women	Men	Women	Men	Women
Normotensive	12.4	5.4	2.7	0.6	6.2	2.6	3.9	3.2
Borderline	24.0	13.7	8.1	6.4	5.9	2.6	6.8	6.3
Hypertensive	28.4	22.1	18.9	16.4	7.0	5.9	18.1	9.7

[a]All trends significant at $p < 0.01$ except for peripheral arterial disease.

TABLE 4. *Hypertensive patients who developed CVD with no prior evidence of target organ involvement: Framingham study, 20-year follow-up*

Age	% with CVD	
	Men	Women
35–44	75	33
45–54	58	56
55–64	48	38
65–74	33	33
All ages	50	39

Target organ involvement: CE x-ray, ECG abnormalities (LVH, NSA, IVB), or albuminuria.

TABLE 5. *5-Year incidence of death and CVD according to ECG LVH: Framingham study, 20-year follow-up, age 65–74*

ECG LVH	Cardiovascular morbidity (%)		Cardiovascular mortality (%)		Total mortality (%)	
	Men	Women	Men	Women	Men	Women
None	13.9	10.6	6.4	4.1	14.2	7.9
Possible	27.3	23.0	20.6	15.4	29.4	20.6
Definite	45.0	43.7	40.6	29.9	53.4	36.2
Risk ratio	3.8	4.6	6.3	7.3	3.8	4.6
t-Value	8.29	9.19	14.50	11.54	12.69	9.76

ogram (ECG) is particularly ominous. Elderly persons who developed ECG evidence of LVH had a 5-year mortality of about 50% for men and about 35% for women. Cardiovascular mortality occurred in 40% of men and 30% of women. A major cardiovascular event of some sort occurred within 5 years in 45% of men and 44% of women (Table 5).

SYSTOLIC HYPERTENSION

Even isolated systolic hypertension proved far from innocuous and was associated with a two- to fivefold excess risk of cardiovascular mortality (Table 6). Cardiovascular morbidity was also increased to almost four times that expected for subjects the same age (Table 6).

The clinical impression that lability indicates a less serious form of hypertension could not be substantiated. Multivariate analysis revealed no evidence that lability affects the level of cardiovascular risk at a given degree of hypertension (10). Thus attention to the lability of the blood pressure and to the diastolic component adds little to the assessment of risk of cardiovascular sequelae associated with blood pressure elevation in the elderly.

SURVIVAL AFTER MYOCARDIAL INFARCTION

The relation of blood pressure to survival after myocardial infarction has been in doubt, particularly in the elderly. Blood pressure after myocardial infarction has been found in Framingham to be unrelated to survival, whereas the blood pressure level before infarction was related to subsequent mortality. This is because a fall in blood pressure is associated with an ominous prognosis, reflecting the damage sustained by the myocardium as a result of the infarction. When those who sustained a fall in blood pressure as a result of infarction are excluded from consideration, there is a distinct relationship of blood pressure status to subsequent survival after infarction as is seen before the event (21).

DISCUSSION

Most population surveys have shown rises in systolic and diastolic blood pressure with age in both sexes (28,30,32). In western society such a rise in pressure with age is usual but not inevitable, as many individuals do not show elevated pressures during advanced age. In some primitive societies rises in pressure with age are not seen at all (33).

TABLE 6. *Two-year morbidity and mortality associated with isolated systolic hypertension: Framingham study, 20-year follow-up, age 55–74[a]*

	Men		Women	
Parameter	Rate per 1,000	Factor of increased risk[b]	Rate per 1,000	Factor of increased risk
Death (all causes)	56	2.0	29	2.0
Cardiovascular mortality	30	1.8	24	4.7
Cardiovascular morbidity	114	3.6	50	3.8

[a]Excludes persons having diastolic blood pressure ≥95 mm Hg at any time over 20 years.
[b]Risk ratio = ratio or rates in isolated systolic HBP and normotensives.

Because a given degree of blood pressure elevation carries the same relative risk and a higher absolute risk in the elderly than in the young, it seems pointless to accept the usual level of pressures in the elderly as "normal." Feinstein (7) pointed out that what is common is not necessarily normal as regards optimal function. Life insurance and epidemiological data have shown consistently that the impact of blood pressure does not diminish as a cause of cardiovascular morbidity and mortality with advancing age (22,28,31,34). Men aged 65 to 74 with hypertension in the Framingham cohort had twice the total mortality per year of those with normal pressures. The difference in mortality was 2.4% per year for this age group compared to only 1.2% for men aged 45 to 54. Furthermore, 25% of older men have hypertension, compared to 11% of younger men; thus the attributable risk is as great or greater in the elderly as in the young. The Framingham Study and other epidemiological population surveys have clearly demonstrated that the cost of hypertension to the community in terms of associated cardiovascular mortality rises with age in both men and women. Thus there is no justification for neglecting high blood pressure among the elderly.

Because systolic blood pressure increases more with age than the diastolic pressure, the prevalence of hypertension characterized primarily by systolic blood pressure elevation is much higher in the elderly (28,30,32). The widened pulse pressure is largely due to the lesser distensibility of the large arterial vessels at higher pressures. Even in normotensive persons, aging tends to displace the arterial pressure-volume curve downward and decrease its slope or arterial capacitance (14,31). Perhaps a more useful index of arterial rigidity than the depth of the dicrotic notch is the ratio of pulse pressure to stroke volume. In hypertensive persons this index correlates significantly with age (43). The frequency of disproportionate systolic pressure elevations, if not isolated systolic hypertension, increases progressively with age (24–26,38). The fact that hypertension in the elderly is predominantly systolic does not make it an innocuous condition (13,24,25). Elevated systolic pressure has been demonstrated to be an important independent contributor to cardiac failure and vascular sequelae of hypertension. Isolated systolic hypertension has been shown at Framingham and elsewhere to be associated with an increased risk of coronary heart disease, stroke, and renal failure (5,11,28).

There is little evidence to support the contention that systolic hypertension is only an index of the degree of atherosclerotic change in the large arteries (24,25). There is no apparent reason why the damage caused to the arterial system by hypertension should derive more from the diastolic than the systolic pressure. Cardiac failure and left ventricular hypertrophy are determined by left ventricular afterload, which in turn derives more from the systolic than the diastolic pressure. Furthermore, one would expect the occurrence of subarachnoid hemorrhage, dissecting aortic aneurysm, or intracerebral hemorrhage to derive more from the peak pressure during each cardiac cycle than the pressure between cardiac beats.

There is still a question as to whether the risk associated with hypertension in the elderly is reversible with treatment. Additionally, treatment is inconvenient and risks major adverse drug effects. The effort and expense are justified only if the quality of life can be improved. It is believed that therapeutic misadventures are more likely in the elderly because in the aged the cardiac output decreases with an increase in arterial pressure (29). The aorta and proximal arteries of old people dilate and the walls of the peripheral arteries thicken (2), increasing cardiac work.

Postural hypotension complicates antihypertensive therapy in the elderly. The blood pressure is regulated by baroreceptor reflexes, which become less sensitive in the aged (8). It seems that the reduced sensitivity of the baroreflex results from the decreased distensibility of the arterial wall in which the baroreceptors are located (2). Postural hypotension is a result of this reduced sensitivity of the baroreflex arc (3,18). Postural hypotension was first clearly delineated as a feature of autonomic damage (37). Autonomic dysfunction can arise from three main causes: (a) isolated damage to the autonomic system, e.g., primary postural hypotension (40); (b) toxic or pharmacological agents which interfere with autonomic reflexes; and (c) systemic disease, of which diabetes mellitus is the most common.

Hypotension in the elderly may also be augmented by a diminished plasma renin response to standing (4), itself due to impaired sympathetic innervation of the juxtaglomerular apparatus. The patient may be asymptomatic despite a large drop in systolic blood pressure, or he or she may have postural weakness, dizziness, faintness, visual impairment, or syncope. These symptoms may be worsened by a variety of drugs, including hypotensive agents, diuretics, and vasodilators.

Caird et al. (3) found that 24% of the ambulant elderly show a systolic drop of 20 mm Hg or more and 5% had a drop of 40 mm Hg or more. Therefore many physicians are uncertain if symptomless hypertensive elderly subjects need treatment and, if so, at what blood pressure level. According to some researchers (23), antihypertensive therapy is indicated for symptomless hypertensive old subjects only when the diastolic pressure is persistently 105 to 110 mm Hg. However, our study showed that systolic hypertension was associated with a two- to fivefold excess risk of cardiovascular mortality.

Although recommendations for the treatment of hypertension in the elderly abound, no objective data based on clinical trials are available. Because cardiac output, glomerular filtration rate, renal blood flow, tubular function, and some hepatic metabolic functions decline in the elderly, the half-life of many drugs is increased and clearance slowed. However, few studies of the pharmacokinetics of antihypertensive drugs in the elderly have been done.

In the elderly, initiation of treatment should be gradual and cautious. Benefits and risks in these individuals need further study, particularly with regard to treatment of isolated systolic hypertension. There is some evidence that we may be making some headway, as the elderly have shared the decline in cardiovascular mortality since 1968. This has been true despite severe undertreatment of hypertension in the elderly. A controlled clinical trial is long overdue to better determine the indications, contraindications, best drugs, side effects, benefits, and hazards of treating hypertension in the elderly. Because of the high morbidity and mortality in this age group, this is a therapeutic and preventive challenge which physicians should accept.

Appropriate management of hypertension in the elderly is still ill-defined. Very little definitive information is available, as only 10% of patients included in 41 published clinical trials of antihypertensive treatment were over 60 (27). Although it is generally agreed that at any age persons with sustained diastolic pressures exceeding 115 mm Hg should be treated, the indication for treatment at lower pressures is controversial. In general, studies of the effectiveness of drug therapy in the elderly, mildly to moderately hypertensive patient contain too few subjects to allow an evaluation. However, the excess mortality and morbidity associated with all varieties of hypertension in the elderly is substantial. Also, results thus far do not indicate any adverse effects, and some evidence suggests benefit. Furthermore, new drugs with fewer such effects and more rational use of old drugs permits treatment with fewer side effects than was possible a decade ago.

Systolic hypertension constitutes a problem, as it is often resistant to therapy (42) and aggressive treatment may lower associated diastolic pressures to an extent which may jeopardize flow to vital organs (24,25). Until proof of efficacy is available, too aggressive management cannot be advocated.

Side effects in the elderly appear to be two to three times as common as in younger persons (15,17,45). Compliance may also be more difficult in elderly patients because of side effects or failing memory, inattentiveness, and complex dosage regimens.

The elderly seem to be more susceptible to unwanted effects of antihypertensive agents which can depress the central nervous system; and hence reserpine, methyldopa, and clonidine are best avoided.

Because the elderly are susceptible to postural hypertension as a result of less-responsive baroreceptors (1,35,39), it is best to avoid adrenergic blockers such as guanethidine, bethanidine, and debrisoquin.

Vasodilators may increase arterial compliance and may be useful because the baroreflex-mediated increase in heart rate which accompanies their use is often less pronounced in the elderly (41). Hence hydralazine is often well tolerated. Although responsiveness is reduced in the elderly, β-blockers are suitable but may cause more adverse reactions (12). Thiazides are economical and effective, and are usually well tolerated in the elderly. Because the elderly may lose potassium, supplementation may be necessary, although hyperkalemia can occur even when supplements are used.

The goal of therapy should be pressures of 150/90 mm Hg. If this is not achieved with thiazide and β-blockers, hydralazine may be added. Although an active approach is justified by the hazards, incomplete information on efficacy mandates caution.

SUMMARY

The controversies surrounding the treatment of hypertension in the elderly are pointed out. The conclusions drawn are based mainly on findings in the Framingham Study. Treatment of hypertension at any age is recommended.

When caring for elderly patients, the physician should:

1. Know the prevalence of hypertension in elderly persons.
2. Understand the role of hypertension in the development of cardiovascular morbidity and mortality in elderly persons.
3. Know how risk factors in hypertension may vary between younger and older patients.
4. Know the principal factors guiding the use of antihypertensive drugs in the management of hypertension in the aged.

REFERENCES

1. Appenzeller, O., and Descarries, L. Circulatory reflexes in patients with cerebrovascular disease. *N. Engl. J. Med.*, 271:820–823, 1964.
2. Bader, H. Dependence of wall stress in the human thoracic aorta on age and pressure. *Cir. Res.*, 20:354, 1967.
3. Caird, F. I., Andrews, G. R., and Kennedy, R. D. Effect of posture on blood pressure in the elderly. *Br. Heart J.*, 35:527–530, 1973.
4. Christlieb, A. R., Munichoodappa, C., and Braaten, J. J. Decrease response of plasma renin activity to orthostasis in diabetic patients with orthostatic hypotension. *Diabetes*, 23:835–840, 1974.
5. Colandrea, M. A., Friedman, G. D., Nichaman, M. Z., and Lynd, C. S. Systolic hypertension in the elderly: an epidemiologic assessment. *Circulation*, 41:239, 1970.
6. Dawber, T. R., Thomas, H. E., Jr., and McNamara, P. M. Characteristics of the dicrotic notch of the arterial pulse wave in coronary heart disease. *Angiology*, 24:244, 1973.
7. Feinstein, A. R. The derangements of the "range of normal." *Clin. Pharmacol. Ther.*, 15:528, 1974.
8. Gibblin, B., Pickering, T. G., Sleight, P., and Peto, R. Effect of age and high blood pressure on baroreflex sensitivity in man. *Circ. Res.*, 29:424, 1971.
9. Gordon, T., and Shurtleff, D. *Means at Each Examination and Inter-examination Variation of Specified Characteristics: The Framingham Study*, edited by W. B. Kannel and T. Gordon. DHEW Publ. No (NIH) 74–478. Government Printing Office, Washington, DC, 1974.
10. Gordon, T., Sorlie, P., and Kannel, W. B. Problems in the assessment of blood pressure: The Framingham Study. *Int. J. Epidemiol.*, 5:327–334, 1972.
11. Goss, L. Z., Rosa, R. M. F., and O'Brien, W. M. Predicting death from renal failure in primary hypertension. *Arch. Intern. Med.*, 124:160, 1969.
12. Greenblatt, D. J., and Koch-Weser, J. Adverse reactions to propranolol in hospitalized medical patients: a report from the Boston collaborative drug surveillance program. *Am. Heart J.*, 86:478–484, 1973.
13. Gubner, R. S. Systolic hypertension: a pathogenetic entity; significance and therapeutic considerations. *Am. J. Cardiol.*, 9:773, 1962.
14. Ho, J. K., Lin, L. Y., and Galysh, F. T. Aortic compliance: studies on its relationship to aortic constituents in man. *Arch. Pathol.*, 94:537, 1972.
15. Hurwitz, N. Predisposing factors in adverse reactions to drugs. *Br. Med. J.*, 1:536–539, 1969.
16. Hypertension in the elderly. *Lancet*, 1:684–685, 1977.
17. Jackson, G., Pierscianowski, T. A., Mahon, W., and Condon, J. Inappropriate antihypertensive therapy in the elderly. *Lancet*, 2:1317–1318, 1976.
18. Johnson, R. H., Smith, A. C., Spalding, J. K. M., and Wollner, L. Effect of posture on blood pressure in elderly patients. *Lancet*, 1:731–733, 1965.
19. Kannel, W. B. Role of blood pressure in cardiovascular morbidity and mortality. *Prog. Cardiovasc. Dis.*, 17:5, 1974.
20. Kannel, W. B., and Sorlie, P. Hypertension in Framingham. In: *Proceedings of the 2nd International Symposium on the Epidemiology of Hypertension*. Chicago Symposia Specialists, Chicago, 1974.
21. Kannel, W. B., Sorlie, P., Castelli, W. P., and McGee, D. Blood pressure and survival following myocardial infarction: the Framingham study. *Am. J. Cardiol.*, 45:326–330, 1980.

22. Kannel, W. B., Wolf, P. A., Verter, J., and McNamara, P. M. Epidemiologic assessment of the role of blood pressure in stroke: the Framingham study. *JAMA*, 214:301, 1970.
23. Kennedy, R. D. High blood pressure and its management. In: *Cardiology in Old Age*, edited by F. I. Caird, J. L. C. Dall, and R. D. Kennedy. Plenum Press, New York, 1976.
24. Koch-Weser, J. Correlation of pathophysiology and pharmacotherapy in primary hypertension. *Am. J. Cardiol.*, 32:499, 1973.
25. Koch-Weser, J. The therapeutic challenge of systolic hypertension. *N. Engl. J. Med.*, 289:481–483, 1973.
26. Koch-Weser, J. Modern approaches to the treatment of hypertension. In: *Clinical Pharmacy and Pharmacology*, edited by W. A. Gouveia, G. Tognoni, and E. V. D. Kleijn. Elsevier/North Holland, Amsterdam, 1976.
27. Koch-Weser, J. Arterial hypertension in old age. *Herz*, 3:235–244, 1978.
28. Lew, E. A. *Build and Blood Pressure Study*. Society of Actuaries, Chicago, 1959.
29. Masoro, E. Other physiologic changes with age. In: *Conference on the Epidemiology of Aging, Elkridge, Maryland, 1972*, edited by A. M. Ostfeld and D. C. Gibson. Government Printing Office, Washington, DC, 1975.
30. Master, A. M., and Lasser, R. P. Blood pressure elevation in the elderly. In: *Hypertension. Recent Advances*, edited by A. N. Brest and J. H. Moyer. Lea & Fibiger, Philadelphia, 1961.
31. Miall, W. E., and Chinn, S. Screening for hypertension: some epidemiologic observations. *Br. Med. J.*, 3:595, 1974.
32. National Center for Health Statistics. *Blood Pressure Levels of Persons 6–74 Years of Age in the United States*, Series II, No. 203. Government Printing Office, Rockville, MD, 1977.
33. Page, L. P., and Sidd, J. J. Medical management of arterial hypertension. *N. Engl. J. Med.*, 287:960, 1972.
34. Paul, O. Risks of mild hypertension: a ten-year report. *Br. Heart J. (Suppl.)*, 33:116, 1970.
35. Pickering, T. G., Gribbin, B., and Oliver, D. O. Baroreflex sensitivity in patients on long term dialysis. *Clin. Sci.*, 43:645–657, 1972.
36. Report of intersociety commission for heart disease resources: the primary prevention of the atherosclerotic diseases. In: *Guidelines for Prevention and Care*, edited by I. S. Wright and D. T. Fredrickson. US GPO, Washington, DC, 1974.
37. Rundles, R. W. Diabetic neuropathy: a general review with report of 125 cases. *Medicine*, 24:111–160, 1945.
38. Seligman, A. W., Alderman, M. H., Engelland, A. L., and Davis, T. K. Treatment of systolic hypertension. *Clin. Res.*, 25:254A, 1977.
39. Sharpey-Schafer, E. P. Effects of Valsalva's manoeuvre on the normal and failing circulation. *Br. Med. J.*, 1:693–695, 1955.
40. Shurtleff, D. *Some Characteristics Related to the Incidence of Cardiovascular Disease and Death: Framingham Study, 18-Year Follow-up*, Sect. 30, edited by W. B. Kannel and T. Gordon. DHEW Publ. No. (NIH) 74-599. US GPO, Washington, DC, 1974.
41. Simon, A. C., Safar, M. A., Levenson, J. A., Kheder, A. M., and Levy, B. I. Systolic hypertension: hemodynamic mechanism and choice of antihypertensive treatment. *Am. J. Cardiol.*, 44:505–511, 1979.
42. Tarazi, R. C., and Gifford, R. W., Jr. Clinical significance and management of systolic hypertension. In: *Hypertension: Mechanisms, Diagnosis, and Treatment*, edited by G. Onesti and A. N. Brest. Davis, Philadelphia, 1978.
43. Tarazi, R. C., Magrini, F., and Dustan, H. P. The role of aortic distensibility in hypertension. In: *Advances in Hypertension*, Vol. 2, edited by P. Milliez and M. Safar. Boehringer Ingelheim, Elmsford, NY, 1975.
44. Walker, S. H., and Duncan, D. B. Estimation of the probability of an event as a function of several independent variables. *Biometrics*, 54:167, 1967.
45. Williamson, J. Adverse reactions to prescribed drugs in the elderly. In: *Drugs and the Elderly*, edited by J. Crooks and I. H. Stevenson. Macmillan, London, 1979.

Fundamentals of Geriatric Medicine, edited by
Ronald D. T. Cape, Rodney M. Coe, and Isadore
Rossman, Raven Press, New York © 1983.

29

Estrogen Replacement Therapy

Kenneth J. Ryan

Consideration of estrogen use as a replacement therapy must be based on some understanding of how and when estrogens normally decline during aging, what estrogen effects if any one should try to maintain after the menopause, and the risks to the patient associated with estrogen therapy. Although more studies are needed, there are sufficient data to help the health care provider and the individual patient make informed choices regarding estrogen use.

ENDOCRINE CHANGES IN AGING WOMEN

By the time a female patient reaches the geriatric stage, she is already postmenopausal, and the question very often is whether to discontinue hormones for those patients who are on estrogens at the time they are first seen (for symptoms or bone loss) or to institute or reinstitute their use. Such considerations require a careful review of the needs of the individual patient.

Endocrine Stages in the Perimenopausal Transition

Women are born with a finite number of ova and follicles, which decrease with age. These follicles become less sensitive to gonadotropin [follicle-stimulating hormone (FSH) and luteinizing hormone (LH)] effects and produce less estrogen even though there may be occasional menstrual periods (hence the occurrence of menopausal signs and symptoms even before the ovaries fail and menstruation stops completely). Gonadotropins may be intermittently elevated. This can occur in women 40 to 50 years of age. At some stage in this depletion of follicles and ova, insufficient levels of estrogen are produced by the ovaries and the menopause ensues.

Endocrine Changes of the Menopause

The menopause is operationally defined as absence of menses for 1 year due to ovarian failure, but the diagnosis can be made whenever complete ovarian failure can be ascertained. It usually occurs between the ages of 48 and 52. As follicles are functionally inactive, little estradiol is produced; ovulation ceases, and no corpora lutea are formed. The gonadotropins rise and remain elevated until late in life, the FSH levels being higher than LH levels in the blood. One can make the diagnosis of ovarian failure by measuring FSH and LH with clinically available assays. As the FSH and LH may be intermittently high and low in the perimenopause transition, one assay taken during this time may not be definitive. Aging affects gonadotropin production, and much later in life levels of gonadotropins may decline.

Women make another estrogen, estrone, in body fat from an androgen produced by the adrenal glands. This nonovarian source of estrogen is present throughout life but increases at the time of menopause and becomes the only, or major, source of estrogen after the menopause. Estrone can also be formed from estradiol in many body tissues, but it is only one-tenth as active as estradiol. This menopausal source of estrogen (i.e., estrone produced in adipose tissue) may cause postmenopausal bleeding and/or may reduce menopausal signs and symptoms of estrogen lack. The amount produced is proportional to the weight (and amount of body fat) of the subject. The estrone produced may therefore be variable in amount, and patients differ with respect to this, just as they vary in symptoms.

Progesterone, which is produced premenopausally by the corpus luteum only in cycles where ovulation occurs, is essentially not present during the postmenopausal period.

Ordinarily, estrogen and progesterone work in concert and sequentially on tissues, with the estrogen inducing the ability of a target cell to respond to progesterone. Normal endometrial development occurs each month as a result of this sequential action of estrogen and progesterone. If ovulation does not occur, only estrogen is secreted. In the absence of progesterone, the endometrial cells may become hyperplastic and develop premalignant changes if stimulated only by estrogens. One of the problems in replacing only estrogen postmenopausally is the absence of the modifying effect of progesterone in tissues such as breast and uterus.

In summary, after the menopause, ovarian estradiol and progesterone disappear, gonadotropins (FSH and LH) rise, and the estrone synthesized in body fat becomes the sole source of estrogen hormone.

SYMPTOMS OF ESTROGEN LACK AFTER THE MENOPAUSE

The only symptoms which seem to be specific for estrogen lack at the time of menopause are hot flashes (vasomotor instability) and vaginal dryness and atrophy. Women vary in the frequency and intensity of hot flashes as well as their reaction to them. The hot flashes may decrease over time, but in some cases they persist and may be disabling.

Estrogens ordinarily relieve these symptoms and in some instances may provide dramatic improvement in the individual's sense of well-being. Hot flashes are also marginally improved with placebo, and recently progestins have been shown to be effective. The etiology of the hot flash is not known, but the condition can be verified by increases in skin temperature synchronous with the feeling of warmth. Hot flashes may result in sweating, insomnia, and other more general menopausal symptoms, all of which are improved when the hot flash is relieved.

Vaginal atrophy is generally progressive due to estrogen lack. It results in pain on coitus, narrowing of the vagina, lack of lubrication, itching, and burning. Although simple lubricants can help with dyspareunia, estrogens will specifically improve the atrophy.

Most other general symptoms (e.g., depression, loss of libido, constipation, irritability, and headache) occur at any age and are not specifically related to estrogen deficiency. Estrogen may seem to alleviate such symptoms, but when tested in carefully controlled studies a specific beneficial effect cannot be demonstrated.

The symptoms of hot flashes and vaginal atrophy may be overwhelming for some women, and relief from low-dose estrogen can be dramatic. If it were not for the cancer risk (see below), there would be little discussion of alternative approaches to care. In the face of the cancer risk, estrogens are recommended in low doses for short periods of time for these nonlife-threatening symptoms.

OSTEOPOROSIS

It has been estimated that 25 to 50% of all women over the age of 60 suffer from osteoporosis, which is a depletion of mineral salts from otherwise normal bone. When sufficiently severe, osteoporosis can result in increased fractures of the forearm, vertebral bodies, and hip, all of which occur more frequently in women than in men as age advances. Twenty percent of women suffer a hip fracture by age 90, and 16% die within 3 months of such an occurrence. Spinal compression fractures occur in 25% of all white women over age 60 usually resulting in a loss of physical height. Osteoporosis is thus a major health problem for the aging woman.

Bone loss can be measured at the rate of approximately 1% per annum over at least the first 10 years postmenopausally, but the rate appears to decline with time. The administration of low doses of mestranol (24.8 µg/day) prevented this loss when compared to placebo. Unfortunately, upon discontinuation of estrogen treatment after 4 years, patients suffered a renewed loss of bone at the rate of 2.5% a year so that by the end of an additional 4 years their bone loss was equivalent to subjects who had never received estrogens.

In case control studies, estrogen use seemed to protect against hip and forearm fractures if taken within 5 years of the menopause or if estrogens were taken for at least 6 years. The risk of fracture was 50 to 60% lower in women taking the estrogens. When estrogen therapy was compared with calcium and placebo, estrogen proved to be most effective, with calcium being intermediate between the hormone and no treatment. There are few objective data on the efficacy of estrogen in the treatment of existing osteoporosis, but it appears that prevention is more successful than therapy after fractures occur.

The challenge for medicine is to try to identify patients most at risk for fractures so that preventive measures can be applied. As cancer risk increases with duration of estrogen therapy (described later), the benefits of preventing fractures must be weighed against the possible development of cancer later in life. There is no simple formula for resolving these conflicting results.

HEART DISEASE

Men ordinarily have a higher incidence of coronary disease early in life than women; the sexes approach parity in this only during old age. It was thought that women were protected by estrogen and that the incidence of heart disease increased after menopause due to its lack. Based on this reasoning, male survivors of a coronary attack were treated with estrogens and in high dose; they surprisingly had more rather than fewer coronary heart problems. Young women on estrogen-containing birth control pills also have a slight increase of coronary heart disease and even death, especially if they smoke. The risk of an estrogen effect increases with the woman's age. This unexpected adverse effect of estrogen is also seen with birth control pills in relation to stroke and thromboembolic disease. With the low dose of estrogen ordinarily taken by postmenopausal women, no increased risk of and no protection against heart disease has thus far been observed.

The one exception is with very young women who are oophorectomized and have a menopause 15 or more years prior to the average age of onset. In such cases, estrogen does seem to be protective against heart disease. Estrogens cause an elevation in some of the serum lipoproteins (high density lipoprotein) that are associated with less atherosclerosis, but estrogens also increase other lipids such as triglycerides. There is no sound basis for estrogen use to protect against heart disease at this time; and other factors such as diet, weight, smoking, and occupation seem to be of greater importance.

PSYCHIATRIC DISEASE AND MENTAL FUNCTION

In limited studies, estrogens do appear to affect the type of sleep and sleep latency, patient mood and self-perception, and memory. It is difficult, however, to relate estrogen lack to psychiatric disease and mental function. There is no specific age or menopausal correlation with psychiatric problems, and cognitive problems with aging may be related more to vascular and degenerative changes in the central nervous system. Much work is needed to define what role, if any, estrogens play in this regard.

ESTROGENS AND CANCER

Breast Cancer

There is extensive literature on the relationships between estrogens and the incidence and age of onset of breast cancer in animals. Estrogens are associated with the induction of breast cancer in female and male animals of susceptible species. Surprisingly, most studies prior to 1975 in humans have shown no ill effect, or even a protective action, of estrogen use. Recently, however, an association of increased risk of breast cancer (twofold) in women taking estrogens for long periods (10 to 15 years) has been reported. Failure to observe this previously may have been due to experimental design or a long latency prior to cancer induction. It has been argued whether estrogens are themselves carcinogenic or predispose a susceptible patient. Estrogens are ordinarily not recommended in the face of a family history of breast cancer. Although the strength of the association between breast cancer and estrogens is still not established, the high natural incidence of breast cancer makes even a small increase in risk worrisome.

Cancer of the Endometrium

Unopposed estrogen can induce hyperplasia and premalignant changes of the endometrium, and there have now been many studies of an increased risk (fourfold) of endometrial cancer with estrogen use over a period of four or more years. The risk seems to increase with dose and length of use. Most such cancers associated with estrogen use appear to be early and of low invasiveness. Treatment by hysterectomy seems to be quite effective, so that although the incidence of endometrial cancer has increased along with increased estrogen use there has been no increase in death from the disease. In one study, decreased estrogen use was associated with a declining incidence of such cancers. Use of progesterone along with the estrogen appears to diminish the risk of hyperplasia and possibly the risk of subsequent cancer.

PHARMACOLOGICAL PROBLEMS WITH ESTROGEN USE

Estradiol is the natural estrogen of premenopausal women, but if it is taken by mouth it is rapidly converted in the liver and intestine to estrone, and hence appears in the blood in that form. The most common estrogen taken by mouth is estrone itself, with or without other conjugated estrogens, rather than estradiol. Other oral forms of estrogen are synthetic derivatives (mestranol and ethinyl estradiol), which may have adverse effects on liver function (jaundice or tumors). In any case, it is difficult to replace the natural hormone estradiol except by injection or subcutaneous implantation of pellets.

When estrogen preparations are taken by mouth, they are cleared by the liver first, and hence the liver may be overdosed relative to other estrogen effects. For example, a dose of estrogen which will not reduce gonadotropins to normal may cause an excessive stimulation of liver synthesis of specific proteins, e.g., thyroid-binding globulin.

To avoid systemic effects, attempts were made to relieve vaginal symptoms by direct application of the estrogen in a vaginal cream. The estrogens, however, are rapidly absorbed into the bloodstream and are largely unchanged. This may provide an alternate route of administration for providing estradiol to the body, but one cannot feel secure in treating the vagina locally without some systemic effect.

In the past, estrogens alone were most frequently given to postmenopausal women, but the apparent protective effect of progesterone with respect to endometrial hyperplasia has prompted use of sequential therapy with both drugs. The disadvantage of progesterone is that when given cyclically after estrogen withdrawal bleeding can occur.

CLINICAL CHOICE IN ESTROGEN USE AND CONCLUSIONS

The earlier concept that women could be treated with estrogen replacement at the time of menopause and continued into old age is flawed by the apparent risks of developing uterine or breast cancer after taking estrogen for more than 4 to 5 years. Treatment of women with estrogen after prior hysterectomy does not alleviate the potential breast cancer problem.

As the major symptoms of menopause (hot flashes and vaginal atrophy) are not life-threatening, some choice and value judgement must be made relative to the needs of individual patients. Short-term therapy may ameliorate specific symptoms, reduce risk of cancer from prolonged exposure, and remain an acceptable form of care.

Osteoporosis and postmenopausal fractures, however, are major health problems, and the true place of estrogen therapy versus diet and exercise is yet to be determined. The problem with estrogen action for bone loss is that the effect is lost on discontinuation of therapy. Whether some estrogen over limited periods will provide longer-range protection from fractures is not known. It would be helpful if techniques were developed to identify subjects most at risk for fractures (accelerated bone loss) so they could be singled out for therapy.

The risk of endometrial cancer from estrogen is fairly well established and that of breast cancer less certain. Whether use of progesterone will protect against malignancy in the breast as well as the endometrium is not known.

Given the uncertainties, prudence dictates that if patients are put on estrogens it should only be for specific symptoms known to be responsive to the hormone. Therapy should be short-term (3 to 5 years) until safer types or routes of hormone replacement are established. A patient on estrogen should be followed by a health care provider who can monitor for breast and uterine cancer, *including periodic endometrial biopsies*, to pick up early lesions. Finally, patients should be fully informed about the effects of estrogen so that they can participate in the judgement of whether, on balance, the use of estrogen is best for them.

When caring for elderly patients, the physician should:

1. Know the principal features of the evolution of female reproductive function with aging.
2. Understand the effects of estrogens, with particular attention to those associated with clinical problems in the aged.
3. Know the risks of prolonged use of estrogens in the postmenopausal patient.
4. Understand the issues, choices, and value judgements which must be examined when the administration of estrogen to the postmenopausal patient is being considered.

SUGGESTED READING

Campbell, S., editor. *The Management of the Menopause and Postmenopausal Years*. MTP Press, Lancaster, England, 1976.

Horsman, A., Gallagher, J. C., Simpson, M., and Nordin, B. E. C. Prospective trial of estrogen and calcium in postmenopausal women. *Br. Med. J.*, 2:789–792, 1977.

Hulka, B. S. Effect of exogenous estrogens on postmenopausal women: the epidemiological evidence. *Obstet. Gynecol. Surv.*, 35:389–399, 1980.

Hutchinson, T. A. Polensky, S. M., and Fernstein, A. R. Postmenopausal estrogens protect against fractures of hip and distal radius. *Lancet*, 2:705–709, 1979.

Kase, N. Perimenopause. In: *Clinical Obstetrics and Gynecology*, edited by N. Kase, Harper & Row, New York, 1976.

Jaffe, R. B. The menopause and perimenopausal period. In: *Reproductive Endocrinology*, edited by S. C. Yen and R. B. Jaffe. Saunders, Philadelphia, 1978.

Lindsay, R., et al. Bone response to termination of oestrogen treatment. *Lancet*, 1:1325–1327, 1978.

Lindsay, R., et al. Long-term prevention of postmenopausal osteoporosis with oestrogen. *Lancet*, 1:1038–1040, 1976.

Ross, R. E., et al. A case control study of menopausal estrogen therapy and breast cancer. *JAMA*, 243:1635–1639, 1980.

Ryan, K. J., et al. Estrogen use and postmenopausal women: a National Institutes of Health consensus conference. *Ann. Intern. Med.*, 91:921–922, 1979.

Schiff, I., and Ryan, K. J. Benefits of estrogen replacement. *Obstet. Gynecol. Surv.*, 35:400–411, 1980.

Schneider, E. L., editor. *The Aging Reproductive System*. Raven Press, New York, 1978.

Weiss, N. S., Ure, C. L., Ballard, J. H., Williams, A. R., and Doling, J. R. Decreased risk of fractures of the hip and lower forearm with postmenopausal use of estrogen. *N. Engl. J. Med.*, 303:1195–1198, 1980.

Fundamentals of Geriatric Medicine, edited by
Ronald D. T. Cape, Rodney M. Coe, and Isadore
Rossman, Raven Press, New York © 1983.

30

Nutrition and the Elderly

Ronald D. T. Cape

There have been and are more fads, fancies, and fashion about diet than about any other aspect of medicine. Physicians and dieticians must be careful of their dietetic advice. Hawkins (13) of Birmingham, England, tells the cautionary tale of a 68-year-old woman who presented herself at his clinic with extensive ecchymoses of her legs and megaloblastic anemia. Thirty years earlier, her revered family doctor had prescribed a carminative and no fruit or vegetables for a bout of flatulent dyspepsia. When he stopped the carminative, he forgot his dietetic instructions. Nothing would persuade the patient to go back on the old doctor's advice, who had long since died. Fortunately, her scurvy responded successfully to vitamin C alone.

Food gathering is a basic biological exercise protected deep in the brain by an appetite center. In modern advanced nations, this activity has been made easy with a plentiful supply of every nutrient. No one need be without food, one would think. However, those who have physical disabilities which impair mobility, economic handicaps which reduce purchasing power, or central nervous problems which reduce appetite and memory may all experience difficulty in securing an adequate diet. These three attributes are most prevalent in the old, and the following recent statements appear to corroborate that many old people are undernourished.

1. Fifty percent of the elderly do not get enough essential nutrients each day.
2. Five to forty percent of the elderly are iron-deficient and often anemic as a result.
3. About one-third of noninstitutionalized elderly suffer from vitamin B_{12} and folate deficiencies.
4. Vitamin and mineral deficiencies seem to account for other symptoms, e.g., loss of appetite, tiredness, delayed wound healing, and confusion.

This chapter demonstrates that the preceding quotes are either exaggerated, untrue, or not supported by available evidence. Ten percent of old people suffer from a variety of disabling conditions which keep them housebound and isolated. This is the cohort in which undernutrition may occur.

AGING

As one ages, changes occur in the function of all bodily systems. The process of development which achieves its peak during the midtwenties continues to produce a series of alterations that are imperceptible from day to day but increasingly obvious from year to year. Wrinkling of skin, shortening of stature, loss of hair, and change in its color are all commonly observed phenomena. Throughout the first five or six decades of life, however, there are few obvious changes in general strength or in one's ability to function fully and independently. From the age of sixty onward, functional decrements become more obvious. Accompanying these overt changes are less obvious ones in body chemistry and organ systems, e.g., urogenital, cardiovascular, or respiratory. The general pattern is illustrated in Fig. 1, with function shown as a band to indicate the variations which occur from one individual to another, the range widening with increasing age.

Lean Body Mass

From a nutritional standpoint, these general changes are important, but even more so are the concurrent alterations in lean body mass. At maturity, the fat-free or lean body mass of men averages 60 kg and that of women about 40 kg (see Section II Overview.) These levels are maintained until the midforties, beyond which there is a slow decrease which speeds up after age 65 (16). By age 75, the average figure for the lean body mass of men is 48 kg and for women 36 kg. The muscular male loses proportionately more of this mass and gains more adipose tissue, which increases by approximately the same amount as is lost by muscle. Accompanying

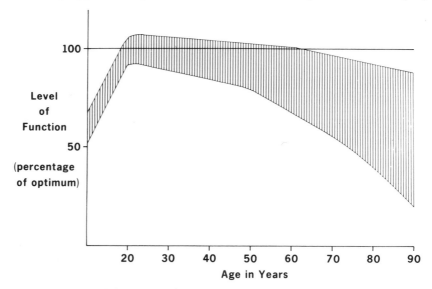

FIG. 1. Effect of aging on function. (From ref. 3.)

these changes, there is an associated but lesser loss of tissue from liver, brain, and kidneys.

Basal Metabolic Rate

A number of workers have demonstrated a reduction in basal metabolic rate (BMR) with age (23). Shock (19) found that the reason for the apparent reduction in BMR was the replacement of muscle by fat, which maintained or even increased the body's surface area but resulted in less-active metabolism. If oxygen consumption is plotted against body water volume (which parallels lean body mass), there is no fall in basal metabolism. The reduction in metabolically active cells reduces caloric requirements for an older person. Concurrent with the loss of lean mass, many elderly individuals exercise less and reduce general activity, further diminishing caloric need. The substantial normal reduction in caloric intake with age is therefore predictable.

Diet Restriction in Experimental Animals

More than 40 years ago, McCay and his co-workers (14) demonstrated that feeding rats a low calorie diet caused them to live longer. In one study, 106 rats were divided into an experimental group of 73 and a control group of 33 animals, respectively. The experimental group was fed a diet which was rich in protein, minerals, and vitamins but deficient in calories, i.e., a diet that would maintain the animals at stationary body weight. The experimental group was then divided into four subgroups and allowed to eat freely after 300, 500, 700, and 1,000 days, respectively.

If the mean survival time of the control animals was taken as 100%, those whose growth was delayed for 300 days had a mean survival of 128%, those delayed until 500 and 700 days 137%, and those retarded at 1,000 days 146%. Not only did the animals live longer but they remained healthier, with fine rather than coarse hair; they were smaller but fitter. Good et al. (12) reviewed the influence of nutrition on immunological aging and disease in studies which confirmed the earlier work by McCay et al. cited above. These workers gave NZB mice a variety of diets with diminished total food intake. If the animals were fed 10 calories/day rather than 20, their life span was dubled. The precise composition of the diet did not affect this result. In all cases autoantibody formation was reduced and lifespan increased. Immunological function deteriorates early in this hybrid strain with reduced numbers of active lymphocytes and diminished output of antibody. These changes were shown to be slowed down by a reduced calorie diet.

NUTRITIONAL SURVEYS

In an age when surveys are a popular research tool, a number of reviews of the dietary habits of elderly people living at home have been carried out. Exton-Smith and Stanton (8) reported an investigation into the dietary habits of elderly women living alone in two North London boroughs, Hornsey and Islington. The average age of the subjects was about 76. When choosing these two boroughs, it was hoped to compare the effect of the presumed disparity in living conditions and therefore in diet. However, contrary to expectation, little difference was found between the two. The authors therefore studied their subjects as one group.

The mean level of calorie intake was 1,890 per day with a range extending from 1,100 to 2,900. Between the ages of 70 and 90, there was a reduction in average caloric intake of 20%. Fifty-seven grams of protein daily was the average intake for the group as a whole, and this too showed a progressive reduction with age, which reached 25% (Figs. 1 and 2). Similar findings were reported for the intake of iron and calcium.

The method used in this study was a meticulous assessment by a trained dietician of the actual food consumed over a period of a week. In two earlier visits to the subjects, the survey was explained, and scales, plastic bags for waste, and charts for recording weights of foods were supplied.

It was possible to relate the amount of protein to the number of main meals (defined as those containing a serving of meat, fish, cheese, or egg). Twenty-eight percent of the subjects had 14 or more main meals during the week, and these individuals averaged an intake of 462 g of protein. On the other hand, 17% had only seven or fewer main meals, and this group averaged 314 g of protein during the week.

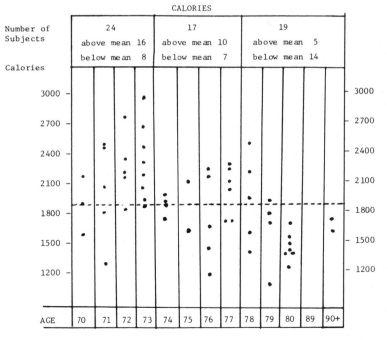

FIG. 2. Calorie intake of 60 elderly females. (Adapted from ref. 8.)

The mean body weight of the subjects in the highest age group (51 kg) was 14% less than that of the subjects in their early seventies (59 kg): The percentage reduction in intake of calories and nutrients was similar in the subgroup that was clinically examined and in the group as a whole. The correlation between diet and health was striking. Only 4 of 21 subjects with better than average diets did not also enjoy better than average health; 17 of 23 with poor diets also had poor health.

This study was carried out in 1962, and the subjects involved were followed up 7 years later (20). By that time, 26 had died or could not be traced, and 7 were in residential or hospital care. This left a total of 27 available for review. Five of those declared themselves unable to participate. Nine of the 22 subjects available for this second study, who represented the elite of the original sample, had reached their late seventies and had done so with little change in their health, physical activities, or amount of food consumed. The remaining 13 consumed less, with a mean decrease in protein intake of 20% and a mean decrease in calorie intake of 17%. The reductions seen in this longitudinal study were similar to those found in the original cross-sectional study. The authors concluded that individuals who maintained their health continued to eat well. They were unable to say whether deterioration in health of the other group caused the reduced intake of food or resulted from it.

Other large-scale surveys have been carried out in randomly selected population groups in Canada (17), Scotland (15), Sweden (21), and the United States (6,11,22), all reaching the same general conclusions. The incidence of signficant undernutrition among the elderly is low, the average consumption of energy producing foods lying between 1,900 and 2,400 calories for men aged 70 to 79 years and between 1,500 and 2,000 calories for women of the same age. Protein intake is usually 70 to 85 g for men and 55 to 65 g for women. There has been little evidence produced of significant lack of vitamins or minerals, although concern has been expressed about calcium and iron, the B vitamins, and ascorbic acid. The known deterioration of renal function has also raised the question of a possible lack of vitamin D metabolites such as dihydrocholecalciferol (Chapter 9).

Protein

The changes that occur in protein metabolism follow a pattern established by the increasing loss of muscle during biosenescence. It is reasonable to postulate that this will result in a reduced need for protein, but it is difficult to arrive at an accurate figure for obligatory demand. For the healthy elderly person, 50 to 70 g of protein in a diet containing 1,800 to 2,400 calories offers an adequate supply of both this substance and the most essential amino acids. There are, of course, patients whose conditions increase the needed quantity, e.g., individuals undergoing surgery, those with chronic wasting disease, or those with slow-healing indolent ulcerations of leg or back. In all of the surveys cited in the previous section, survivors in longitudinal studies continued to ingest adequate or even quite large quantities of protein.

Calcium

There is a 12% loss of bone tissue in men and a 25% loss in women between the fifth and ninth decades. This appears to represent a true aging phenomenon which occurs concurrently with the loss of muscle tissue already described. Also, according to Garn (10), populations continue to lose bone irrespective of the calcium intake. It follows that an inadequate intake of the element is not the cause of the bone loss phenomenon, but it may have relevance to the degree of loss.

The importance of calcium in the diet of elderly subjects lies in its relation to the inevitable loss of bone which accompanies aging. The human body adapts well to a wide variation in calcium intake. Population surveys in many countries produce no evidence that a high calcium intake prevents the universal loss of bone that occurs with aging or that low calcium intake promotes such bone loss. At the present time, there is no known dietary regimen that prevents adult bone loss or osteoporosis.

Iron

There are a large number of studies from different countries describing the prevalence of anemia in old people. The serum ferritin concentration in healthy persons has been measured in more than 1,000 randomly selected Canadians between the ages of 1 and 90. Valberg and co-workers (24) found no evidence to support the view that iron stores were less adequate in elderly subjects than younger ones on the basis of estimates of serum ferritin. They state that a highly significant correlation has been found between serum ferritin concentration and three other indices of body iron status: hemosiderin content of bone marrow, percentage absorption of iron, and size of body iron stores as measured by quantitative phlebotomy.

It has been suggested that both hemoglobin levels and iron stores may be low in elderly subjects. The consensus of evidence from most studies indicates that there is no reason to postulate such age-related changes. It may in fact be dangerous to do so because a low hemoglobin or inadequate iron stores is almost certainly an indication of morbidity. Appropriate investigation for sites of bleeding, particularly in the alimentary tract, are required. When such are pursued thoroughly, a site of blood loss will be found in 50 to 70% of cases.

Of 247 consecutive female admissions to one ward in Birmingham, England, 192 individuals showed evidence of sideropenia, low serum iron levels (<70 mg/dl), and 89 were anemic (hemoglobin <11.7 g/dl) (Figs. 3 and 4). At first glance, this suggests that there may be a considerable number of cases of nutritional anemia in the population. Reports on the incidence of anemia (7), however, demonstrate that old people who are admitted to hospital have a higher proportion of low hemoglobin levels than do old people in the general population, the reason being that anemia is an indicator of morbidity.

One hundred and ten cases of moderate to severe anemia encountered in practice at Selly Oak Hospital in Birmingham were studied from an etiological standpoint (7). Included were 83 with evidence of iron deficiency which divided into seven

PROTEIN

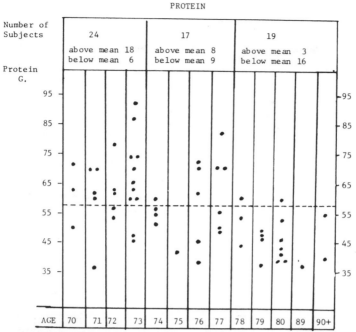

FIG. 3. Protein intake of 60 elderly females. (Adapted from ref. 8.)

main groups. The first were those in which there was obvious blood loss: 19 with positive occult blood tests, 4 with demonstrable intestinal lesions, 2 with urinary blood loss, and 1 with bleeding varicose ulcers; in seven groups the deficiency was associated with other conditions (Table 1). In 25 cases there was no evidence of blood loss or other obvious disease responsible for the anemia. In this group two patients had no therapy, and their hemoglobin rose to normal levels on the hospital diet, presumptive evidence of undernutrition. In the other cases, treatment consisted of blood transfusion in 2 and iron therapy in 21. As a result of this treatment, 17 reached normal hemoglobin levels and 13 were discharged from hospital. Two points should be emphasized: (a) The 110 cases were geriatric patients whose ages ranged from 62 to 92 with a preponderance of the very old. The relatively good response to treatment is supporting evidence of a prior nutritional deficiency. (b) Less than one-third of iron deficiency is nutritional.

Fortification of foods with iron is to be deprecated because it will result in concealment of a potential clue to the diagnosis of gastrointestinal cancer, which is notoriously symptomless in its early stages. The discovery of a mild anemia on a routine check is a vital pointer to the need for appropriate investigation for such conditions. This is particularly true for the elderly, in whom the prevalence of cancer of the colon or rectum increases markedly. There are thus two good reasons for avoiding such fortification of foods. Firstly, surveys cited previously indicate that there are few, if any, old people lacking adequate iron intake in their diet, and

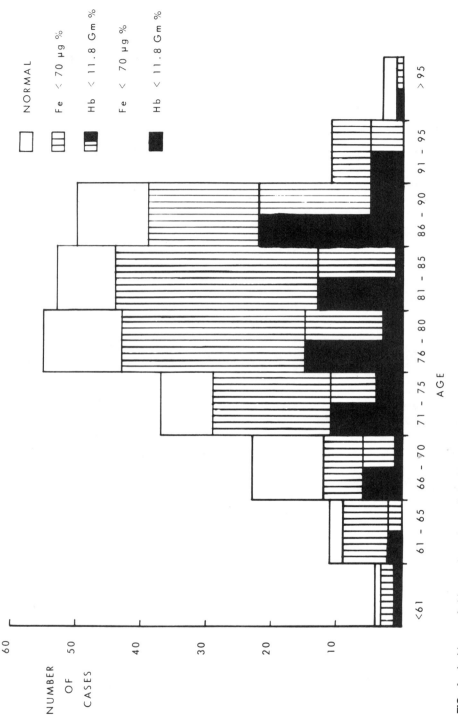

FIG. 4. Incidence of sideropenia and anemia in 247 consecutive female patients admitted to Selly Oak Hospital, Birmingham, England. (Data from ref 7)

TABLE 1. *Lone iron deficiency*[a]

Cause	No.
Blood loss	25
Chronic infection	7
Malignant diseases	9
Renal failure	3
Chronic arthritis and analgesic consumption	3
Analgesic consumption	3
Hypothyroidism	1
Concurrent vitamin B_{12} deficiency	5
Concurrent folate deficiency	8
"Nutritional" (idiopathic)	25
Total	83

Data from ref. 7.
[a]Serum iron less than 70 μg/100 ml and/or saturation less than 16%.

secondly there is a danger of masking lethal conditions by unnecessary attempts at overprotection.

Vitamins

A number of claims have been made about lack of vitamins in the elderly person's diet. A recent study by Baker et al. (2) stated that levels of thiamine, vitamin C, and vitamin B_{12} were "strikingly depressed" in noninstitutionalized elderly, and over 30% of the institutionalized old had pyridoxine and nicotinate hypovitaminemia. Both groups showed depressed levels of folate and vitamin B_{12}. Unfortunately, all the results are expressed as a range about a mean, and it is difficult to know what the actual individual data were. There were some misleading statements made suggesting that fatigue, mental confusion, and anemia frequently result from B_{12} deficiency. The latter is, of course, true, and cases of dementia have been attributed to cerebral manifestations of vitamin B_{12} deficiency. However, in a study of B_{12} levels published in 1961 (5), there was no observable connection between low B_{12} levels and confusion. One must therefore have some reservations about accepting the conclusions of Baker and his colleagues.

More interesting than the apparent deficiencies were the vitamins found in plentiful supply. These included vitamins A and E, which underlines the lack of rationale for elderly patients to take this substance as a supplement. Baker and his co-workers (1) later gave their institutionalized subjects oral vitamin supplements and found that these did not significantly affect the serum levels. When they gave a single intramuscular dose of a multivitamin preparation and re-estimated the levels after 3 months, however, there was significant improvement in the serum vitamin levels. This is an interesting and possibly highly important finding. If these results are confirmed and little benefit is found to result from regular oral vitamin supplements, an enormous amount of money is currently being poured down the drain to provide such additives.

NUTRITION AND DISABILITY

Any consideration of nutrition must revolve around two questions: (a) Are there dietary deficiencies, as yet unrecognized, which are responsible for disease? (b) Can better nutrition prevent or reduce the incidence of morbidity? To examine these questions in relation to elderly people, the clearest evidence comes from a further study by Exton-Smith et al. (9). In 1970 the Department of Health and Social Security in the United Kingdom published the first Report of the Panel on the Nutrition of the Elderly. This pointed out certain factors which were likely to lead to malnutrition in the elderly: limited mobility, loneliness, and social isolation. Exton-Smith and his colleagues set out, therefore, to study the diets of a group of housebound elderly people and to compare these with the diets of residents of old age homes and active old people living in their own homes.

The housebound group included 44 women and 10 men with a mean age of 83. The residents of the homes for the aged, 25 women and 15 men, had a mean age of 81, and the 68 women and 37 men living in their own homes had a mean age of 75.6. The data collection methods were the same as in these researchers' nutrition survey cited above. Three of the main findings of this study were:

1. The weekly consumption of main foods demonstrated that, for most items, the active groups consumed more than the housebound, the only exception being milk for the men.
2. The significance of main meals has already been mentioned. The active groups ate more cooked evening meals than did the housebound.
3. Finally, the mean nutrient intakes for each group were estimated for the persons 70 to 79 years old (Table 2) and for those aged 80 and over (Table 3). Note that for virtually all foods the housebound had a smaller intake. Again the one exception is calcium (from milk) in the 70 to 79-year-old men.

Exton-Smith and his colleagues concluded: "The study of the housebound adds further evidence that low intakes of nutrients are associated with deterioration in

TABLE 2. *Mean nutrient intakes of those aged 70 to 79 in three residential groups*

Nutrient	Men			Women		
	Residential homes	Active	House-bound	Residential homes	Active	House-bound
No. of people	8	32	2	6	53	10
Calories	1,846	2,345	1,406	1,715	1,745	1,190
Protein (g)	55·8	87·0	64·0	52·4	57·6	38·5
Protein (% calories)	12	14·8	18	12	13	13
Fat (g)	80	102	59	76	82	56
Carbohydrates (g)	245	261	160	217	199	137
Calcium (mg)	835	922	944	747	778	634
Iron (mg)	8·6	11·5	8·3	8·3	9·3	5·6
Vitamin C (mg)	30	46	27	39	50	27
Vitamin D (IU)	85	123	73	75	99	68

From ref. 9.

TABLE 3. *Mean nutrient intakes of those over 80 years in three residential groups*

	Men			Women		
Nutrient	Residential homes	Active	House-bound	Residential homes	Active	House-bound
No. of people	6	5	8	17	15	32
Calories	1,858	2,535	1,816	1,496	1,656	1,320
Protein (g)	50·9	70·3	55·0	46·4	54·0	42·0
Protein (% calories)	11	11	12	12	13	13
Fat (g)	69	91	87·6	68	77	60
Carbohydrates (g)	274	340	208	187	188	160
Calcium (mg)	920	944	810	688	807	660
Iron (mg)	6·7	11·8	8·0	7·2	8·2	6·0
Vitamin C (mg)	16	49	32	37	37	31
Vitamin D (IU)	100	89	83	58	76	47

From ref. 9.

physical and mental health in old people. There is no decline in intake with age, indeed the youngest people often had the lowest intakes. This is because, for the housebound, in contrast with the active group, disability was just as severe and as frequent in the younger as in the older people. Thus decline in intakes is to be attributed to disease rather than to the effects of age alone."

I would like to stress this point. We hear and read many statements about the dangers of undernutrition of elderly people. None of the properly constructed sample surveys have confirmed them. What has been demonstrated is that those at particular risk are the housebound, a potentially identifiable group. In the study by Exton-Smith et al., the cause of their confinement "in 80% of cases is immobility due to osteoarthritis, blindness, heart disease, mental disturbance, strokes, fractured femora, deafness, chronic bronchitis, and obesity." There was a further small group, the remaining 20%, who were "fearful of venturing out of doors alone." This type of crisis of confidence is a familiar occurrence among elderly people, and a deeper understanding of its nature and causes is urgently required.

The answer to both the questions posed above—Are there dietary deficiencies, as yet unrecognized, which are responsible for disease? and Can better nutrition prevent or reduce the incidence of morbidity?—is: "Not as far as we know." This does not mean that in the future the importance of new food factors may not emerge. There is, for example, significant evidence now available which associates senile dementia of the Alzheimer's type with deficiency of choline acetyltransferase, a low-affinity enzyme necessary for the biosynthesis of acetylcholine. Attempts are already being made to counter this deficiency by raising the levels of circulating precursors by dietary manipulation. To date results have not been encouraging, but that does not alter the fact that, in time, appropriate dietary additives may play a role in preventing or treating this condition.

There is therefore no justification for the four statements with which this chapter began. The statements are not only untrue but encourage the giving of a variety of food supplements which are quite unnecessary and discourage proper medical review of the vague symptoms that could frequently be due to significant disease.

In 1948 Sheldon (18) pointed out that decline in food intake accompanied deterioration of health, often about the middle of the eighth decade. This association has since been confirmed and reinforced by the studies of Exton-Smith and his colleagues. Cape and Henschke (4) have shown that the incidence of disability rises slowly between the ages of 65 and 80, from 5 to 10%, and beyond that more dramatically to 30% or more by age 90. It is this 10% of old people who are at particular risk of undernutrition, and our efforts to develop preventive programs should be concentrated on them.

The more one studies the problems of the old, the more one comes back to the fact that failing health is the key factor which causes immobility; the person then becomes housebound and suffers the associated social isolation. From whatever angle one views the established facts, one always returns to the need for better medical care and management to reduce dependence. Better diagnosis, more discriminating therapeutics, and improved rehabilitation will do more for the nutrition of the elderly than anything else.

SUMMARY

Commonly held myths regarding nutrition in the elderly are refuted here by citing data from carefully conducted studies. The use of dietary supplements is discussed. It is noted that the elderly do better nutritionally when they are active, and not housebound.

When caring for elderly patients, the physician should:

1. Know the incidence and prevalence of malnutrition in the elderly.
2. Know the dietetic needs of the elderly.
3. Have sufficient understanding and knowledge of the nutritional needs of the elderly to be able to advise patients on this subject.

REFERENCES

1. Baker, H., Frank, O., and Jaslow, S. P. Oral versus intramuscular vitamin supplementation for hypovitaminosis in the elderly. *J. Am. Geriatr. Soc.*, 28:42–45, 1980.
2. Baker, H., Frank, O., Thind, I. S., Jaslow, S. P., and Louria, D. B. Vitamin profiles in elderly persons living at home or in nursing homes versus profile in healthy young subjects. *J. Am. Geriatr. Soc.*, 27:444–450, 1979.
3. Cape, R. D. T. The aging human. In: *Aging and Immunity*, edited by K. Singhal, N. R. Sinclair, and C. R. Stiller, pp. 213–224. Elsevier/North Holland, New York, 1979.
4. Cape, R. D. T., and Henschke, P. J. Perspective of health in the elderly. *J. Am. Geriatr. Soc.*, 28:295–299, 1980.
5. Cape, R. D. T., and Shinton, N. K. Serum-vitamin B_{12} concentration in the elderly. *Gerontol. Clin.*, 3:163–172, 1961.
6. Chope, H. D., and Breslow, L. Nutritional status of the aging. *Am. J. Public Health*, 46:61–67, 1957.
7. Ehtisham, M., and Cape, R. D. T. Protocol for diagnosing and treating anemia. *Geriatrics*, 32:91–99, 1977.
8. Exton-Smith, A. N., and Stanton, B. R. *Report of an Investigation into the Dietary of Elderly Women Living Alone.* King Edward's Hospital Fund, London, 1965.

9. Exton-Smith, A. N., Stanton, B., and Windsor, A. C. M. *Nutrition of Housebound Old People.* King Edward's Hospital Fund, London, 1972.
10. Garn, S. M. Bone loss and ageing. In: *Nutrition of the Aged*, edited by W. W. Hawkins, pp. 73–90. The Nutrition Society of Canada, Quebec City, 1978.
11. Gillum, H. L., and Morgan, A. F. Nutritional status of the aging. *J. Nutr.*, 55:265–303, 1955.
12. Good, R. A., Fernandes, G., and West, A. Nutrition, immunologic aging and disease. In: *Aging and Immunity*, edited by S. K. Singhal, N. R. Sinclair, and C. R. Stiller, pp. 141–164. Elsevier/North Holland, New York, 1979.
13. Hawkins, C. Megaloblastic anemia in old age. In: *Medicine in Old Age*, edited by J. N. Agate. Pitman, London, 1966.
14. McCay, C. M., Maynard, L. A., Sperling, G., and Barnes, L. L. Retarded growth, life span, ultimate body size and age changes in the Albino rat after feeding diets restricted in calories. *J. Nutr.*, 18:1–13, 1939.
15. McLeod, C. C., Judge, T. G., and Caird, F. I. Nutrition of the elderly at home. *Age Ageing*, 1:158–166, 1974.
16. Novak, L. P. Aging total body potassium fat-free mass, and cell mass in males and females between ages 18 and 85 years. *J. Gerontol.*, 27:438–443, 1972.
17. *Nutrition Canada. National Survey*, Chap. 8, pp. 76–83, 97–102. Health and Welfare Canada, Ottawa, 1973.
18. Sheldon, J. *The Social Medicine of Old Age.* Nuffield Foundation, Oxford, 1948.
19. Shock, N. W. System integration. In: *Handbook of the Biology of Aging*, edited by C. E. Finch and L. Hayflick, pp. 639–665. Van Nostrand Rheinhold, New York, 1977.
20. Stanton, B. R., and Exton-Smith, A. N. *A Longitudinal Study of the Dietary of Elderly Women.* King Edward's Hospital Fund, London, 1970.
21. Steen, B., Isaksson, B., and Svanborg, A. Intake of energy and nutrients and meal habits in 70 year old males and females in Gothenburg, Sweden: a population study. *Acta Med. Scand.*, [*Suppl.*], 611–39–86, 1977.
22. Steinkamp, R. C., Cohen, N. L., and Walsh, H. E. Resurvey of an aging population: fourteen-year follow-up. *J. Am. Diet. Assoc.*, 46:103–110, 1965.
23. Tremolieres, J., and Geissler-Blum, C. Nutrition and metabolism. In: *Practical Geriatrics*, edited by H. P. Von Hahn, pp. 55–75. Karger, Basel, 1975.
24. Valberg, L., Sorbie, J., Laudnig, J., and Pelletier, O. Serum ferritin and the iron status of Canadians. *Can. Med. Assoc. J.*, 114:417–421, 1976.

Fundamentals of Geriatric Medicine, edited by
Ronald D. T. Cape, Rodney M. Coe, and Isadore
Rossman, Raven Press, New York © 1983.

31

Surgery and the Elderly Patient

Bernard S. Linn

Surgical controversy arises when therapeutic operations are either withheld from
or initiated for elderly patients solely because of their age. Usually surgeons have
taken a cautious approach to operating on the elderly in the belief that older age
per se carries increased surgical risk. At the same time, there is undoubtedly some
excess surgery in the elderly resulting from underestimation or ignorance of specific
risks. In either extreme, increasing knowledge about aging and the older person's
response to surgery can provide a basis for making more appropriate decisions.

Some judgments leading to inappropriate surgery fall in the ethical, rather than
the clinical, realm. Deciding what is ethically correct can be very difficult, especially
when approaching mortality prompts value judgments concerning how little might
be gained or lost. If old age provokes poor surgical decisions, data must be collected
and practices corrected, just as excess hysterectomies for women and unnecessary
tonsillectomies for children must be controlled. A broader approach, however, might
be that of uniformly ensuring the right to elective operations, regardless of age.

This chapter provides some information that may be helpful in making rational
decisions for or against surgery in older patients. Studies on age and surgical
outcomes are reviewed, and the variability of operative risk in older patients is
documented. Finally, specific management strategies for the elderly surgical patient
are discussed.

CHRONOLOGICAL AGE AS A FACTOR IN
SURGICAL DECISION-MAKING

The surgical literature contains many studies of the effect of age on surgical
results in thousands of patients aged 60 to 100. Table 1 summarizes mortality rates
by type of operation in elderly patients. Two-thirds of these studies included multiple
surgical procedures, and the remainder examined one particular operation or type
of surgery for the elderly. Outcome comparisons among these studies or with the
general surgical literature are difficult as there are differences in patient populations,
indications for surgery, and definitions of operative morbidity and mortality. How-

TABLE 1. *Mortality rates in reported studies of the elderly undergoing surgery*

Author and year	Lowest age studied	Total sample	Percent mortality		
			Elective	Emergency	Overall
GENERAL SURGERY					
Brooks (1938)	70	293	—	—	19.0
Hay (1940)	70	—	—	—	16.6
Welch (1948)	70	—	—	—	20.7
Estes (1949)	60	400	5.0	16.4	6.5
Carp (1951)	70	—	—	32.0	—
Haug and Dale (1952)	60	354	5.7	21.9	9.0
Bosch et al. (1952)	60	500	8.8	17.4	9.6
Gilchrist and dePeyster (1956)	70	—	—	—	11.1
Cutler (1956)	70	—	—	44.0	—
Limbosch (1956)	70	1,000	—	39.5	—
Cohn et al. (1957)	70	—	4.0	23.0	—
Meyer et al. (1958)	80	66	—	—	0
Klug and McPherson (1959)	60	1,706	—	—	8.5
Ryan (1960)		—	7.4	29.3	—
Bolt (1960)	70	—	—	29.0	—
Wilder and Fishbein (1961)	80	—	—	36.0	19.4
Scott (1961)	70	180	—	—	13.8
Gemählich and Krautwing (1961)	70	—	—	—	14.0
Arkins et al. (1964)	70	1,148	—	—	10.8
Marshall and Fahey (1964)	80	207	—	23.2	—
Aubry et al. (1965)	80	500	—	—	20.0
Anderson et al. (1965)	70	3,703	—	—	10.5
Bonus and Dorsey (1965)	75	—	5.8	24.0	—
Mitty and Echemendia (1965)	75	549	7.7	15.2	—
Lorhan (1967)	80	710	—	—	22.3
Cole and Mason (1968)	60	3,656	—	—	5.1
Randall (1968)	65	6,731	—	—	4.8
Brander et al. (1970)	70	206	—	—	11.0
Ziffren and Hartford (1972)	80	—	—	—	7.1
Burnett and McCaffrey (1972)	70	608	—	—	13.3
Griffiths (1972)	70	487	6.4	16.9	—
Anderson and Østberg (1972)	70	7,922	—	—	8.0
Kohn et al. (1973)	80	599	—	—	11.8
Albano et al. (1975)	60	93	—	—	15.0
Santos and Gelperin (1975)	70	2,186	—	—	4.9
Djokovic and Hedley-White (1975)	80	500	—	—	6.2
ANEURYSMECTOMY					
O'Donnell et al. (1976)	80	111			
Purely elective			2.0	—	—
Expanding			10.0	—	—
Ruptured			—	74.0	—
HEART					
Bowles et al. (1969)	60	54	—	—	20.0
Austen et al. (1970)	70	40	—	—	20.0
Oh et al. (1973)	60	114			
Aortic valve			—	—	15.0
Mitral			—	—	18.0
Multiple			—	—	60.0
Mitral valve			—	—	0.0
Berman et al. (1980)	70	27	—	—	17.6
ABDOMINAL					
Stahlgren (1961)	70	—	—	18.0	—
Hormozi and Mahringer (1965)	80	—	—	21.4	—
Rzepiela (1973)	65	267	8.0	21.3	21.3

ever, two conclusions from the literature on the elderly surgical patient can be made: (a) Surgical morbidity and mortality are higher in older as compared with younger patients. (b) Outcomes for even the most difficult operations in the elderly are favorable if appropriate attention is given to all factors which affect the degree of operative risk.

Surgical Outcomes in Elderly versus Young Patients

Surgical results depend on patient risk due to severity of presenting and cumulative disease coupled with the quality of care provided to that patient (42). For example, if severity of illness were constant in comparable patients, better outcomes would indicate better quality of care. Conversely, if quality of care is constant, better outcomes would indicate less severely ill patients with lower risks. Unfortunately, there are no universal standards for assessing either the severity of illness or the quality of care.

Emergency surgery for all ages carries a two- to eightfold greater risk than operating electively for the same disease (21). Emergency repair of an incarcerated hernia, for example, produces poorer outcomes than elective herniorrhaphy of a similar reducible hernia. Additionally, operative risk increases with both more advanced primary disease and more associated pathology (52). Hence a patient with a ruptured appendix has greater surgical risk than one whose appendix is intact. Likewise, the patient needing a cholecystectomy who also has cardiopulmonary problems is at greater risk than a comparable patient without associated disease. Kohn (39) has suggested that diseases which increase the risk of death can be grouped into those that occur to varying degrees in all aging individuals (e.g., arteriosclerosis), those that are not universally present but increase with age (e.g., neoplasia) (some of which peak at earlier ages, reflecting age variations in susceptibility), and those that are not related to aging but have more serious consequences in older persons (e.g., pneumonia or influenza).

Surgeons have always been concerned about coexisting disease, and as the elderly frequently appear to have multiple conditions, particularly cardiac and respiratory problems, such factors must be assessed carefully in terms of additional risk. Anderson and Ostberg (4) found the number of coexisting diseases to be a gross measure of surgical risk, with each additional disorder increasing the risk by a factor of four. As the elderly often have associated multiple pathology and higher incidence of emergency surgery, outcome in the elderly is often poor compared with that in younger patients. Thus increased surgical risk with age can in part be attributed to multiple pathology, more advanced diseases, and more frequent emergency surgery.

Operative risk in the elderly is still more complex. Although there is no completely satisfactory way to measure operative risk accurately, an overall framework can be provided for thinking about older patients. Older people can be assigned a biological, psychological, and chronological age. Even though chronological age is easiest to measure, it is perhaps the least useful in predicting surgical risk. Measurement of biological age is a highly desirable but not yet attainable goal, and at present one has to rely on clinical assessments of the extent of disease and physical reserve. Biological variability increases over time, so that overall individual capacity is not predictable by chronological age (Chapter 30). Bafitis and Sargent (9) reviewed data on changes in organ function from birth to old age. They found that variability increased with age, indicating that the functions of various organs and the general adaptability of the body changed at differing rates in different individuals. In terms of reserve and experience with illness, there are indications that many individuals who live into extreme old age are more biologically elite and have been more physically resistant to illness (43,45). Other factors that influence physiological and psychological functioning may be attitudes about age and being old. Linn and Hunter (44) found that older persons who did not view themselves as old functioned better physically and were better adjusted psychologically.

There are both positive and negative factors to be considered in patients as a consequence of their age. On the negative side, consider an 80-year-old with a lifetime of good health. Although physiologically the person may look 10, 20, or even more years younger, there is still no question that he or she has aged over a lifetime and looks "older" than as a young adult, even a young person with a severe illness. In Rowe's discussion (56) of clinical research on aging, he has outlined some of the physiological changes that occur with normal aging. Renal function, as measured by creatinine clearance (57) and glucose tolerance (5) both decline with age in the absence of renal disease or diabetes (Chapters 9 and 10). Crane and Harris (23) illustrated that the decreased renin levels that occurred with aging, which might be interpreted as indicative of disease, were actually normal; that the plasma renin concentration and activity were reduced by 30 to 50% in the elderly; and that this occurred even when levels of renin substrate were normal. These differences between young and old could be magnified by salt restriction, diuretic therapy, or upright posture. Other biological functions which decline with age include cardiac output, vital capacity of the lung, lean muscle mass, and cellular immunity (27). The negative factor then is that aging does take its physiological toll. Rowe's discussion pointed out that even though some changes occur and may be normal for the elderly, other functions do not change. He suggested the importance of recognizing that findings on many common laboratory tests (e.g., hematocrit, serum electrolytes, and urinalysis) are not influenced by age in clinically important ways, and that a treatable disease may be overlooked if an abnormal finding on such a test is attributed to old age alone. (For a more detailed discussion of physiological aging, the reader is referred to Section II of this book.)

One positive aspect regarding surgery in the elderly is the individual's own longevity. Some would assume that when a person reaches the age of life expectancy little effort needs to be made to extend life further. Survival to advanced age, however, in and of itself predicts more years of survival. Although life expectancy at birth is 71.9 years, at 65 it is 15.6 more years, at 75 it is 9.8, and even at 80 it is 7.6 years (64). Wangensteen believed that no patient who required a life-saving operation should be permitted to die simply because of chronological age (63).

Anyone who gets past the mortal diseases of middle age and early old age has demonstrated durability and resilience. The conclusion expressed at the 1964 meeting of the American College of Surgeons was that "a vigorous, optimistic octagenarian is a better surgical risk than a feeble, pessimistic younger patient" (2).

Surgical Outcomes in the Elderly

The literature on surgery in the elderly verifies good results with proper management. Surgical outcomes in the elderly must be compared carefully because of uncontrolled differences, both described and undescribed, among different reports. Nevertheless, surgical mortality in the elderly is somewhat higher than the 1.5% figure for those under 70 years of age. Meyer and co-workers (49) reported no mortality in 66 consecutive 80-year-old patients undergoing major surgical operations. The gross operative mortality rates in the four largest series in the elderly since 1968 were 4.8% for 6,731 patients (55); 5.1% for 3,656 patients (22); 8% for 7,922 patients (4); and 4.9% for 2,186 patients (60). Elective abdominal aortic aneurysmectomy mortality for 111 patients 80 years and over ranged from 2 to 10%, as compared with 74% for emergency postrupture operations (53). Bowles et al. (14) reported an open-heart surgery mortality rate of 20% in 54 patients over 60 compared with 19% in younger groups. Recently the better-anesthesia-risk group among 500 patients over age 80 undergoing major surgery for elective and emergency procedures had operative mortality rates of 1% with no increased mortality up to age 95 (25). These studies, along with others, have made thoughtful surgical leaders more willing to operate on elderly patients. Ochsner (51) said it best: "In 1927, as a young professor of surgery at the Tulane Medical School, I taught and practiced that an elective operation for inguinal hernia in a patient older than 50 years of age was not justified.... Today age is in no way a surgical contraindication."

The other extreme is the possibility of excess surgery. McCarthy and Widmer (48) reported that in 30% of persons who voluntarily sought a second opinion about proposed surgery the need was not confirmed by a board-certified consultant. Congressional committees quickly extrapolated this to mean that millions in the United States, particularly those on Medicare and Medicaid, were having unnecessary surgery. Mandatory programs in some states were instituted to provide second opinions, but state courts declared some unconstitutional because a negative second opinion denied reimbursement. Gertman and his associates (30) pointed out that, although negative second opinions for elective surgery often implied unwarranted surgery, studies showed that two-thirds of the negative second opinions were reversed when they were submitted to a third, thus indicating reasonable disagreement among physicians. Data on utilization of surgical operations in short-term hospitals (65) showed that surgery was lowest for patients over age 65. Patients aged 15 to 44 had the highest surgical rate (47% of all discharges, including deaths), and those 65 and above had the lowest rate (32%).

The use of heroic measures to extend life through surgery for patients who are terminally ill is a slightly different category of what might be considered excess surgery. Often the motive is not monetary or experimental but is done without enough thought as to whether the result will enhance the overall quality of life left to the individual. Surgery may in fact make the time left less rewarding. Glenn (32) suggests that operations in the elderly can be classified as those expected to result in complete restoration of health, those aimed at diminishing disability, and those aimed at achieving a limited postponement of inevitable death. When considering operations that postpone inevitable death, the chance of improving quality of life, as well as length of survival, should be carefully evaluated.

SURGICAL MANAGEMENT OF THE ELDERLY PATIENT

The surgical management of elderly patients is not the responsibility of the surgeon alone. The referring physician, anesthesiologist, medical consultant, patient, and family participate in surgical decisions. Principles of good surgical care are not specific to the elderly but apply to patients of all ages. In this sense, elderly patients are not different from the young, but rather have accumulated more age-related change and disease which must be considered. One can therefore define comprehensive management for elderly patients in terms of underlying age-related physiological losses which have gradually but progressively accrued, aggravated by the superimposed cumulative damage done by past and present disease. The net result is a loss of adaptability and physiological reserve to cope with further insults. It is evident that surgical results will be poorer in individuals who, as a result of these combined effects of aging and disease, have less reserve of adaptability to additional stress.

Although one should obviously prepare all patients maximally for surgery in order to minimize the trauma, it is particularly critical in the elderly because of their loss of adaptive reserve. Special attention should be given to helping the patient and family understand the surgical problem. Questions should be encouraged and answered. The surgeon must be alert for signs that the older person may not be able to give a truly informed consent and be ready to involve the family in this respect. Cassileth et al. (19) studied 200 patients who gave informed consent about treatment and found that 60% understood what they had signed but that only 40% had read the consent form carefully. They did not find age a factor in determining who read or understood the forms. Being bedridden or not reading the form carefully were the primary reasons for lack of understanding. Grundner (34) studied surgical consent forms from five large hospitals and found four were written at the level of a scientific journal and the other at the level of a specialized academic magazine. He suggested analysis of all consent forms for readability. If the elderly person shows signs of confusion, has poor eyesight, or has little formal education, it may be necessary to give extensive verbal explanation at a very simple level to both the patient and the family. It is important for any patient approaching surgery to have an understanding of what is going to happen, not merely for medicolegal reasons but, more importantly, to allay fears about the unknown, either real or imagined. Once the patient and family have been informed, management can conveniently be divided into preoperative, operative, and postoperative periods.

Preoperative Management

Preoperative management is perhaps the most important of the three stages, and careful assessment and planning in this stage can avoid many later problems (51).

1. Assess the patient comprehensively, considering the presenting illness in the context of coexisting disease and age-related changes. Although less time is available before emergency surgery, preoperative assessment is still essential. Think of vital organs, particularly heart, lungs, liver, and kidneys. Regardless of whether abnormalities of function are due to age or to disease, each organ system must be evaluated and deficiencies considered in planning surgery. A good physician will have an idea of overall function after an adequate history and physical examination, coupled with standard tests such as complete blood count (CBC), urinalysis, chest x-ray, and electrocardiogram (ECG). In addition, certain deviations from youthful function must be anticipated in the absence of laboratory abnormalities, e.g., diminished creatinine clearance in spite of normal urea nitrogen and creatinine levels.

2. Treat systems that can be improved before surgery. For some elderly patients admitted to the hospital, the surgical problems are urgent. Conditions such as ruptured aorta, rapidly deteriorating intracranial hematoma, massive continuing bleeding due to ruptured organ, and traumatic injuries require early recognition and prompt operative intervention before irreversible damage occurs. The opportunity to salvage the patient could be lost if preoperative preparation is unduly prolonged in the hope of achieving optimal conditions. Under such urgent conditions, the operative procedure should be initiated swiftly and limited to controlling the condition which will save the patient's life. Unless an absolute emergency exists, treatment for imbalances in blood, electrolytes, and fluids, as well as for congestive failure and respiratory insufficiency, needs to be started before going to the operating room. In purely elective situations, all vital organs should be restored to maximal possible function before the operation. Even if it takes a week, the time spent in active therapy to compensate for congestive cardiac failure, control hypertension, achieve optimal pulmonary and excretory function, restore fluids, electrolytes, and blood deficiencies, improve nutritional status, and prepare the gastrointestinal tract is of more value preoperatively than later, when the patient may be in trouble.

3. Estimate the risk for development of emergency surgical problems. Because of the greater risk in emergency operations on older persons, it becomes increasingly important to anticipate and correct surgical problems which might lead to an emergency. Questions to be asked are: Will the elective surgery offer improved quality of life or increased survival? Will postponement risk later and more hazardous emergency surgery (patient with a small but reducible inguinal hernia which incarcerates more easily than a bigger defect)? Would postponing surgery until excessive obesity is reduced decrease overall operative risk? Is there irreversible impairment of a vital organ that results in even relatively simple surgery presenting excessive risk? (For example, severe pulmonary fibrosis and emphysema in an elderly patient with recently discovered asymptomatic gallstones usually contraindicates elective surgery.) Is it likely that the patient will succumb to another disease

before the surgical problem becomes clinically significant? These and similar questions should sound familiar, as they are often asked when considering surgery for patients of all ages; but they are particularly important in the elderly.

4. Keep the patient mobile and out of bed as much as possible. In addition to maintaining positive nitrogen balance, the many other salutary effects of mobility include prevention of musculoskeletal atrophy of disuse, sodium retention, respiratory and venous stasis, skin pressure sores, and bladder dysfunction.

5. Prepare the patient for postoperative events. Respiratory and exercise regimens should be rehearsed; and elderly patients need even more than usual mental preparation for possible intravenous therapy, respirators, or colostomy.

Operative Management

In one sense, the patient is at least risk during surgery when all vital functions are under constant surveillance and immediate direct control. Catastrophes as severe as cardiac arrest, pneumothorax, or hemorrhage are better handled in the operating room than anywhere else. Foldes (28) pointed out that the ultimate success or failure of the surgical operation often depends more on the quality of the pre- and postoperative care than on the skill of the surgeon. Yet, certain intraoperative considerations can reduce postoperative complications in the elderly (21).

1. Plan and supervise anesthesia management. The surgeon and anesthesiologist should work in close cooperation to plan the operation with a view to handling possible problems and avoiding overtaxing the patient. The range of possible anesthetic techniques and agents enables one to adapt appropriately to the specific needs of each patient. Careful supervision during the anesthetic period is essential at all times. Due to normal aging changes which can diminish circulation to the heart and other vital organs, older patients are even more sensitive than others to hypovolemia, hypoxia, or lower than normal perfusion pressures. Any potential causes of inadequate perfusion, even for the briefest periods, should be anticipated and prevented.

2. Minimize operating time. Neither undue haste nor cutting corners is suggested, but it is essential to plan ahead so that the surgical team can refrain from excess discussions during the operative procedure and quickly proceed to completion.

3. Handle tissues gently. Care with tissues is always important but particularly so in the elderly where aging reduces the vascular supply and diminishes the ability to heal and regenerate after surgical trauma. Handling includes incision, exposure, excision, anastomosis, suturing, and closure. Dr. Richard Shackleford of Johns Hopkins used to tell his residents, "every stitch a masterpiece."

4. Consider staged procedures. There are patients (e.g., those with diverticular abscess or perforated colon cancer) in whom simple diverting proximal colostomy followed later by excision at the second stage, and even a third stage for colostomy closure, may be safer than a single but unduly long or traumatic operation.

5. Watch body temperature. This vital sign, though easily monitored, is often neglected. Longer operations are more likely to produce hypothermia.

Postoperative Management

The postoperative period may well be the time of greatest risk for the patient because of confidence and relaxation of attentiveness after "the worst" (i.e., the surgery) is over.

1. Check vital signs frequently—more often during the early postoperative days, tapering off gradually as the patient improves. These checks take little time and provide important information about common postoperative complications, e.g., wound infection, pneumonia, phlebitis, urinary retention, and ileus. Reactions may develop more slowly in the elderly, and clues of distress may be less obvious and occur later. During the immediate postoperative period, any trend should be noted. A rising pulse rate, a slight fall in blood pressure, less urine output—all require attention. Complications are best dealt with by preventing their development.
2. Avoid extremes of therapy. For example, postoperative fluids and electrolytes should be given at levels calculated to be best for each patient rather than at arbitrary predetermined levels. Administering too much fluid (congestive failure), as well as too little (atelectasis, clotting), is dangerous. The patient's position during intravenous infusions is of major importance. Remember again that elderly patients have, in general, less reserve capacity to adapt to change. Necessary drugs should always be given; but dosages, particularly of analgesics and hypnotics, frequently need to be much lower for elderly patients. When in doubt about dosage, give less medication more frequently, observing the effects closely.
3. Be alert for signs of mental confusion. Patients who do not regain preoperative mental capacities rapidly are always a concern. Altered mental status is a very common manifestation of systemic postoperative problems and should never be attributed to old age and overlooked. Anoxia, stroke, or excess medication are much more likely causes than simply a delayed recovery from anesthesia.
4. Initiate progressive activity, coughing exercises, respiratory physiotherapy, and any indicated rehabilitative measures. Just as in the preoperative stage, ambulation is very important, helping to reduce the likelihood of atelectasis, pneumonia, phlebothrombosis, thrombophlebitis, and other complications. Some contraindications to ambulation are bleeding, insecure wound closure, high fever, cardiac decompensation, peritonitis, pneumonia, or acute thrombophlebitis.

EPILOGUE

It is true that aging leads slowly and inexorably to a decline in overall capacity and function. However, those individuals who become our older patients are generally tougher than average, having survived killer diseases of youth and middle age. Furthermore, elderly survivors are living into extremes of old age. Operative risks, although greater than for a younger patient, are *not* prohibitive. Numerous recent reports studying thousands of cases have documented the relative safety of properly managed surgery in the elderly. Elderly surgical patients deserve the same careful evaluation for surgical care as younger patients. Consider the risks and benefits of surgery for each patient individually and decide to operate based on these considerations and not on the patient's age.

When caring for elderly patients, the physician should:

1. Know how the morbidity and mortality of surgery in elderly patients differ from those in younger patients.
2. Know the factors that are more important than chronological age in the assessment of surgical risk in elderly patients.
3. Know the ways in which the increased variability of functional capacity in the aged demands more highly individualized care of the aged than of younger persons.
5. Know the features of preoperative, operative, and postoperative care which are responsive to the particular needs of elderly patients.

REFERENCES

1. Albano, W. A., Zielinski, C. M., and Organ, C. H. Is appendicitis in the aged really different? *Geriatrics*, 30:81–88, 1975.
2. American College of Surgeons. Editorial. *Bull. Coll. Surg.*, 20:5, 1964.
3. Anderson, B., Genster, H., and Langberg, K. Geriatric surgery in a community. *Acta Chir. Scand. [Suppl.]*, 354:1–103, 1965.
4. Anderson, B., and Ostberg, J. Long-term prognosis in geriatric surgery: 2–17 year follow-up of 7922 patients. *J. Am. Geriatr. Soc.*, 20:255–258, 1972.
5. Andres, R. Aging and diabetes. *Med. Clin. North Am.*, 55:835–846, 1971.
6. Arkins, R., Gmessaert, A. A., and Hicks, R. G. Mortality and morbidity in surgical patients with coronary artery disease. *JAMA*, 190:485–488, 1964.
7. Aubry, V., Renis, R., Kuri-Szanto, M., and Paout, M. Factors affecting survival of the geriatric patient after major surgery. *Can. Anaesth. Soc. J.*, 12:510–520, 1965.
8. Austen, W. G., DeSanctis, R. W., Buckley, M. J., Mundth, E. D., and Scannell, J. G. Surgical management of aortic valve disease in the elderly. *JAMA*, 211:624–626, 1970.
9. Bafitis, H., and Sargent, F. Human physiological adaptability through the life sequences. *J. Gerontol.*, 32:402–410, 1977.
10. Berman, V. D., David, T. E., Lipton, I. H., and Lenhei, S. C. Surgical procedures involving cardiopulmonary bypass in patients aged 70 or older. *J. Am. Geriatr. Soc.*, 28:29–32, 1980.
11. Bolt, D. E. Geriatric surgical emergencies. *Br. Med. J.*, 1:832–836, 1960.
12. Bonus, R. L., and Dorsey, J. M. Major surgery in aged patients. *Arch. Surg.*, 90:95–96, 1965.
13. Bosch, D. T., Islani, A., Tarr, C. T. C., and Beling, C. A. The elderly surgical patient. *Arch. Surg.*, 64:269–277, 1952.
14. Bowles, T., Hallman, G. L., and Cooley, D. A. Open-heart surgery in patients over sixty years of age. *J. Am. Geriatr. Soc.*, 17:817–821, 1969.
15. Brander, P., Kjellberg, M., and Tammisto, T. The effects of anaesthesia and general surgery on geriatric patients. *Ann. Chir. Pyraec. Fenn.*, 59:138–145, 1970.
16. Brooks, B. Surgery in patients of advanced age. *J. Tenn. Med. Assoc.*, 31:128–135, 1938.
17. Burnett, W., and McCaffrey, J. Surgical procedures in the elderly. *Surg. Gynecol. Obstet.*, 134:221–226, 1972.
18. Carp, L. Common problems in geriatric surgery. *Geriatrics*, 6:100–111, 1951.

19. Cassileth, B. R., Zupkis, R. V., Sutton-Smith, K., and March, V. Informed consent—why are its goals imperfectly realized? *N. Engl. J. Med.*, 302:869–899, 1980.
20. Cohn, R., Close, M. B., and Mathewson, C. Operations upon the aged. *Calif. Med.*, 86:299–301, 1957.
21. Cole, W. H. Medical differences between the young and the aged. *J. Geriatr. Soc.*, 28:589–614, 1970.
22. Cole, W. H., and Mason, J. H. Surgical aspects in the care of the geriatric patient. In: *The Care of the Geriatric Patient*, edited by E. V. Cowdry. Mosby, St. Louis, 1968.
23. Crane, M. G., and Harris, J. J. Effect of aging on renin activity and aldosterone excretion. *J. Lab. Clin. Med.*, 87:947–959, 1976.
24. Cutler, C. W., Jr. Management of surgical emergencies in the aged. *Bull. NY Acad. Med.*, 32:495–501, 1956.
25. Djokovic, J. L., and Hedley-Whyte, J. Prediction of outcome of surgery and anesthesia in patients over 80. *JAMA*, 242:2301–2306, 1979.
26. Estes, W. L. Reduction of mortality in surgery of the aged. *Penn. Med. J.*, 52:937–943, 1949.
27. Finch, C. E., and Hayflick, L. *Handbook of the Biology of Aging*. Van Nostrand Reinhold, New York, 1977.
28. Foldes, F. F. Preoperative preparation and postoperative care of the aged. *Geriatrics*, 7:165–169, 1952.
29. Gemählich, M., and Krautwing, K. Experiences in surgery on the aged. *Z. Altersforsch.*, 15:106–110, 1961.
30. Gertman, P. M., Stackpole, D. A., Levenson, D. K., Manuel, B. M., Brennan, R. J., and Janko, G. M. Second opinions for elective surgery: the mandatory medicaid program in Massachusetts. *N. Engl. J. Med.*, 302:1169–1173, 1980.
31. Gilchrist, R. K., and dePeyster, F. A. Abdominal surgery of the aged. *JAMA*, 160:1375–1378, 1956.
32. Glenn, F. Pre- and postoperative management of elderly surgical patients. *J. Am. Geriatr. Soc.*, 21:385–393, 1973.
33. Griffiths, J. M. T. Surgical policy in the over-seventies. *Gerontol. Clin.*, 14:282–296, 1972.
34. Grundner, T. M. On the readability of surgical consent forms. *N. Engl. J. Med.*, 302:900–902, 1980.
35. Haug, C. A., and Dale, W. A. Major surgery in old people. *Arch. Surg.*, 64:421–427, 1952.
36. Hay, A. W. S. Surgery in the aged. *J. Can. Med. Assoc.*, 43:531–537, 1940.
37. Hormozi, A., and Mahringer, W. Zur Chirugie des holeren Lebensaeters unter besonderer Berucksichtigung der Notfalle. *Med. Wochenschr.*, 19:174–177, 1965.
38. Klug, T. J., and McPherson, R. C. Postoperative complications in the elderly surgical patient. *Am. J. Surg.*, 97:713–717, 1959.
39. Kohn, R. P. Human aging and disease. *J. Chronic Dis.*, 16:5–21, 1963.
40. Kohn, R. P., Zehart, F., Vormittag, E., and Grabner, H. Risks of operation in patients over 80. *Geriatrics*, 28:100–105, 1973.
41. Limbosch, J. Experiences with more than 1000 elderly surgical patients. *Arch. Surg.*, 73:124–132, 1956.
42. Linn, B. S. The impact of continuing education on the process and outcome of emergency room burn care. *JAMA*, 244:565–570, 1980.
43. Linn, B. S., Linn, M. W., and Gurel, L. Physical resistance and longevity. *Gerontol. Clin.*, 11:362–370, 1969.
44. Linn, M. W., and Hunter, K. I. Perceptions of age in the elderly. *J. Gerontol.*, 34:46–52, 1979.
45. Linn, M. W., Linn, B. S., and Gurel, L. Patterns of illness in persons who lived to extreme old age. *Geriatrics*, 27:67–70, 1972.
46. Lorhan, T. Surgery and anesthesia in the octogenarian. *Am. J. Surg.*, 114:665–671, 1967.
47. Marshall, W. H., and Fahey, P. J. Operative complications and mortality in patients over 80 years of age. *Arch. Surg.*, 88:896–904, 1964.
46. McCarthy, E. G., and Widmer, G. W. Effects of screening by consultants on recommended elective surgical procedures. *N. Engl. J. Med.*, 291:1331–1335, 1974.
49. Meyer, K. A., Jacobson, H. A., and Beaconsfield, P. Surgical treatment of the octogenarian. *J. Int. Coll. Surg.*, 29:263–269, 1958.
50. Mitty, W. F., and Echemendia, E. Surgery in the aged. *GP*, 31:122–130, 1965.
51. Ochsner, A. Is risk of indicated operation too great in the elderly? *Geriatrics*, 22:121–130, 1967.

52. Ochsner, A. Aging. *J. Am. Geriatr. Soc.*, 24:385–393, 1976.
53. O'Donnell, T. F., Jr., Darling, R. C., and Linton, R. R. Is 80 years too old for aneurysmectomy? *Arch. Surg.*, 111:1250–1257, 1976.
54. Oh, W., Hickman, R., Emanuel, R., McDonald, L., Somerville, J., Ross, D., Ross, K., and Gonzaleg-Lavin, L. Heart value surgery in 114 patients over the age of 60. *Br. Heart H.*, 35:174–180, 1973.
55. Randall, H. T. The treatment of cancer in older patients. In: *Surgery of the Aged and Debilitated Patient*, edited by H. Powers. Saunders, Philadelphia, 1968.
56. Rowe, J. W. Clinical research on aging: strategies and directions. *N. Engl. J. Med.*, 297:1332–1336, 1977.
57. Rowe, J. W., Andres, R., Tobin, J. D., Norris, A. H., and Shock, N. W. The effect of age on creatinine clearance in men: a cross-sectional and longitudinal study. *J. Gerontol.*, 31:155–163, 1976.
58. Ryan, P. Surgery for abdominal emergencies. *Geriatrics*, 15:73–89, 1960.
59. Rzepiela, E. Early postoperative complications of acute abdominal diseases in elderly patients. *Gerontol. Clin.*, 15:92–112, 1973.
60. Santos, A. L., and Gelperin, A. Surgical mortality in the elderly. *J. Am. Geriatr. Soc.*, 23:42–46, 1975.
61. Scott, D. Anaesthetic experience in 1300 major geriatric operations. *Br. J. Anaesthesiol.*, 33:354–370, 1961.
62. Stahlgren, L. H. An analysis of factors which influence mortality following extensive operations upon geriatric patients. *Surg. Gynecol. Obstet.*, 113:283–292, 1961.
63. Suarez, R. M. Cardiovascular evaluation in geriatric surgery. *Postgrad. Med.*, 31:395–400, 1962.
64. U.S. Dept. of Health, Education, and Welfare, Public Health Services, National Center for Health Statistics. Life tables. *Monthly Vital Statistics Report*, Series 24, No. 11, 1974.
65. U.S. Dept. of Health, Education, and Welfare, Public Health Services, National Center for Health Statistics. Utilization of short-stay hospitals. *Vital and Health Statistics*, Series 13, No. 41, 1977.
66. Welch, C. S. Surgery in the aged. *N. Engl. J. Med.*, 238:821–832, 1948.
67. Wilder, R. J., and Fishbein, R. H. Operative experience with patients over 80 years of age. *Surg. Gynecol. Obstet.*, 113:205–212, 1961.
68. Ziffren, S. E., and Hartford, C. E. Comparative mortality for various surgical operations in older versus younger groups. *J. Am. Geriatr. Soc.*, 20:485–489, 1972.

Fundamentals of Geriatric Medicine, edited by
Ronald D.T. Cape, Rodney M. Coe, and Isadore
Rossman, Raven Press, New York © 1983.

32

Ordinary Versus Extraordinary Measures in Care of the Elderly

Ian R. Lawson

"Ordinary" and "extraordinary" are words which are more provocative than accurate with respect to the issues and which derive from one overpublicized area of hospital care. Clarifying the semantics of elderly care constitutes much of what geriatric medicine has been about. It has ambiguous official standing as yet (8); and with the exception of a few Veterans Administration hospitals and faith-related long-term care facilities, it lacks any distinctive area of clinical practice. Hence its present impetus in the United States remains the attempt to reconceptualize care of the elderly in circumstances in which it has neither standing nor control. That it tries to do so around the distinct biological focus of the very elderly is more antithetical than complementary to conventional medical approaches.

Geriatric medicine is more than merely adapting the techniques used in other areas of adult medical care to the elderly. To the degree that practitioners of this discipline are prepared to make the biology of old age of overriding importance and the use of diagnostic and therapeutic techniques subservient, they will run countercurrent, as we shall see, to much of medical process and trends. Certainly, therefore, controversy about the role and extent of medical activism in care of the disabled elderly, especially in its high technology pursuits, should be assured a steady place in the professional literature. Why, then, has there been so little evidence of it compared to the extensive debate, for instance, about appropriate care for irretrievably brain-damaged young adults (e.g., the Miss Quinlans) or multi-afflicted newborns (5), both of which cases are outnumbered by the problematic morbidities of the elderly? Indeed, some of our false notions of prolonged "medicated survival" of the elderly are derived from the profession's experience and thinking about the moribund young rather than about the morbid old. Hence, as earlier implied, the controversy cannot begin until there are those prepared to address the elderly case in its own right and, both at the individual case and general level, take up a sturdy advocacy in the antithetical debate which must follow.

It was almost 20 years ago that what remains a typical controversy emerged in the *Lancet* between a general internist and geriatric physicians about the kind of medical care appropriate for disabled elderly. The generalist (as disappearing a breed on the British hospital scene as on the American) argued for a friendly counselor role, one that would eschew the restorative, scientific activism then being promoted by the emergent career geriatricians (10). Paradoxically, he also complained about the inappropriate use of his own acute medical wards, blocked by an occupancy of dependent, undischargeable elderly people who had somehow found their way there. Geriatric physicians found in his dual complaint a vindication of their position: that such elderly benefited from an observant and discretionary activism, one which would also promote the appropriate use of hospital resources, and from using the specially developed facilities in geriatric care, which are still "extraordinary" in comparison to those available in the United States (1,24).

The controversy is typical because it remains bivalent: What kind of inactivism or activism is appropriate for care of the elderly? The scene has changed in that the hospital is now dominated by the activities of high-technology specialists whose activism, rather than inactivism, toward the elderly contributes to the modern dilemma. The scene remains the same in that geriatric medicine is still a stand for a stratagem of activism which is biologically rather than procedurally determined. Like the British scene of 20 years ago, we in the United States now have our own demographic tide of elderly overflowing hospital and nursing home walls. So too, the "unblocking" of "acute care beds" (by depositing disabled elderly somewhere else) has now become many physicians' sole perception of geriatric need. That restricted view has been reinforced rather than corrected by the formal systems of utilization review and Professional Standard Review Organizations, which make effective alternatives in geriatric care that much more difficult to practice and demonstrate (11).

CRITICAL CARE

Left unexplored and largely undebated, the "ordinary versus extraordinary" issue in critical care remains to surface in subtle ways, in particular by an uncomfortable ambivalence in practices of care that should be done with confidence or not at all. One senior medical resident told me recently that, after training, he intended to relate to a small hospital without resident house staff, where he believed he could serve the elderly more helpfully, for, as a member of a university house staff program, "I've seen too much of the other side." The most profound phenomenon I faced later, as a Vice-President for Medical Affairs (V.P.M.A.) of one of Connecticut's large teaching hospitals, was the sense of alienation, expressed by many of its attending staff physicians, from the very institution and technologies over which the public at large assumed they had total dominance! That alienation is frequently most discomforting in the intensive care units, where the attending physician feels at the periphery of the scene, a bystander to acts and processes whose details, he knows, require a competence he does not possess, whose activators (house staff, full-time subspecialists, highly specialized nurses and technicians) he uneasily defers to.

That these activators themselves may be more confident about the "how" and "what" than the "why" and "whether" of what they do for particular patients is rarely voiced, except as an after-the-experience reminiscence, similar to that of the medical resident earlier quoted. I made the administrative practice, when V.P.M.A., of visiting the hospital in the wee sma' hours of the early morning. There was often a lull of nursing activities that permitted one to talk and reflect on a day that had been too busy to permit the same. Nurses in a critical care unit once asked me, in particular regard to their many elderly patients, whether there should not be an explanation of the "whys" and "whethers" of such care, as there was already in-service education as to procedures and pathophysiology. I have no doubt that such needs, left unmet, make for an inarticulate sense of unease. Certainly house staff were eager to involve me in cases where the attending physician had prescribed excessive activism in care. By and large, however, that unvoiced sense of unease or self-doubting seems only to impel the participants to perform their tasks of patient care more urgently and more routinely, permitting display of neither questioning nor feeling.

The overall appearance to the recipients of care (or more often their observant family members) can be appalling. Netsky (18) has written about it as a physician-teacher becoming for the time being a bedside relative and an aghast spectator of his demented mother's intensive care (her earlier and his current wishes notwith-standing). This occurred in a major teaching hospital and became for him "a night-mare of depersonalized institutionalization." He makes an important remark about the attending physician role: "He listened sympathetically...but nothing changed. He who should have been in control of the system was dominated by it." Poe (20), writing as an attending geriatric physician, sees severe tensions between dictates of conscience and judgment and the context and processes of the modern hospital. The case has been argued by the Director General of the World Health Organization, no less, that the enormous costs engendered by the "doctor-hospital complex" about terminal care, worldwide, is starving preventive and primary care services of the resources that they need and with which they could show demonstrably better yield in human life and well-being (15). In a reply to this, it has been argued that an examination of the excessive investment in types of hospital care of the elderly might explain the concomitant deprivation of alternative geriatric services, both institutional and community (12,16). Such considerations receive additional force from critical care units. Cullen and his colleagues (4) reported only a 27% survival after 1 year, with only 27 of 62 survivors fully recovered, at an average cost per patient (in 1972) of over $14,000. Few very elderly were included in the study, but the older patients were disproportionately represented among the nonsurvivors (4). That a large part of many elderly persons' lifelong medical costs are engendered in hospital during the last year of life may represent a gross imbalance of investment (6). Personal audit of to-and-fro transfer from nursing homes to intensive care areas of hospitals has shown costs exceeding $16,000 per hospital stay.

The situation is not made easier by the fact that nursing home care is hardly able to provide the basic life support services necessary for terminal care, compelling doctor, patient, and relatives to acquiesce in reluctant transfers to the general hospital and to submit to resuscitative care rather than comfort-supporting care (as in the case of Netsky's mother). It is from such discordance, between what may be wanted on a limited scale of intervention and what is compulsively supplied, that the hospice movement has emerged. However, highly interactive care for the articulate (mostly younger) dying patient is still care for a minority. What of the much larger number of very elderly dying from a terminal illness that commonly has them incommunicado for weeks or months or years by reason of confusion, dementia, or aphasia? Altogether, the doctor's choices are not easy, and they become less easy as the doctor becomes more experienced. In the case of those severely or irrecoverably ill elderly persons who do not have (as the majority do not) access to the few, faith-related, high-caliber geriatric institutions, patient and doctor have choices limited by the kind of undifferentiated institutional services available, both hospital and long term. Furthermore, when the patient's needs exceed or inconvenience these services, the operating conditions of the institutions have a perverse way of making the patient's biology and occupancy deemed inappropriate rather than vice versa. Rossman (21) has explored "the environments of geriatric care." As he describes the hazards of submitting fragile and multiply ill elderly to the uncomprehending environment of hospital on the one hand, or to the inadequate environment of the standard nursing home on the other, the tone is very much that of "how to survive unfriendly waters, written by a master mariner"!

ENDS AND MEANS

In the idea of "ordinary versus extraordinary measures" we may be submitting to the technological fix that only complicated hardware constitutes exceptional care. In fact, there is nothing ordinary about any form of medical care, just as there is nothing very extraordinary about the particular kind of instruments it employs. The one end is as artificial as the other. The real questions are: What is meant by one's "therapeutic intentions"? Are the type and scale of medical intervention appropriate for the support of those intents? Spicker (22) focuses on the confusion between ends and means in his discussion of the "right to a natural death." He writes (22):

> The powerful image is one of a debilitated, dying person, usually elderly, whose condition is incurable; the person is abandoned, multiply betubed, sedated, suffering intractable, chronic pain; the medical professionals appear unconscionably doing more and more with the medical armamentarium available to them in the modern hospital, and so forth. The cry for a "natural death" is a form of public outrage in reaction to this inhumane care setting made incomprehensible to us in the presence of complex life-sustaining machinery. So the cry is for the removal of all of the apparatus, all the so-called "artificial" means of prolonging life or dying, however you construe this scenario. Regrettably, the public's image is distorted. Moreover, the public lens is focussed in the wrong corner of the room, so to speak. The problem is not the technology of modern medicine nor the tubes and pharmacopoeia. The issue of dignity rests with the realization of the patient's

will; that he or she be the final authority in the treatment decisions during the final days and weeks of life.

Spicker also asks

...what can one name in the mundane events of everyday living that is not in some way artificial? The entire pharmacopoeia and even the so-called "natural foods" are shot through with human artifice. Even the "food" sustaining the life of Ms. Karen Ann Quinlan is not natural [and] is fed through plastic nasogastric tubes which enable the nutriment to reach the upper absorption area of the stomach and intestines....

The real issues are professional discretion and judgment as well as patient consent, not the scale or complexity of our resuscitative technology. Problems in their application apply at any age where, as Jonas (9) writes:

...the treatment does nothing but keep the organism going without in any sense being ameliorative...In addition, when treatment becomes identical with keeping alive, there arises for physician and hospital the spectre of killing with discontinuance, for the patient the spectre of suicide with demanding it, for others that of complicity in one or the other with mercifully facilitating or not resisting it...The worrisome cases are those of the more or less captive, viz., hospitalized patients with terminal illness, whose helplessness necessarily casts others in the role of accessories to realizing his option for death, even to the point of substituting for him in making the option.

More commonly than not, however, such *ultimum moriens* in the case of the elderly is a product of several interacting major pathologies and multiple systems failure. In aggregate (as the well-publicized case of President Tito showed) it will exceed the capacities of even the most aggressive and elaborate use of "life support" systems of critical care technology. It is the younger adult with an irretrievably damaged brain but healthy other systems who is the costly long-term problem.

The elderly who are dying with the meager provisions of the nursing home should not be classified with the young dying slowly in costlier circumstances, as a similar kind of expensive, medicated survivalism. As the hospice movement shows, decent professional care of the dying need not be so expensive as standard hospital care but, on the other hand, will never be as cheap as the standard skilled nursing facility. Agate's advocacy for the dying elderly in Britian (2) has yet to be made here: "Because their death rates are so high, geriatric departments must have first class equipment and amenities to help their terminal patients to die with dignity, free from suffering, and with peace of mind." Extraordinary arguments for extraordinary measures indeed!

EXTRAORDINARY CARE IN ITS PRECRITICAL DIMENSIONS

Often the physician can implement measures that would prevent the elderly from entering that phase of multiple system decompensation that intensive hospital care, although inevitable, may still fail to correct. The calamity of nursing home care, judged from its high rehospitalization rate, is that it is ill-equipped and only peripherally served by the physician whose alacrity of response could perhaps save the day. Following are several examples of presenting symptomatology that will invariably progress to multisystem crisis if left untended. Commonly and even more dangerously, the mode of presentation is insidious. My early treatment is controversial!

1. Heavy glycosuria in the very elderly diabetic can lead to a nonketotic hyperosmolar syndrome. *Prompt* treatment of any precipitating infection by intramuscular or oral antibiotic; *gentle* replacement of fluids by subcutaneous clysis (minimizing thereby the risks of overloading the intravascular compartment by directly using it); and short-term regular insulin on a t.i.d. sliding scale—all are more effective in the early case than the massive interventions of the late. However, just try introducing clysis to a hospital conditioned to the "bigger is better" of venous-arterial cannulation!

2. Gram-negative septicemia is common in the nursing home population. If suspected (by rigors, high fever, limb mottling, or low blood pressure with any fever), is it automatically a case for transfer to critical care? I became impressed by the delay between early diagnosis made in the nursing home and the initiation of treatment in the adjoining hospital. The patient negotiates the emergency room and admitting process, is seen by doubting house staff, has blood drawn (again) for CBC, cultures, etc. Having regularly seen hours go by before the belated start of antibiotics (then "piggyback" by intravenous infusion of course), I introduced a protocol for the immediate start of intramuscular antibiotics after blood culturing (13) and kept the patient in the nursing home. Profound septic shock thereafter became a rarity.

3. Ultrasonography and Doppler sonography enable a noninvasive, early diagnosis of correctible aneurysm of the aorta before rupture and of ileofemoral stenosis before gangrene. Why do we listen to the heart sounds so intently and to the arteries so much less so? And why is our examination of the feet so cursory when the information of incipient insufficiency is so plainly there in the loss of dorsal hair, dermal atrophy, the loss of pedal pulses? Short of corrective arterial surgery, there is still much to do. If only we treated preventively the arterially incompetent foot as Paul Brand of Vellore eventually promoted for the leprosy foot. Even in advanced arterial disease, gangrene is less often spontaneous than precipitated, as in the leper's foot, by trauma to which the patient is insensitive. In addition to making the above observations, grip the Achilles tendon and note the absence of deep pain. Then regard the footwear or the nail-cutting habits. Why are so many gangrenous legs still being taken off above the knee, making prosthetic fitting and the energy costs of ambulation so much more penalizing (3)? Why has cardiology trapped physicians into regarding pacemakers as the only form of prosthetic instrument, calling for their awareness and advocacy?

EXTRAORDINARY MEASURES OF ELECTIVE TYPE

The combination of modern anesthesia, implant prosthetics, and surgical skill has seen a revolution in care for the very elderly. However, this underpublicized aspect of extraordinary measures suffers severely from the departmentalized type of continuing medical education in hospitals. In departments of medicine, the forum is dominated by physician subspecialists presenting pathophysiological exquisites about some peculiarly ill people, leading trainees to produce a plethora of data rather than therapeutic elucidation. Where do the internist and family practitioner hear case presentations on cataract surgery and lens replacement, hearing deficits and their surgical and prosthetic correction, joint replacement, oral and dental interactions with drugs and mood state, anesthesiology and the compromised cardiopulmonary system, or electroshock treatment versus tricyclics for depression?

Without such interdisciplinary awareness, the physician is still a novice in the field of extraordinary measures. Without this, the physician is advising about elective procedures on which he or she is not fully informed—whose benefits and risks to the total patient, considering the overall pathophysiological status of the multiply diseased person, both postoperatively and in the long term, he cannot assess.

Sometimes advanced old age is actually a positive indication for prosthetic implants. For implantable devices whose long-term durability has not been determined, the elderly patient's limited life expectancy reduces the impact of long-term stress failure. The multiple pathologies of elderly patients, including incipient brain dysfunction, also may make a stronger case for some types of elective surgery than would their absence! Following cataract extraction, elderly people can have profound problems of visual-perceptual adjustment from external replacement lenses, which confer such magnification and peripheral field distortion that both distance judgment and equilibrium are permanently upset (19). What such lenses rely on is, of course, the capacity of the intact brain to circumvent the resultant image distortions. Some elderly brains may not have this capacity. Contact lenses are difficult enough for the nimble fingers and wits of the teenager to maintain; arthritic hands or proprioceptive blunting make them impossible. Hence, for all these reasons, lens implantation (whatever its 5- or 10-year durability or risks) may be the optimal choice for a 90-year-old with mild memory failure and osteoarthritic fingers (17). Furthermore, restoration of vision with elective procedures does not have to be total (as with younger patients) to be satisfactory. When severe dependency and distress are present, partial improvements in each enhance both patient and family well-being (23).

All these procedures require the support and referral of physicians, who understand the true basis of "fitness" for the elective surgery involved and the extraordinary range of procedures and materials increasingly available. [Hench (7) lists 50 implantable devices made from more than 40 different materials.] The current capacity for pathophysiological monitoring and evaluation has been developed more for critical care of multisystem failure (or for "stress testing" the middle-aged executive) than for assessing elective procedures for the elderly who are ambulant but restricted. To an elderly person who can get about even with restricting symptoms, elective measures may represent smaller risk and larger potential gain relative to waiting for such catastrophes as fall, fracture, progressive immobility, or vascular episode. For example, a recent study of walking after total hip replacement shows that considerable gains in efficiency result, suggesting reduced stress on the compromised heart (14) and possibly better and longer life.

SUMMARY

Determination of what constitutes ordinary or extraordinary diagnostic or therapeutic interventions for truly frail elderly individuals demands an individualized, comprehensive assessment of clinical, ethical, and life quality issues, with and without the measure under consideration. Using criteria that recognize effect on the quality of life and expected duration of life may often convert the active and hitherto even extraordinary treatment into the conservative and ordinary course. Only when clinical decisions concerning elderly patients include the relevant individual and general geriatric data—free of ageist biases—can we comfortably welcome care of the elderly into the mainstream of American health care.

When caring for elderly patients, the physician should:

1. Know the ethical issues raised by the need to consider possible use of high-technology interventions in elderly persons with limited biological reserves or life expectancy.
2. Know how an overreliance on high technology may divert attention from other measures which may prevent multisystem failures in elderly patients with limited physiological reserves.
3. Know how terminal care can be given its own positive values.
4. Know how an understanding of the preterminal personality and wishes of the terminal patient can be important to the management of his or her dying and death.
5. Know how the needs can be identified and met of other health care personnel involved in the care of the desperately ill or dying elderly patient.

REFERENCES

1. Agate, J. N. Letter. *Lancet*, 2:658, 1962.
2. Agate, J. N. Care of dying in geriatric departments. *Lancet*, 1:364–366, 1973.
3. Committee on Prosthetic-Orthotic Education. *The Geriatric Amputee. Principles of Management.* National Academy of Sciences, Washington, D.C., 1971.
4. Cullen, D. J., Ferrara, L. C., Briggs, B. A., Walker, P. F., and Gilbert, J. Survival, hospitalization charges and follow-up results in critically ill patients. *N. Eng. J. Med.*, 294:982–987, 1976.
5. Duff, R. S., and Campbell, A. G. M. Moral and ethical dilemmas in the special care nursery. *N. Eng. J. Med.*, 289:890–894, 1973.
6. Gornick, M. Ten years of Medicaid: Impact on the covered population. *Social Security Bull.*, 40:8–9, 1976.
7. Hench, L. L. Biomaterials. *Science*, 208:826–831, 1980.
8. Institute of Medicine. *Aging and Medical Education.* National Academy of Sciences, Washington, D.C., 1978.

9. Jonas, H. The right to die. *Conn. Med. (Suppl.)*, 43:35–42, 1979.
10. Kemp, R. The diagnosis of old age. *Lancet*, 2:515, 1962.
11. Lawson, I. R. Professional Standards Review Organization and care of the elderly. *JAMA*, 229:311–313, 1974.
12. Lawson, I. R. Letter, *Lancet*, 1:481, 1976.
13. Lawson, I. R., and Chapron, D. A basic pharmacopoeia for geriatric practice. In: *Clinical Aspects of Aging*, edited by W. Reichel. Williams & Wilkins, Baltimore, 1978.
14. McBeath, A. A., Bahrke, M. S., and Balke, B. Walking efficiency before and after total hip replacement as determined by oxygen consumption. *J. Bone Joint Sur.*, 62A:807–810. 1980.
15. Mahler, H. Health—A demystification of medical technology. *Lancet*, 2:829–833, 1975.
16. Moore, F. D. Letter. *Lancet*, 1:83, 1976.
17. National Institutes of Health consensus development conference: intraocular lens implantation. Sept.:10–11, 1979.
18. Netsky, M. G. Dying in a system of "good care": case report and analysis. *Conn. Med.*, 41:33–36, 1977.
19. Paton, D., and Craig, J. A. Aphakic vision. *Clin. Symp.*, 26:21–23, 1974.
20. Poe, W. D. The physician's dilemma: when to let go. *Forum Med.*, 3:163–166, 1980.
21. Rossman, I. Environments of geriatric care. In: *Clinical Geriatrics*, 2nd ed., edited by I. Rossman, Lippincott, Philadelphia, 1979.
22. Spicker, S. F. Do we have a right to a natural death—ethical, legal and medical considerations. *Conn. Med. (Suppl.)*, 43:42–45, 1979.
23. Wilcock, G. K. Benefits of total hip replacement to older patients and the community. *Br. Med. J.*, 2:37–39, 1978.
24. Wilson, L. A., and Lawson, I. R. Letter. *Lancet*, 2:658, 1962.

Fundamentals of Geriatric Medicine, edited by
Ronald D. T. Cape, Rodney M. Coe, and Isadore
Rossman, Raven Press, New York © 1982.

Questions for Self-Assessment

DIRECTIONS: In questions 1–9, only *one* alternative is correct. Select the one
best answer and blacken the corresponding lettered box on the
answer sheet.

1. Menopause occurs because of:

   (A) Depletion of gonadotropins
   (B) Failure of the endometrium to respond to hormones
   (C) Aging of the hypothalamus
   (D) Depletion of follicles and ova
   (E) Vascular changes

2. In elderly patients:

   (A) Staging of surgery so that two or three small procedures are done instead
       of one large operation markedly increases the risk to the patient
   (B) It is advisable to operate more slowly than in younger patients to avoid
       tissue damage
   (C) Healing is usually slower than in younger patients
   (D) Surgical risk roughly doubles every 5 years after the age of 75
   (E) Elective surgery is generally not indicated for benign conditions unless
       the patient is having symptoms

3. Of the following, the *most* likely cause of malnutrition in the elderly is:

   (A) Eating an unbalanced diet of convenience foods
   (B) Failure to maintain an adequate intake of fruit and vegetables
   (C) Illness or disability resulting in loss of mobility
   (D) Failure to absorb nutriments adequately
   (E) Loss of teeth resulting in inability to eat meat

4. The administration of high doses of estrogen:
   - (A) Helps to prevent coronary disease in men who are at high risk
   - (B) Lowers the level of serum lipids
   - (C) Lowers the level of triglycerides
   - (D) Increases the incidence of coronary disease in men who are at high risk
   - (E) Is appropriate for men who have had a myocardial infarction

5. An elderly patient whose blood pressure has been rising over the years is considered to have hypertension warranting intervention when the blood pressure first reaches:
   - (A) 150/100 mm Hg
   - (B) 160/85 mm Hg
   - (C) 160/95 mm Hg
   - (D) 180/100 mm Hg
   - (E) None of the above

6. An 82-year-old man has an asymptomatic adenocarcinoma of the rectum near the anal verge without evidence of bone or hepatic metastases. The remainder of the physical examination is within normal limits. The *most* appropriate management at this time is:
   - (A) Medical palliation alone
   - (B) Abdominoperineal resection with permanent colostomy
   - (C) Palliative transverse colostomy without resection
   - (D) Local resection
   - (E) Chemotherapy alone

7. After menopause, estrogen is:
   - (A) Not produced
   - (B) Synthesized mainly in the ovarian tissue
   - (C) Secreted mainly by the adrenal glands
   - (D) Produced by the uterus
   - (E) Derived from the conversion of an adrenal androgen in body fat

8. In an older woman in whom pregnancy has been ruled out, a diagnosis of menopause can be made when there is:
   - (A) An absence of menses for 6 months
   - (B) Persistent elevation of the serum follicle-stimulating hormone and luteinizing hormone levels
   - (C) A low estrogen level
   - (D) A low progesterone level
   - (E) No change in the basal body temperature on a monthly cycle

9. Hypertension in elderly patients:

(A) Predominantly involves systolic pressure
(B) Predominantly involves diastolic pressure
(C) Generally involves both systolic and diastolic pressure proportionately
(D) Is generally labile, with systolic and diastolic pressures variable
(E) Is generally indistinguishable in clinical features from hypertension in younger persons

DIRECTIONS: In questions 10–20, *one or more* of the alternatives may be correct. You are to respond either *yes* (Y) or *no* (N) to *each* of the alternatives. For every alternative you think is correct, blacken the corresponding lettered box on the answer sheet in the column labeled "Y". For every alternative you think is incorrect, blacken the corresponding lettered box in the column labeled "N".

10. Elevation of systolic blood pressure without elevation of diastolic blood pressure is associated with an increased risk of:

(A) Renal failure
(B) Congestive heart failure
(C) Myocardial infarction
(D) Stroke
(E) Death

11. Reasons that octogenarians require fewer calories in their diets than younger persons include:

(A) Basal metabolic rate is reduced by 40%
(B) Lean body mass is reduced by 15 to 20%
(C) Total body water is increased by 7%
(D) Muscular activity is reduced
(E) Total amount of sleep in 24 hours is increased

12. Confusion in an elderly patient that develops 24 hours after an apparently successful operation:

(A) Is often a first sign of a complication
(B) Is more common than in younger patients
(C) Suggests a delayed effect of the anesthetic agent
(D) May be an indication of underlying brain atrophy
(E) Requires psychiatric evaluation

13. It is claimed that iron deficiency anemia occurs commonly in elderly patients. True statements on this subject include:

(A)   Forty percent of the elderly are iron-deficient and often anemic as a result

(B)   A Canadian study found that iron stores were less adequate in elderly subjects than younger ones

(C)   Occult bleeding is the most common cause of iron deficiency anemia in old people

(D)   Less than one-third of all cases of iron deficiency anemia in the elderly are nutritional in origin

(E)   A low hemoglobin and inadequate iron stores are good indicators of morbidity

14.   Administration of estrogen after menopause is associated with:

(A)   Retardation of osteoporotic changes
(B)   Lowering the blood level of gonadotropic hormone
(C)   Increasing muscle mass
(D)   Improvement of symptoms of arthritis
(E)   Increased production of progesterone

15.   Preoperative laboratory test results that are influenced by the age or the patient include:

(A)   Serum electrolyte levels
(B)   Serum creatinine clearance
(C)   Blood urea nitrogen (BUN) levels
(D)   Hematocrit
(E)   Urinalysis

16.   True statements concerning the blood pressures of elderly persons include:

(A)   Systolic blood pressure rises almost linearly with increasing age
(B)   Women are more responsive than men to treatment of hypertension
(C)   Women have more complications of hypertension than men
(D)   Elevated blood pressure levels in patients who have had a myocardial infarction are associated with an increased risk of death

17.   Early postoperative ambulation in the elderly surgical patient:

(A)   Reduces the frequency of atelectasis
(B)   Has important psychological effects
(C)   Helps maintain nitrogen balance
(D)   Reduces the frequency of thromboembolic episodes
(E)   Helps maintain calcium balance

18.   There is evidence of some vitamin deficiencies reported in elderly subjects. The most common deficiencies include:

(A) Vitamin A
(B) Vitamin B$_1$
(C) Vitamin C
(C) Vitamin D
(E) Vitamin E

19. Postural hypotension in elderly patients can result from:

(A) Reduced sensitivity of the baroreflex receptor
(B) Migraine headaches
(C) Administration of phenothiazines
(D) Systemic disease
(E) Arterial rigidity

20. True statements about proper diet for old people include:

(A) The ideal diet for the octogenarian is a mixed one with adequate protein, fruit, vegetables, and fibers
(B) All foods for old people should be sieved or puréed to ensure adequate absorption
(C) Milk is a most useful source of both protein and calcium and should form a staple of the elderly person's diet
(D) Iron supplementation is essential to maintain adequate stores in the elderly
(E) Because of its calorie-producing nature, fat should be avoided by the old

Answers to Self-Assessment Questions

Section	Question number	Correct answer(s)	Author reference(s)
Biology of Aging	1	A	Shock
	2	C	Davis and Davis
	3	C	Rowe
	4	E	Rowe
	5	B	Shock
	6	A	Rowe
	7	E	Rowe
	8	D	Davis and Davis
	9	A	Davis and Davis
	10	C	Rowe
	11	A	Davis and Davis
	12	D	Hayflick
	13	B	Shock
	14	C	Davis and Davis
	15	B	Rowe
	16	C	Rowe
	17	C	Shock
	18	E	Davis and Davis
	19	A	Shock
	20	B	Hayflick
	21	A,D,E	Beard
	22	B,D	Beard
	23	A,B,C,D	Gilchrest
	24	A,C,E	Hayflick
	25	A,B,C,D,E	Beard
	26	B,D	Beard
	27	C,D	Gilchrest
	28	B,E	Gilchrest
	29	A,D,E	Gilchrest
	30	A,B,D	Beard
	31	A,C	Gilchrest
	32	A,B,C	Beard
	33	A,B,D	Hayflick
Diagnosis	1	A	Grotta and Fields
	2	D	Levenson
	3	C	Seimon
	4	C	Seimon
	5	D	Levenson
	6	D	Willington
	7	C	Grotta and Fields
	8	D	Seimon
	9	A	Seimon

Section	Question number	Correct answer(s)	Author reference(s)
	10	C	Levenson
	11	A	Levenson
	12	A	Grotta and Fields
	13	D	Willington
	14	B	Grotta and Fields
	15	E	Levenson
	16	C	Moore and Whanger
	17	D	Rodstein
	18	B	Seimon
	19	D	Seimon
	20	A,B,C,D	Moore and Whanger
	21	A,B,C,D	Willington
	22	B	Levenson
	23	A,B,C,D,E	Rodstein
	24	A,C,E	Willington
	25	B,C,D	Willington
	26	A,C,D	Grotta and Fields
	27	A,B,D	Moore and Whanger
	28	A,B,C,D,E	Rodstein
	29	A,B,C,D	Grotta and Fields
	30	A,B,C,D,E	Moore and Whanger
	31	A,B,E	Levenson
	32	A,C,D,E	Rodstein
	33	C	Willington
	34	A,B,C,D,E	Rodstein
Management	1	E	Kepes
	2	B	Pollak
	3	B	Patterson
	4	A	Patterson
	5	C	Patterson
	6	D	Levenson
	7	B	Moscovitz
	8	E	Kepes
	9	E	Bentley
	10	A	Levenson
	11	E	Levenson
	12	B	Patterson
	13	A	Moscovitz
	14	B	Moscovitz
	15	C	Kepes
	16	E	Levenson
	17	B	Levenson
	18	A,D,E	Levenson
	19	A,B,D,E	Pollak
	20	A,C,E	Moscovitz
	21	A,B,D	Bentley
	22	A,B,C	Carruthers
	23	A,B,C,D,E	Carruthers
	24	B,D	Pollak

Section	Question number	Correct answer(s)	Author reference(s)
	25	B,D,E	Carruthers
	26	A,B,D,E	Pollak
	27	A,E	Kepes
	28	A,C	Bentley
	29	A,B,C	Patterson
	30	A,B,D	Carruthers
	31	A,B,D	Moscovitz
	32	A,C,E	Bentley
	33	B,C	Pollak
	34	A,B,C,E	Kepes
	35	A,B,E	Carruthers
	36	A,C	Bentley
Controversies	1	D	Ryan
	2	C	Linn
	3	C	Cape
	4	D	Ryan
	5	C	Kannel et al.
	6	B	Linn
	7	E	Ryan
	8	B	Ryan
	9	A	Kannel et al.
	10	A,B,C,D,E	Kannel et al.
	11	B,D	Cape
	12	A,B	Linn
	13	C,D,E	Cape
	14	A,B	Ryan
	15	B,D	Linn
	16	A,D	Kannel et al.
	17	A,B,C,D,E	Linn
	18	B,C	Cape
	19	A,C,D	Kannel et al.
	20	A,C	Cape

Patient Management Problems

INSTRUCTIONS

A *patient management problem* (PMP) is a written simulation of the types of problems physicians actually encounter in clinical practice. As in real life, you are presented a case and then required to make a series of inquiries, decisions, and actions aimed toward diagnosis and appropriate management. Each decision you make supplies new information that you must incorporate in subsequent decisions until you have worked through the whole problem. Upon completion of the PMP, explanations for each possible step taken and a score for each option will enable you to assess your ability to evaluate, diagnose, and manage particular clinical problems.

The PMP begins with a brief description of a patient whose condition you are called upon to diagnose and treat. Following this is a series of subproblems or "decision points," focused on such things as history taking, physical examination, laboratory tests, and management. At each decision point you are asked to choose, from a list of possibilities, the tests, procedures, or actions you believe most appropriate for dealing with your patient's situation. Feedback is provided for each option you choose.

In working through the PMP, your challenge is to request all the needed information and order the correct procedures without asking for information or ordering tests and treatments that are noncontributory.

TO MAXIMIZE YOUR PERFORMANCE ON THE PMPs, FOLLOW THESE GUIDELINES:

1. Proceed through the decision points in the order in which they are presented.
2. Read the lead-in to each decision point carefully and determine the strategy you would employ if actually presented with the situation described.
3. Read all the options for a decision point before making *any* selections (the options are listed in random order).
4. Select options in the order of clinical importance—routines, if called for, first; then others in normal clinical sequence. Within each decision point, choose *as many* options as you think necessary.
5. Keep in mind that selection of options should include attention to substantiating your preliminary diagnosis, risk to the patient, invasiveness, and cost-effectiveness. These factors will be the basis for scoring.

6. Record your answers on the appropriate answer sheet. For *each* option you select, blacken the box beneath the YES. For each option you do not select, blacken the box beneath NO.

7. Find the outcome for each option you select by turning to the answer page and reading (only) the entry with the corresponding number. Do not read the outcome to options you do not select, since the information revealed might be confusing or misleading.

8. Keep in mind that you may not find among the options listed the precise step you would take in your own practice. Your choice is limited to those options that are listed. On the other hand, you may find studies or techniques offered that are not available to you in your practice. For the PMP, assume that all listed options are available and that it is up to you to choose which will be employed (possibly by a consultant).

9. Let the feedback to each option guide you to the choice of the next most logical one. When you have completed a section to your satisfaction—having selected as many options as you think are relevant or indicated—proceed to the next decision point.

10. When you have completed the last decision point, turn to the Critique. This will indicate with numerical scores which options were correct and provide an explanation for each.

CRITIQUE

The critique on the pages following each problem presents explanations for each of the various options. The reasons given for the accuracy or prudence of each option represent the consensus of a team of geriatric clinicians.

The critique also provides you an opportunity to assess your performance on each step of the PMP. A score ranging from $+5$ to -5 is indicated beside the explanation for each option. The basis for scoring is as follows:

$+5$ *essential*—the resolution of the problem is unlikely or impossible if this option is not chosen

$+3$ *important*—will contribute substantially to diagnosis or management; should usually be done in rendering prudent care

$+1$ *useful*—routine; can be done without undue expense and will give useful confirmatory or exclusional information

  0   *optional*—an examination that may or may not be helpful or timely, depending on aspects of the clinical context, including aspects that may not be known; generally, not expensive or intrusive

-1 *nonproductive*—including intrusive or distracting questions or examinations or treatments, which, without being harmful, impede or retard the efficient management of a problem through consumption of time or expense

-3 *harmful or contraindicated*—invasive questions or procedures likely to create problems or to consume expensive resources; includes unnecessary exposure to radiation, to dangerous medication, and so on

-5 *life-threatening or grossly inappropriate*—producing a major increase in risk to life or health; strongly contraindicated

PROBLEM A

Falling, Not Due to Accidents in a 79-Year-Old Woman

Ronald D. T. Cape

GENERAL INFORMATION

A 79-year-old woman is admitted to the hospital following a fall with one week's history of nausea and vomiting. In the past several weeks, she has had a number of unexplained falls not apparently due to accidents. The patient is being treated for atherosclerotic heart disease by digoxin and hydrochlorothiazide. She has had diabetes mellitus for 4 years, which has been managed by diet and an oral hypoglycemic drug (tolbutamide).

DECISION POINT A-1

In your evaluation of the cause of this patient's falls, and with the understanding that a thorough history will be taken, to which of the following points would you wish to give particular importance at this time?

1. Were the falls associated with blackouts?
2. Has there been any sensation of palpitation?
3. Has the patient recognized any prodromal features immediately prior to falling?
4. Was recovery succeeded by a period of unusual drowsiness or blankness?
5. Was there any dizziness associated with the falls?
6. Did the patient experience any excessive sweating or feeling of chill at the time of the falls?
7. Did the falls have a discernible relationship to meals?
8. Was there any associated incontinence?
9. Was there any amnesia following the falls?
10. Were any other symptoms experienced concurrently or immediately following the falls?
11. Was there any association between the falls and specific neck movements?
12. Was the patient able to rise from the floor unaided following the fall?
13. Have falls occurred when the patient is wearing a scarf or collar around her neck?
14. Have falls occurred immediately after assuming the erect position?
15. Has there been noticeable increase in polydipsia and polyuria associated with episodes of falling?
16. Has there been a relationship between the time of taking antidiabetic medication and the falls?

17. Has the patient been taking medications as prescribed?
18. Is there a history of alcohol intake?
19. Is the patient taking any drugs besides those prescribed?

Turn to page 348 for answers

DECISION POINT A-2

On admission to the hospital, physical examination revealed a regular heart rhythm at 60 beats per minute. Blood pressure was 130/80 mm Hg. There were a few basal lung crackles and 1 to 2 + pitting edema. Roentgenogram of the chest demonstrated some cardiac enlargement and Kerley B lines. Hemoglobin level was 12.1 g/dl. Blood urea nitrogen (BUN) level was 15 mg/dl. Serum creatinine level was 1.0 mg/dl. Urinalysis demonstrated glucose + + and a trace of protein. Serum digoxin level was 3.5 ng/ml (therapeutic level, 1 to 2 ng/ml).

Digoxin was discontinued, and there was some improvement in her nausea and vomiting. Another fall occurred 10 days after admission. The patient was examined a few minutes after the fall. To which of the following items of physical examination would you now wish to give special attention in your effort to determine the cause of the falls?

20. Examination of the deep tendon reflexes
21. Examination of the heart
22. Blood pressure supine and standing
23. Examination of lungs
24. Examination of neck movements
25. Examination of eye movements
26. Presence of rombergism
27. Examination of cerebellar function
28. Examination for primitive reflexes
29. Auscultation of carotids
30. Palpation of carotids
31. Examination of mental status

Turn to page 348 for answers

DECISION POINT A-3

With the information you now have, consider the following investigative procedures and choose those that are thought to be most appropriate at this time.

32. Electrocardiogram (ECG)
33. 24-hr cardiac monitoring
34. Serum electrolyte levels
35. Echocardiography
36. Nystagmography
37. Liver enzyme levels
38. Serum calcium level
39. Serum protein levels
40. Pneumoencephalography

41. Fasting glucose concentration
42. 5-hr glucose tolerance test
43. Roentgenogram of skull
44. Computed tomography (CT scan) of head
45. Cerebrospinal fluid (CSF) flow studies
46. Examination of CSF
47. Electroencephalogram (EEG)
48. Doppler screening of carotids
49. Carotid angiography
50. Serum digoxin level

Turn to page 348 for answers

DECISION POINT A-4

With the information you now have, which of the following do you wish to include for management of this patient?

51. Reassurance only; no indications of serious condition
52. Advise avoidance of any ties around the neck
53. Order treatment with antiplatelet agents
54. Order treatment with anticoagulants
55. Restart digoxin at reduced dosage
56. Cardiologic consultation to consider insertion of on-demand pacemaker
57. Provide cervical collar
58. Order dilantin
59. Advise rising slowly from bed
60. Order compression support garment to legs and lower limbs to be pulled on before rising
61. Advise regular meals according to diabetic diet

Turn to page 348 for answers

ANSWERS

DECISION POINT A-1

1. Yes; falls associated with unconsciousness lasting ½ to 2 min
2. No
3. No
4. No
5. No
6. No
7. No
8. No
9. No
10. No
11. No
12. Yes
13. No
14. No
15. No
16. No
17. Patient and daughter agree that compliance is good
18. Occasional glass of sherry (3 a week)
19. No

DECISION POINT A-2

20. Present and equal bilaterally
21. Regular rhythm; normal S1 and S2
22. 130/80; 115/80; no symptoms associated
23. Poor movement, equal bilaterally; a few crackles at both bases
24. Somewhat limited; no pain; no dizziness or faintness elicited with movement in any direction
25. Full; no nystagmus
26. No
27. Within normal limits
28. Face-hand, snout, palmomental, and glabellar tap reflexes: normal responses
29. No carotid bruit heard
30. Bilaterally symmetrical carotid pulses
31. Patient fully oriented

DECISION POINT A-3

32. Sinus rhythm, left bundle branch block
33. Two episodes of paroxysmal atrial tachycardia (180/min); one prolonged (1-hr) spell of bradycardia (40/min); a blackout occurred during period of tachycardia
34. Na, 135 mEq/Liter; K, 4.0 mEq/Liter; Cl, 100 mEq/Liter; CO_2, 23 mEq/Liter
35. Some left atrial enlargement; otherwise normal anatomy
36. Within normal limits
37. SGOT 30 μU/ml; alkaline phosphatase, 150; lactic dehydrogenase (LDH) normal
38. 8.6 mg/dl
39. Albumin, 3.2 g/dl; globulin, 3.0 g/dl
40. Normal for age
41. Fasting level 150 mg/dl
42. Diabetic curve
43. Within normal limits
44. Normal for age
45. Normal for age
46. Protein, 40 mg/dl; glucose, 90 mg/dl; no cells seen
47. A little slow theta activity, otherwise within normal limits
48. No evidence of stenosis
49. Ordered
50. 0.25 ng/ml

DECISION POINT A-4

51. Given
52. Advice given
53. Ordered
54. Ordered
55. Ordered
56. Requested
57. Done
58. Ordered
59. Advice given
60. Ordered
61. Advice given

CRITIQUE

CASE SUMMARY

This 79-year-old woman, like many geriatric patients, has multiple problems, including falling, which is one of the most common. In addition to the falls, she has ischemic heart disease, diabetes mellitus, and evidence of cardiac arrhythmias; and she is receiving treatment with more than one drug. The presenting problem is falling, and this is the focus of this patient management problem. An attempt has been made to indicate the particular questions and examinations that have to be undertaken in order to assess this problem. This PMP is modeled after an actual patient in whom eventual response to the combination of antiarrhythmic drugs (digoxin) and an on-demand pacemaker were successful in preventing the blackouts and falls.

DECISION POINT A-1   Score

In your evaluation of the cause of this patient's falls, and with the understanding that a thorough history will be taken, to which of the following points would you wish to give particular importance at this time?

1. Were the falls associated with blackouts?
   It is important to determine whether falls are associated with transient loss of consciousness or not. If they are, the later investigation will focus upon the cause of the blackout rather than the circumstances of the fall itself. It is important to know the duration of periods of unconsciousness, if possible. Periods of unconsciousness lasting more than a minute or two would suggest epilepsy, with postictal somnolence or sleep, or diabetic or hypoglycemic coma.
   If you had selected this option your score would be . . . .   +3

2. Has there been any sensation of palpitation?
   If the patient has experienced palpitations, this would suggest a cardiac arrhythmia, such as paroxysmal tachycardia.
   If you had selected this option your score would be . . . .   +1

3. Has the patient recognized any prodromal features immediately prior to falling?
   An aura would indicate the high likelihood of seizure, as would the occurrence of drowsiness following the unconscious period.
   If you had selected this option your score would be . . . .   +1

4   Was recovery succeeded by a period of unusual drowsiness or   **Score**
blankness?
(See critique 3.)
If you had selected this option your score would be . . . .   +1

5.   Was there any dizziness associated with the falls?
Questions regarding dizziness often fail to differentiate sensations of light-headedness, such as may be associated with postural hypotension, from vertigo. A positive answer will need to be followed by other questions to distinguish between these two.
If you had selected this option your score would be   0

6.   Did the patient experience any excessive sweating or feeling of chill at the time of the falls?
Excessive sweating or a feeling of chill may be associated either with a vasovagal attack or with hypoglycemia.
If you had selected this option your score would be . . . .   +1

7.   Did the falls have a discernible relationship to meals?
Dizziness or loss of consciousness due to hypoglycemia classically occurs after a period of fasting (before meals).
If you had selected this option your score would be . . . .   +1

8.   Was there any associated incontinence?
The occurrence of incontinence with falls would suggest their association with a convulsive disorder.
If you had selected this option your score would be . . . .   +1

9.   Was there any amnesia following the falls?
A retrograde amnesia following the fall might be associated either with a transient ischemic attack or with epilepsy, but in this case the question is probably of doubtful value.
If you had selected this option your score would be . . . .   +1

10.   Were any other symptoms experienced concurrently or immediately following the falls?
Questions phrased in this open-ended manner are useful. They give the patient an opportunity to review the episode or problem under discussion and may help jog the memory of significant events or experiences. In this case, no further information is elicited.
If you had selected this option your score would be   0

11. Was there any association between the falls and specific neck movements?
   Episodes of drop-attacks and of syncope due to carotid sinus syndrome might both be stimulated by movements of the neck.
   If you had selected this option your score would be . . . .   + 3

12. Was the patient able to rise from the floor unaided following the fall?
   Following drop-attacks, patients are often quite unable to rise from the floor unaided.
   If you had selected this option your score would be . . . .   + 1

13. Do falls occur when the patient is wearing a scarf or collar around her neck?
   Falls due to the bradycardia of the carotid sinus syndrome are more common in men than in women; this is thought to be due to their wearing of more constrictive collars. For a female patient, this question yields information of probably limited value.
   If you had selected this option your score would be . . . .   − 1

14. Have falls occurred immediately after assuming the erect position?
   When falls occur on rising from a sitting or reclining position, the probability of postural hypotension is clearly indicated.
   If you had selected this option your score would be . . . .   + 3

15. Has there been noticeable increase in polydipsia and polyuria associated with episodes of falling?
   Diabetic coma or an increase in diabetic symptoms is unlikely to bear any relationship to this patient's recurrent falls. On the other hand, given the acute conditions with which this patient presented, the possibility of hyperosmolar coma would need to be given consideration. The most recent fall might reflect a change in the patient's diabetic state.
   If you had selected this option your score would be . . . .   + 1

16. Has there been a relationship between the time of taking anti-diabetic medication and the falls?
   It is unlikely that the time of taking of drugs would be related to the occurrence of the falls described in this patient.
   If you had selected this option your score would be   0

17. Has the patient been taking medications as prescribed?
   It is appropriate to know whether the patient's symptoms are in any way related to any of the drugs that she may be taking, whether for diabetes mellitus or for other problems.
   If you had selected this option your score would be . . . .   + 3

351

18. Is there a history of alcohol intake? Score

It is sometimes ignored that alcoholism occurs among the elderly, as among younger persons. Lethargy, confusion, and falls may be associated. For this patient, alcoholism does not contribute to her problems.

If you had selected this option your score would be . . . .   +1

19. Is the patient taking any drugs besides those prescribed?

It is useful to know what other drugs, such as tranquilizers, sedatives, laxatives, aspirin, or proprietary decongestants, the patient may be taking.

If you had selected this option your score would be . . . .   +1

DECISION POINT A-2 Score

To which of the following items of physical examination would you wish to give special attention in your effort to determine the cause of the falls?

20. Examination of the deep tendon reflexes

The fact that deep tendon reflexes are all present and equal bilaterally suggests that this patient does not have a localizing neurologic defect; this information helps to exclude the possibility that her falls have been due to transient ischemic attacks.

If you had selected this option your score would be . . . .   +1

21. Examination of the heart

Examination of the heart is clearly an important part of the evaluation of the patient. She has a regular rate of 60/min, with normal heart sounds and no murmur. These findings do not exclude the possibility that she may have arrhythmias from time to time.

If you had selected this option your score would be . . . .   +3

22. Blood pressure supine and standing

This is an important examination, which would determine whether postural hypotension is present. Findings diagnostic of postural hypotension would ordinarily require that the systolic pressure must fall by at least 20 mm Hg, with an equivalent drop in the diastolic pressure, on rising from the supine to the standing position. In this patient, no evidence of postural hypotension is found.

If you had selected this option your score would be . . . .   +3

23. Examination of lungs

Abnormalities in examination of the lungs are not at all likely

to be related to the complaint of blackouts or falls in this patient. **Score**
If you had selected this option your score would be . . . . -1

24. Examination of neck movements
It is useful to know the response of the patient to controlled movements of the neck, to ascertain whether such movements cause any dizziness or suggestion of fainting. Either of these findings would suggest vertebrobasilar ischemia or the possibility of drop-attacks.
If you had selected this option your score would be . . . .   · $+1$

25. Examination of eye movements
Examination of eye movements in some patients who have had cerebral vascular incidents such as transient ischemic attacks show limitation of movement in one or another direction.
If you had selected this option your score would be . . . . $+1$

26. Presence of rombergism
The finding of rombergism is unlikely to be of any particular value in this situation, where we are concerned with isolated falls associated with blackout spells.
If you had selected this option your score would be . . . . -1

27. Examination of cerebellar function
Signs of cerebellar function are not likely to be helpful in the differential diagnosis of falls in this patient, and more than routine attention to them would be unwarranted.
If you had selected this option your score would be . . . . -1

28. Examination for primitive reflexes
Primitive reflexes, such as face-hand, snout, palmomental, or glabellar tap reflexes, are usually thought to be indicators of frontal or parietal lobe damage, and they may be associated with dementia; but in this patient they are unlikely to be of significance or of value and special attention given to them would be unwarranted with the information at hand.
If you had selected this option your score would be . . . . -1

29. Auscultation of carotids
Auscultation over the carotid arteries is an important element of the assessment of a patient who has had falls or other episodes that might represent transient ischemic attacks due to emboli originating in plaques within the carotid arteries. Murmurs due to narrowing of the arteries will need to be differentiated from murmurs transmitted from the aortic valve area. Sonographic

examination of the carotids may locate areas of involvement. **Score**
If you had selected this option your score would be . . . . +3

30. Palpation of carotids
Palpation of the carotid arteries may yield useful information regarding the strength and symmetry of the pulses or the presence of a thrill at the site of narrowing. Pressure (always *unilateral*) over the carotid sinus may indicate undue sensitivity (marked bradycardia or a period of asystole) and point to a possible reason for falls.
If you had selected this option your score would be . . . . +1

31. Examination of mental status
In an elderly person who has been falling without explanation, an assessment of mental status is needed. This is an essential element of the adequate neurologic examination. In this case, the mental status of the patient does not suggest confusion or dementia.
If you had selected this option your score would be . . . . +3

DECISION POINT A-3 Score

With the information you now have, consider the following investigative procedures and choose those which are thought to be most appropriate at this time.

32. Electrocardiogram (ECG)
Examination of the ECG is strongly indicated for any situation in which arrhythmias are likely to be present. In this patient, left bundle branch block suggests that she has significant heart disease.
If you had selected this option your score would be . . . . +5

33. 24-hr cardiac monitoring
Twenty-four-hour cardiac monitoring is the procedure of choice in determining whether a patient is suffering from significant paroxysmal arrhythmias. In this case, episodic arrhythmias are noted, and the relationship of one of them to a blackout spell helps to pinpoint the cause of her falls. It should be noted that 24-hr monitoring may give normal results on one occasion in patients who have significant arrhythmias. A negative result is not, therefore, to be regarded as definitive. The test should be repeated when symptoms suggest the need.
If you had selected this option your score would be . . . . +5

34. Serum electrolyte levels
   The examination of serum electrolyte levels may be regarded
   as more or less routine, but the possibility exists that a severely
   reduced serum sodium level might indicate the basis for postural
   hypotension.
   If you had selected this option your score would be   0

35. Echocardiography
   Echocardiography is a useful, noninvasive method of examining
   various aspects of the anatomy and function of the heart. It will
   sometimes demonstrate aortic stenosis in patients with murmurs
   who have syncopal episodes with exercise. It is not likely,
   however, to be of particular relevance to the present situation.
   If you had selected this option your score would be   0

36. Nystagmography
   Nystagmography may be helpful in the investigation of the
   possibility of cerebellar lesions; in a patient who has no cerebellar signs, such as ataxia or other gait disturbance, it is not
   likely to be helpful.
   If you had selected this option your score would be ....   −3

37. Liver enzyme levels
   There is no reason to believe that a disturbance of hepatic
   function is related to falling spells in this patient. The examination would be irrelevant and expensive.
   If you had selected this option your score would be ....   −1

38. Serum calcium level
   This examination has little to offer in the investigation of a
   patient with falling episodes.
   If you had selected this option your score would be ....   −1

39. Serum protein levels
   This examination has little to offer in the investigation of a
   patient with falling episodes.
   If you had selected this option your score would be ....   −1

40. Pneumoencephalography
   Pneumoencephalography has largely been superseded by other
   tests and is nearly obsolete in the examination of patients with
   possible central nervous disorders. Echoencephalography, computed tomography (CT scan), radionuclide scans, and cerebral
   angiography have proved to be much more satisfactory ways
   of investigating the anatomy of the brain and of the ventricular
   system than pneumoencephalography. No basis has been laid

for the use of any of these examinations in this patient as yet. **Score**
If you had selected this option your score would be . . . . −5

41. Fasting glucose concentration
A measurement of the patient's fasting blood glucose level will give useful information regarding the level of control of her diabetes mellitus, and perhaps indicate the possibility that hypoglycemia may contribute to her falls. The latter is unlikely, however, in the case of falls unaccompanied by any premonitory or postfall disturbances in the sensorium.
If you had selected this option your score would be . . . . +3

42. 5-hr glucose tolerance test
The patient can be presumed to have had the diagnosis of diabetes mellitus adequately established in the past. There is no need to put her through the time-consuming, uncomfortable, and expensive procedure associated with a glucose tolerance test.
If you had selected this option your score would be . . . . −3

43. Roentgenogram of the skull
There is no substantial basis for this expensive investigation. (See critique 40.)
If you had selected this option your score would be 0

44. Computed tomography (CT scan) of head
(See critique 40.)
If you had selected this option your score would be . . . . −3

45. Cerebrospinal fluid (CSF) flow studies
Studies of the dynamics of CSF flow would be of particular interest in patients suspected of having normal pressure hydrocephalus. This problem is not under consideration in this patient, and such studies would be of no value here.
If you had selected this option your score would be . . . . −5

46. Examination of CSF
The examination of CSF might have been appropriate at the time of the patient's *first* fall, but hardly needs to be done now. In an elderly person, a fall may be the first recognized sign of a cerebrovascular accident, hemorrhage, or meningitis. It may be difficult to exclude these as diagnostic possibilities and examination of the CSF may be crucial to their recognition. In this patient, however, there is no indication that falls are the result of an active primary intracranial process, and examination of the CSF is unwarranted at this time.
If you had selected this option your score would be . . . . −3

47. Electroencephalogram (EEG)   **Score**
    An EEG would help to assess the possibility of epilepsy in this
    patient; on the other hand, her history has made epilepsy un-
    likely, and this expensive and time-consuming procedure is not
    likely to be of value.
    If you had selected this option your score would be   0

48. Doppler screening of carotids
    Sonographic examination of the carotid arteries is a simple
    noninvasive procedure, which can give useful information re-
    garding their caliber and the possibility of calcification within
    the walls. For a patient in whom falling spells might be the
    result of transient ischemic attacks of carotid plaque origin, this
    examination might give very useful information. In this case,
    no stenosis or calcification was noted.
    If you had selected this option your score would be . . . .   +1

49. Carotid angiography
    Carotid angiography is unnecessary and potentially dangerous
    in this patient, in whom it may have been rendered irrelevant
    by the results of sonographic examination of the carotid arteries.
    There is no indication, as yet, that the patient's falling has any
    relationship to cerebral vasculature. (See critique 48.)
    If you had selected this option your score would be . . . .   −5

50. Serum digoxin level
    The patient has had a high serum level of digoxin on admission
    to the hospital. A low level of digoxin with the new fall indicated
    that digoxin toxicity was not involved and opens the way to
    reconsideration of the patient's need for digoxin.
    If you had selected this option your score would be . . . .   +1

DECISION POINT A-4   **Score**

With the information you now have, which of the following do you
wish to include for management of this patient?

51. Reassurance only; no indications of serious condition
    At this stage in the investigation of this patient, any simple or
    casual reassurance would not be helpful and might be potentially
    harmful. A clearer idea of the cause of the falls must be estab-
    lished. The investigation can surely move forward in a climate
    of frankness and realistic optimism without the patient being
    told that "everything is going to be alright" or "there doesn't
    seem to be anything serious the matter."
    If you had selected this option your score would be . . . .   −3

52. Advise avoidance of any ties around the neck **Score**
We have no evidence here that this advice should be given. In any case, the materials that elderly ladies are likely to wear around their necks are ordinarily loose-fitting.
If you had selected this option your score would be . . . .   −1

53. Order treatment with antiplatelet agents
No evidence of transient ischemic attacks has been found that would warrant the administration of antiplatelet drugs to this patient. Moreover, the evidence for the effectiveness of aspirin in preventing such attacks so far indicates its usefulness only in males.
If you had selected this option your score would be . . . .   −1

54. Order treatment with anticoagulants
(See critique 53.) Anticoagulants fall into the same category. These agents are potentially much more dangerous than the antiplatelet agents and should not be used under the present circumstances.
If you had selected this option your score would be . . . .   −5

55. Restart digoxin at reduced dosage
When episodes of tachycardia have been demonstrated by 24-hr cardiac monitoring, the administration of digoxin is clearly indicated. This patient had been receiving digoxin on admission to the hospital, presumably because of a history of paroxysmal tachycardia.
If you had selected this option your score would be . . . .   +5

56. Cardiologic consultation to consider insertion of on-demand pacemaker
At this stage, there may not be enough clinical evidence that this woman has a sick sinus syndrome to account for her episodes of tachycardia or bradycardia; on the other hand, there is clearly some form of bradytachycardia syndrome present. Until a firm diagnosis can be made, the use of a pacemaker should be postponed.
If you had selected this option your score would be . . . .   +5

57. Provide cervical collar
Nothing in the patient's history, physical examination, or investigative studies has suggested that her falls are cataplectic or related to carotid sinus syndrome; accordingly, the use of a cervical collar is unlikely to be helpful.
If you had selected this option your score would be . . . .   −1

58. Order dilantin   **Score**

Since there is no clinical evidence of epilepsy, the administration of dilantin would be inappropriate. Moreover, dilantin appears to be a more dangerous drug in older persons than in younger persons.

If you had selected this option your score would be ....   −3

59. Advise rising slowly from bed

Patients with postural hypotension are usually advised to rise slowly from supine or sitting positions; postural hypotension is not a factor in this case.

If you had selected this option your score would be ....   −1

60. Order compression support garment to legs and lower limbs to be pulled on before rising

(See critique 59.) The same considerations apply to the use of support garments.

If you had selected this option your score would be ....   −3

61. Advise regular meals according to diabetic diet

There is no evidence that less-than-satisfactory regulation of this patient's diabetes mellitus has anything to do with her falls. She should be encouraged to continue with whatever adequate regimen she has found comfortable in the past.

If you had selected this option your score would be ....   −1

SUMMARY

The case described has been that of a 79-year-old woman who has multiple problems, which included heart disease, digoxin intoxication, and falling. At times, she was mentally confused and lethargic. By focusing on the cause of the falls, it was possible to develop a management program that offered her a resolution of her major problems. The description was based on a specific patient who enjoyed 2 years of independent living in the home of her son and daughter-in-law following the sequence of events related.

Falls were the critical element in a person whose ability to remain in a domestic environment was threatened by them. The initial presence of nausea and vomiting was due to digoxin overdosage, which might have played a role in the cause of the falls, but proved to be only a complication in a typical clinical situation encountered in an elderly patient. Having resolved these features, a further fall confirmed that these had no direct etiologic association with the iatrogenic upset. The key investigation proved to be the 24-hr cardiac monitoring, which revealed the presence of relatively long periods of tachyarrhythmia with an hour-long episode of bradycardia.

The name of sick sinus syndrome for this situation is correctly being abandoned, and it is now more commonly referred to as a tachybradycardia syndrome. While this situation is probably not common, it emphasizes the role of sudden arrhythmias, both fast and slow, as the cause of an abrupt change in cardiac output resulting in transient loss of consciousness and falling.

Falling, in itself, is a debilitating feature of illness in elderly patients, resulting in fear first of venturing out of doors and then even of walking about in the home. The resulting inactivity will lead to loss of muscle strength, and the resulting weakness will increase the likelihood of further falls. Thus, a vicious circle may be established that can be broken only by a determination of the cause of the falls and by a systematic approach to the problem, such as that portrayed in this particular case.

BIBLIOGRAPHY

Cape, R. D. T. (1978): *Aging: Its Complex Management*, pp. 113–136. Hagerstown, Md., Harper & Row.

Ferer, M. I. (1974): *The Sick Sinus Syndrome*. Mt. Kisco, N.Y. Futura Publishing Company.

Kaplan, B. M., Langendorf, R., Leo, M., and Pick, A. (1973): Tachycardia-bradycardia syndrome (so-called "sick sinus syndrome"). *Am. J. Cardiol.*, 31:497.

Marriott, H. J. L., and Myerburg, R. J. (1978): Sick sinus syndrome. In: *The Heart*, edited by J. W. Hurst, pp. 678–679. New York, McGraw-Hill.

Moss, A. J., and Davis, R. J. (1974): Brady-tachy syndrome. *Prog. Cardiovasc. Dis.*, 16:439.

Rubinstein, J. J., Schulman, C. L., Yurchak, P. M., and DeSanctis, R. M. (1972): Clinical spectrum of the sick sinus syndrome. *Circulation*, 46:5.

PROBLEM B

Persistent Fever in a 72-Year-Old Physician

Joan I. Casey

GENERAL INFORMATION

A 72-year-old general practitioner consults you, an internist, about a persistent fever. You obtain from him a history of fever of three weeks' duration with frequent spikes to 38.3°C (101°F). He says that he has some shortness of breath and malaise, and he is pretty sure that he has several times seen some blood tingeing to the urine.

On physical examination, you note that he is thin and quite anxious. His temperature is 38.9°C (102.0°F). His pulse rate is 100/min. You decide that he needs hospitalization for a complete workup to determine the etiology of his fever.

On admission to the hospital, his blood pressure is 160/70 mm Hg, pulse rate 112, temperature 38.9°C (102.0°F) rectally, and respiratory rate 18/min.

DECISION POINT B-1

With the understanding that a thorough history will be taken in the evaluation of this patient, to which of the following points would you give particular attention as important to his current problem?

1. Was the hematuria present at the start, at the end, or throughout urination?
2. Family history of tuberculosis
3. History of positive PPD skin test
4. History of night sweats
5. History of urinary frequency or dysuria
6. History of flank pain
7. Loss of weight
8. History of cough
9. History of alcohol intake
10. History of heart disease
11. History of smoking
12. History of recent dental procedures
13. History of recent urinary tract manipulations
14. History of recent urinary tract infections
15. Presence of shaking chills
16. History of diabetes mellitus
17. Use of aspirin or anticoagulants
18. History of recent travel

19. Presence of phlebitis in past few months
20. History of nausea, vomiting, or diarrhea
21. Recent sexual contacts
22. History of headaches
23. History of myalgias or arthralgias
24. History of myocardial infarctions
25. Presence of skin lesions
26. History of visual disturbances

Turn to page 364 for answers

DECISION POINT B-2

With the understanding that a thorough physical examination will be done, to which of the following points would you wish to give particular attention as germane to this patient's presenting complaint?

27. Palpation of abdomen
28. Auscultation of abdomen
29. Examination of lungs
30. Neurologic examination of limbs
31. Examination of temporal vessels
32. Examination of eyes
33. Examination of scrotum
34. Cardiac examination
35. Examination of lymph nodes
36. Examination of texture of hair
37. Examination of skin
38. Examination of oropharynx

Turn to page 364 for answers

DECISION POINT B-3

With the information that you now have, which of the following laboratory tests would you now order? Include everything you think is appropriate for diagnosis.

39. Hematocrit
40. Leukocyte count
41. Differential blood count
42. Urinalysis
43. Culture of specimen of urine
44. Specimen of urine for culture for tuberculosis
45. Specimen of urine for acid-fast stain
46. Erythrocyte sedimentation rate (Westergren)
47. Serum alkaline phosphatase level
48. Specimen of urine for cytologic examination
49. PPD skin test
50. Serum calcium level
51. Blood cultures

52. Serum haptoglobin level
53. Latex fixation test
54. Nephrotomogram
55. Intravenous pyelogram (IVP)
56. Sonogram
57. Renal aspirate
58. Renal angiography
59. Renal biopsy
60. Biopsy of liver

Turn to page 364 for answers

DECISION POINT B-4

With the information you now have, which of the following should be initiated for the management of this patient?

61. Order treatment with 40 mg of prednisone daily
62. Order antimicrobial therapy
63. Request surgical consultation for nephrectomy
64. Request surgical consultation for valve replacement
65. Order treatment by radiotherapy
66. Order treatment with appropriate hormones
67. Order skin testing of family members
68. Order bone scan
69. Order serum α-2 globulin level
70. Roentgenogram of chest

Turn to page 364 for answers

ANSWERS

DECISION POINT B-1

1. Throughout urination
2. One brother had tuberculosis years ago
3. No
4. Yes, occasionally
5. No
6. No
7. Eight pounds in six weeks
8. No
9. Drinks one to two cocktails a week
10. No
11. Nonsmoker
12. No, patient is edentulous
13. No
14. No
15. No
16. No
17. No
18. None
19. One episode 10 weeks ago
20. Occasionally
21. Only with wife of 40 years
22. No
23. No
24. No
25. No
26. No

DECISION POINT B-2

27. No tenderness, guarding, or masses
28. No bruits or rubs
29. Minimal rales at both lung bases
30. Reflexes normal; sensation is decreased bilaterally in lower limbs
31. Within normal limits
32. Within normal limits
33. No masses or inflammation
34. No murmurs or gallops
35. No adenopathy
36. Within normal limits
37. No lesions
38. Healthy teeth, gums, and tongue

DECISION POINT B-3

39. 38%
40. 14,000/mm³
41. 75% PMNs, 20% lymphocytes, 4% monocytes, 1% eosinophils
42. 3 to 5 RBC/HPF
43. No growth
44. Results available in three weeks
45. Negative
46. 100 mm/hr (normal 0 to 15)
47. 225 IU (normal, 30 to 85)
48. Negative
49. Negative
50. 12 mg/dl (normal, 9.0 to 10.5)
51. One of four cultures positive for *Staphylococcus epidermidis*
52. Elevated (normal, 53 to 150 mg/dl hemoglobin-binding capacity)
53. Minimal elevation
54. Caliceal blunting of right kidney, with nonradiolucent mass on tomogram
55. Caliceal blunting of right kidney
56. Internal echoes and poor transmission through upper pole of right kidney
57. No fluid obtained
58. Numerous corkscrew vessels; no response to epinephrine; some arteriovenous shunting
59. Within normal limits
60. Within normal limits

DECISION POINT B-4

61. Ordered
62. Ordered
63. Requested
64. Requested
65. Ordered
66. Ordered
67. Ordered
68. Ordered
69. Ordered
70. Ordered

CRITIQUE

CASE SUMMARY

Fevers in elderly persons have substantially the same causes as in younger persons.

Fever of unknown origin (FUO) is one of the most challenging diagnostic problems. This patient, 72 years of age, who complains of fever of several weeks' duration with daily spikes to 38.3°C (101.0°F) fulfills the major criteria for defining his illness as an FUO. It is necessary for the physician dealing with such patients to have knowledge of the various possible causes of FUOs in order to proceed in methodical fashion, rather than initiate invasive procedures or examinations that may do more harm than good.

Fevers of unknown origin should always call to mind three possible major causes: infection, malignant disease, and metabolic disturbances. Infections may be chronic or occult (tuberculosis or endocarditis); malignant diseases may have fever as their only initial symptom (lymphoma or renal cell carcinoma); and fever may be the prime signal for metabolic disturbances (hyperthyroidism or drug fevers, for example). In the elderly patient, FUOs are proportionately more likely to represent malignant disease than in the younger patient.

In this patient, hematuria has been noted, and it might well represent either infection (renal tuberculosis or cystitis) or malignant disease (renal cell carcinoma or bladder tumor).

DECISION POINT B-1   Score

With the understanding that a thorough history will be taken in the evaluation of this patient, to which of the following points would you give particular attention as important to his current problem?

1. Is the hematuria present at the start, at the end, or throughout urination?
   The observation that the urine contains blood throughout the period of bladder emptying suggests that the blood has a renal, rather than urethral, origin. In the latter case, the red cell content of urine might vary with the phase of micturition.
   If you had selected this option your score would be . . . .   +1

2. Family history of tuberculosis
   This question should be routine in the evaluation of elderly patients and is particularly appropriate in patients with FUOs. Tuberculosis is one of the most common causes of unexplained fever in elderly patients.
   If you had selected this option your score would be . . . .   +1

3. History of positive PPD skin test   **Score**

   This examination is highly appropriate (see critique 2). Interpretation of the PPD skin test must be cautious, inasmuch as some patients with advanced tuberculosis may be in a state of anergy, with false-negative results.

   If you had selected this option your score would be . . . .   +1

4. History of night sweats

   The history of night sweats is not very specific to tuberculosis and will not differentiate that infection from a variety of others.

   If you had selected this option your score would be . . . .   +1

5. History of urinary frequency or dysuria

   A question regarding frequency or dysuria is important. Frequency of urination and dysuria are common in patients with urinary tract infections, tuberculosis, renal abscess, prostatism, or carcinoma of the prostate.

   If you had selected this option your score would be . . . .   +3

6. History of flank pain

   This important question explores the possibility of urinary tract infection, perinephric abscess, renal tuberculosis, renal carcinoma, nephrolithiasis, or renal vein thrombosis with all of which flank pain may be associated; such pain would not likely be associated with other causes of hematuria.

   If you had selected this option your score would be . . . .   +3

7. Loss of weight

   A history of recent loss of weight concurrent with the fever is an important finding, reflecting that there is likely to be a serious underlying process, such as infection or malignant disease.

   If you had selected this option your score would be . . . .   +3

8. History of cough

   A history of cough would suggest the possibility of reactivation of pulmonary tuberculosis or disease metastatic to the lung; the negative answer does not exclude the possibility of renal tuberculosis.

   If you had selected this option your score would be . . . .   +3

9. History of alcohol intake

   A question regarding history of alcohol intake is appropriate. Alcoholism and tuberculosis are strongly associated; alcoholism is a common problem among elderly persons and particularly among elderly physicians.

   If you had selected this option your score would be . . . .   +1

10. History of heart disease
This question regarding prior heart disease is appropriate. A history of congenital or acquired heart lesions would suggest that the patient was at increased risk of bacterial endocarditis.
If you had selected this option your score would be . . . .   +1

11. History of smoking
As with carcinoma of the lung and the larynx, carcinoma of the bladder has been clearly shown to have a higher frequency among cigarette smokers than among nonsmokers. Frequency, dysuria, and hematuria may be early signs. In this patient, the discovery that the patient does not smoke makes the likelihood of carcinoma of the bladder a little less likely, but does not exclude it altogether.
If you had selected this option your score would be . . . .   +1

12. History of recent dental procedures
This question is appropriate. Dental procedures may initiate the bacteremia, which results in bacterial endocarditis.
If you had selected this option your score would be . . . .   +3

13. History of recent urinary tract manipulations
As with dental procedures, manipulations of the urinary tract (prostatic massage or surgery) may be common antecedents to bacterial endocarditis in elderly men.
If you had selected this option your score would be . . . .   +3

14. History of recent urinary tract infections
It is appropriate to inquire as to the possibility of urinary tract infection; renal and perirenal abscesses have increased incidence in patients with recurrent urinary tract infections, and prostatitis and carcinoma of the prostate may present as recurrent urinary tract infections.
If you had selected this option your score would be . . . .   +1

15. Presence of shaking chills
The occurrence of shaking chills is particularly likely to suggest infectious origin for fever rather than malignant or metabolic origin. The absence of chills is less useful as a diagnostic point.
If you had selected this option your score would be . . . .   +1

16. History of diabetes mellitus
A question regarding diabetes mellitus is appropriate; patients with diabetes are particularly susceptible to infection, and especially to renal abscess.
If you had selected this option your score would be . . . .   +1

367

17. Use of aspirin or anticoagulants   **Score**
    A question regarding the use of aspirin or anticoagulant drugs
    is appropriate. Either may cause hematuria in elderly patients.
    If you had selected this option your score would be . . . .   +1

18. History of recent travel
    A question regarding recent travel should be routine. Diseases
    endemic in any locality recently visited should be considered
    for the possibility that they may be responsible for an FUO
    (schistosomiasis, for example).
    If you had selected this option your score would be . . . .   +1

19. Presence of phlebitis in past few months
    Phlebitis in elderly patients is sometimes the first sign of an
    underlying malignancy and is not uncommon in patients with
    renal carcinoma or pulmonary carcinoma. Thrombophlebitis of
    the legs with extension upward could also result in renal vein
    thrombosis.
    If you had selected this option your score would be . . . .   +3

20. History of nausea, vomiting, or diarrhea
    It is appropriate to ask what symptoms, mild or otherwise, may
    be associated with an FUO. Nausea and vomiting are not un-
    usual findings in patients with renal carcinoma.
    If you had selected this option your score would be . . . .   +3

21. Recent sexual contacts
    A history of recent sexual contacts is not likely to elucidate the
    cause of an FUO or hematuria in this patient; this invasive type
    of question should generally be omitted.
    If you had selected this option your score would be   0

22. History of headaches
    The occurrence of headaches in a patient who has an FUO may
    suggest the diagnosis of temporal arteritis.
    If you had selected this option your score would be . . . .   +1

23. History of myalgias or arthralgias
    Temporal arteritis may be suggested by myalgias or arthralgias
    in some patients in whom the findings in the temporal artery
    itself can be minimal.
    If you had selected this option your score would be . . . .   +1

24. History of myocardial infarctions
    The history of myocardial infarction is not likely to be relevant
    to the present problem of fever of unknown origin. The question

may be appropriate in establishing the baseline physiologic status of the patient, but will not contribute to the differential diagnosis.
If you had selected this option your score would be .... −3

25. Presence of skin lesions
The presence of skin lesions could be an important finding. Petechiae would suggest bacterial endocarditis or other infection; an eczematoid eruption may be seen in patients who have renal cell carcinoma.
If you had selected this option your score would be .... +1

26. History of visual disturbances
The history of visual disturbances might suggest temporal arteritis, with which transient episodes of monocular blindness may occur. Sometimes these become permanent.
If you had selected this option your score would be .... +1

DECISION POINT B-2   Score

With the understanding that a thorough physical examination will be done, to which of the following points would you wish to give particular attention as germane to this patient's presenting complaint?

27. Palpation of abdomen
Abdominal examination is a most important part of the physical evaluation of the patient. It should not exclude examination of the flanks for tenderness or masses or observation for protective muscular spasm (guarding). Enlargement of the spleen occurs with bacterial endocarditis.
If you had selected this option your score would be .... +3

28. Auscultation of abdomen
Ausculation of the abdomen is at least as important as palpation. The presence of bruits or rubs would suggest aneurysm (atherosclerotic, mycotic, etc.), infection involving serous surfaces, or other cardiovascular abnormalities. These findings may be demonstrated even when palpation of the abdomen has revealed no abnormality.
If you had selected this option your score would be .... +3

29. Examination of lungs
Examination of the lungs will be an important part of the physical examination. Arteriovenous malformations are occasionally associated with renal carcinoma. Patients with such arteriovenous malformations may have cardiac failure because of high

cardiac output; this is suggested by your patient's blood pressure of 160/70 mm Hg.   **Score**

If you had selected this option your score would be . . . .   +1

30. Neurologic examination of limbs
The neurologic examination should not be limited to testing the deep tendon reflexes, but should include a sensory evaluation as well. Peripheral neuropathy, giving decreased sensation in the lower limbs, may be the only physical clue to malignant disease, including renal carcinoma.
If you had selected this option your score would be . . . .   +1

31. Examination of temporal vessels
Tortuosity of the temporal vessels would suggest the possibility of temporal arteritis as the cause of fever of unknown origin.
If you had selected this option your score would be . . . .   +1

32. Examination of eyes
Important clues to the diagnosis of fever of unknown origin may be found in the eyes or eyegrounds. Tuberculosis (miliary), endocarditis (Roth spots), and, less frequently, renal tumors may produce lesions in the retina.
If you had selected this option your score would be . . . .   +1

33. Examination of scrotum
The examination of the contents of the scrotum is important. Renal tuberculosis may be accompanied by tuberculous epididymitis. Varicocele or thrombosis of the left spermatic vein is a classic, though rare, finding in hypernephroma of the left kidney.
If you had selected this option your score would be . . . .   +3

34. Cardiac examination
An examination of the cardiovascular status should be done routinely. The finding of a murmur will suggest the possibility of bacterial endocarditis, particularly if the murmur is of recent origin.
If you had selected this option your score would be . . . .   +1

35. Examination of lymph nodes
Examination of the lymph nodes should be a routine part of the evaluation of a patient with fever of unknown origin. Adenopathy may occur in conjunction with renal cell carcinoma.
If you had selected this option your score would be . . . .   +1

36. Examination of texture of hair
Examination of the texture of the hair is not likely to be useful

in this patient. Thyrotoxicosis may produce fine, soft hair, along with fever, but it cannot account for hematuria. Accordingly, the examination is irrelevant to this patient.

If you had selected this option your score would be ....   −1

37. Examination of skin
Skin lesions may be present in patients who have renal cell carcinoma or bacterial endocarditis. The patient is frequently unaware of these lesions, so the physician must take the initiative in making the examination.
If you had selected this option your score would be ....   +1

38. Examination of oropharynx
Evidence of carious or abscessed teeth or gingivitis might indicate a basis for subacute bacterial endocarditis. Negative findings are less helpful than positive findings. An abnormal tongue might suggest a vitamin deficiency, possibly with peripheral neuritis as a finding. In this case, the tongue is within normal limits.
If you had selected this option your score would be ....   +1

DECISION POINT B-3

Score

With the information that you now have, which of the following laboratory tests would you now order? Include everything you think is appropriate for diagnosis.

39. Hematocrit
The screening test for anemia should be routine, but it is not likely to provide much help in the differential diagnosis. It may indicate whether the patient has had significant blood loss or is suffering from bone marrow depression due to infection.
If you had selected this option your score would be   0

40. Leukocyte count
(See critique 41.)
If you had selected this option your score would be   0

41. Differential blood count
The leukocyte count and differential are routine; the differential is the more helpful of the two, especially if abnormal. Leukocytosis with shift to the left will suggest infection; the differential is frequently normal despite infection.
If you had selected this option your score would be ....   +1

42. Urinalysis
This routine examination must be done here to confirm that the

urine contains blood, and it may give other useful information. If you had selected this option your score would be . . . .   **Score**

+1

43. Culture of specimen of urine
(See critique 44.)
If you had selected this option your score would be . . . .   +1

44. Specimen of urine for culture for tuberculosis
Examination of the urine for infection is appropriate. Not only the usual pathogens, but *Mycobacterium tuberculosis* should be looked for. Unfortunately, the results of culture for tuberculosis will not be known for several weeks.
If you had selected this option your score would be . . . .   +1

45. Specimen of urine for acid-fast stain
Acid-fast stain of the urine is not likely to be helpful and may be more misleading than useful, since organisms such as *Mycobacterium smegmatis* may be found.
If you had selected this option your score would be . . . .   −3

46. Erythrocyte sedimentation rate (Westergren)
The sedimentation rate is a nonspecific indicator of disease, without often indicating the nature of the morbid process.
If you had selected this option your score would be   0

47. Serum alkaline phosphatase level
Measurement of the alkaline phosphatase level is an important examination and may be helpful in establishing the differential diagnosis. The serum alkaline phosphatase level may be evaluated in patients who have renal cell carcinoma or who have renal tuberculosis. It would not be elevated in patients who have bacterial endocarditis, temporal arteritis, or renal abscess.
If you had selected this option your score would be . . . .   +3

48. Specimen of urine for cytologic examination
Cytologic examination of the urine has not proved to be very helpful; there are many false-positive and false-negative results of the examination.
If you had selected this option your score would be . . . .   −3

49. PPD skin test
An intermediate-strength PPD skin test is appropriate; if that is negative, a second-strength PPD skin test should be done in a patient with FUO. If both tests are negative, the diagnosis of active tuberculosis is unlikely; occasionally, however, ill pa-

tients are anergic to PPD, though they may have been positive reactors in the past.

If you had selected this option your score would be . . . .   +1

50. Serum calcium level
    The serum calcium level may be elevated in both renal cell carcinoma and renal tuberculosis.
    If you had selected this option your score would be . . . .   +3

51. Blood cultures
    Blood culture is an important part of the evaluation of patients who have FUO. Several cultures (three or more) should always be taken, and sometimes a larger number of cultures will be necessary before a significant pathogen is recovered from a patient with endocarditis or endarteritis. The finding of a single positive culture, out of four, for *Staphylococcus epidermidis* would rarely indicate an infection due to this organism; it would more frequently be a contaminant. If it is found, further blood cultures should be done.
    If you had selected this option your score would be . . . .   +1

52. Serum haptoglobin level
    Elevations of the serum haptoglobin level may be found in a variety of disorders; the test is of little value in differential diagnosis (see critique 69).
    If you had selected this option your score would be   0

53. Latex fixation test
    The latex fixation titer may be somewhat elevated in elderly patients generally, but a very high titer would suggest either temporal arteritis or endocarditis.
    If you had selected this option your score would be . . . .   +1

54. Nephrotomogram
    The nephrotomogram is a crucial test in patients with renal cell carcinoma. An intravenous pyelogram (IVP) may suggest the diagnosis, but often enough caliceal blunting is seen without the tumor being demonstrated. When a renal cell carcinoma is suspected, the IVP and nephrotomogram should be ordered together so that both tests could be done at the same time.
    If you had selected this option your score would be . . . .   +5

55. Intravenous pyelogram (IVP)
    (See critique 54.)
    If you had selected this option your score would be . . . .   +3

56. Sonogram Score

When a lesion has been found in the kidney by nephrotomography, the nature of the lesion can be clarified by sonography, which is able to distinguish solid tumor from a septic lesion such as abscess. In this patient, the findings of internal echoes and poor transmission through the upper pole of the right kidney suggest a solid tumor.

If you had selected this option your score would be ....   +1

57. Renal aspirate

There is no need to aspirate a lesion having the characteristics demonstrated on nephrotomography and sonography in this patient. The likelihood of abscess is negligible.

If you had selected this option your score would be ....   −3

58. Renal angiography

Angiography may help the surgeon to know the extent of the lesion and the nature of its blood supply. In this patient, numerous corkscrew vessels feeding the mass were shown, and these showed no response to the injection of epinephrine. There appeared to be some arteriovenous shunting within the lesion.

If you had selected this option your score would be ....   +3

59. Renal biopsy

Renal biopsy is not indicated in this patient. The findings so far elucidated are sufficiently characteristic of renal cell carcinoma that the appropriate management would be to go directly to the removal of the involved kidney.

If you had selected this option your score would be ....   −5

60. Biopsy of liver

No basis has been laid for biopsy of the liver in this patient. Biopsy of the liver is sometimes helpful in the workup of patients who have FUO and may reveal the miliary lesions of tuberculosis or the granulomas of sarcoid; it is not, however, indicated in this patient.

If you had selected this option your score would be ....   −3

DECISION POINT B-4 Score

With the information you now have, which of the following should be initiated for the management of this patient?

61. Order treatment with 40 mg of prednisone daily

Treatment with high doses of corticosteroids might have been helpful for a patient with temporal arteritis, but no basis has been laid for its use in this patient.

If you had selected this option your score would be . . . . −5

62. Order antimicrobial therapy
    No basis exists for antimicrobial therapy in this patient. The
    finding of *Staphylococcus epidermidis* in the blood apparently
    represents contamination.
    If you had selected this option your score would be . . . . −3

63. Request surgical consultation for nephrectomy of right kidney
    Nephrectomy is the only therapy appropriate to the diagnosis
    of renal cell carcinoma in this patient.
    If you had selected this option your score would be . . . . +5

64. Request surgical consultation for valve replacement
    Valve replacement might have been appropriate if a diagnosis
    of bacterial endocarditis were established, but it is not indicated
    in this patient.
    If you had selected this option your score would be . . . . −5

65. Order treatment by radiotherapy
    Some of the tumors responsible for FUO are sensitive to ra-
    diation; renal cell carcinoma is not. Accordingly, radiotherapy
    is inappropriate in this patient.
    If you had selected this option your score would be . . . . −5

66. Order treatment with appropriate hormones
    Hormonal treatment has been helpful in the management of
    some malignant tumors of organs under endocrine influence
    (breasts, for example), but has not proved to be useful in patients
    with renal cell carcinoma.
    If you had selected this option your score would be . . . . −1

67. Order skin testing of family members
    Skin testing of family members would be appropriate if tuber-
    culosis had been demonstrated in this patient, but that is not
    the case here.
    If you had selected this option your score would be . . . . −5

68. Order bone scan
    Bone scan is an appropriate part of the management of renal
    carcinoma, as should be a roentgenogram of the chest, in order
    to determine if metastases have occurred.
    If you had selected this option your score would be . . . . +5

69. Order serum α-2 globulin level   **Score**
As with the haptoglobin level (see critique 52), the level of α-2 globulins may be a useful, though not specific, index of the prognosis for patients with renal carcinoma.
If you had selected this option your score would be . . . .   +3

70. Roentgenogram of chest
(See critique 68.)
If you had selected this option your score would be . . . .   +3

SUMMARY

In summary, we have a 72-year-old physician who has had daily fever spikes of 38.3°C (101.0°F) for six weeks, with hematuria and loss of weight. Initial history and physical examinations were not strikingly abnormal; however, several diagnostic possibilities could be ruled out by these procedures, and some results were helpful in leading to or supporting the final diagnosis. These latter included the history of phlebitis and the finding of sensory changes in the lower limbs. When the calcium and alkaline phosphatase levels were found to be elevated in this patient, tuberculosis and renal cell carcinoma were very likely possibilities. Subsequently, more invasive laboratory tests revealed a mass in the right kidney, which by sonography and angiography was thought to be a malignant tumor. In managing such tumors, bone scans and roentgenograms of the chest should be done to discover the extent of metastases, if present.

Nephrectomy is the treatment of choice for renal cell carcinoma, and results can be very good even in cases in which metastasis has occurred to one or more areas. Radiotherapy is not recommended, and chemotherapy and hormonal therapy have been disappointing to date.

BIBLIOGRAPHY

Christensen, W. I. (1974): Genitorurinary tuberculosis: Review of 102 cases. *Medicine*, 53:377–390.
Clayman, R. Y., Williams, R. O., and Fraley, E. L. (1979): The pursuit of a renal mass. *N. Engl. J. Med.*, 300:72–79.
Cronin, R. E., Kaelney, W. D., Miller, P. D., Stabler, D. P., Gabow, P. A., Ostroy, P. R., and Schrier, R. W. (1976): Renal cell carcinoma: Unusual systemic manifestations. *Medicine*, 55:291–311.
Jacoby, G. A., and Swartz, M. N. (1973): Fever of unknown origin. *N. Engl. J. Med.*, 289:1407–1410.
Petersdorf, R. G., and Beeson, P. B. (1961): Fever of unexplained origin: Report on 100 cases. *Medicine*, 40:1–30.

PROBLEM C

Complications of Hip Fracture in a 79-Year-Old Widow

Franz U. Steinberg

GENERAL INFORMATION

You are notified that your patient, a 79-year-old widow, has been brought by ambulance to the hospital emergency room. One hour earlier, she had stumbled over a throw rug and fallen. She experienced immediate sharp pain in her right thigh, and she was unable to get up. Her cries for help were heard by a neighbor who called the ambulance.

The patient's health has been adequate. Her only medications are eye drops for glaucoma and occasional aspirin for low-back pain.

On physical examination you find the patient to be alert, but she is apprehensive and in pain. The heart rate is 88/min with occasional ectopic beats. Her blood pressure is 160/88 mm Hg. The right lower extremity is shortened by 2 cm, as measured from the anterior superior iliac spine to the medial malleolus. The hip is in external rotation. Attempts to gently manipulate the hip cause the patient severe pain. Roentgenogram of the hip demonstrates an intertrochanteric fracture of the femur. You request a consultation with an orthopedic surgeon. On the following morning, under spinal anesthesia, the fracture is repaired by insertion of a compression hip screw. The patient tolerates the procedure without complications. An indwelling catheter was inserted before the operation and removed 48 hours later.

Three days after the operation, you are notified that your patient is incontinent of small amounts of urine, and she is unable to void on the toilet or the bedpan.

DECISION POINT C-1

Assuming that a thorough history will be taken, to which of the following points in the history would you give particular importance in the evaluation of this complication?

1. Is the patient aware of bladder distention?
2. The patient's sensation of having to have a bowel movement
3. Sensation of "burning" or pain during urination
4. History of previous incontinence
5. History of kidney stones
6. Family history of bladder problems
7. Presence of bulging into the vagina when bearing down
8. Number of childbirths
9. Numbness or weakness of legs

Turn to page 382 for answers

DECISION POINT C-2

With the understanding that a thorough physical examination will be done, to which of the following items of the physical examination would you wish to give particular emphasis with regard to the present complication?

10. Palpation of abdomen for masses
11. Palpation of abdomen for tenderness
12. Palpation of abdomen for rebound tenderness
13. Examination for bowel sounds
14. Rectal examination
15. Vaginal examination
16. Sensory examination of lower limbs
17. Motor examination of lower limbs
18. Examination of reflexes of lower limbs
19. Examination of perianal sensation

Turn to page 382 for answers

DECISION POINT C-3

With the information you now have, which among the following further examinations would you order as important to the diagnosis of the patient's problem?

20. Urinalysis
21. Culture of urine
22. Catheterization for residual urine
23. Catheterization; then, fill bladder through catheter with water and ask patient to cough
24. Blood urea nitrogen (BUN)
25. Serum creatinine level
26. Serum potassium level
27. Plain roentgenogram of abdomen
28. Intravenous pyelogram (IVP)
29. Roentgenogram of lumbosacral spine
30. Cystogram
31. Proctoscopy
32. Roentgenogram of bowel with barium enema
33. Urodynamic studies
34. Myelogram

Turn to page 382 for answers

DECISION POINT C-4

With the information you now have, which of the following would you choose for the management of this patient?

35. Therapy with nitrofurantoin
36. Insert indwelling catheter for 72 hr; then remove and observe if patient can now void

37. Have patient void every 2 hr during day and once at night; nurse must see that bladder is emptied completely each time
38. Therapy with bethanecol chloride

Turn to page 382 for answers

DECISION POINT C-5

On the seventh postoperative day the patient complains of chest pain located in the left side of the chest. The pain started while she was eating. She has been sitting in a chair much of the time, and she has attended physical therapy once daily. Assuming that a complete interval history will be taken, to which symptoms would you give particular importance for the evaluation of the present complaint?

39. Location of pain
40. Is pain aggravated by breathing?
41. Character of pain
42. Presence of shortness of breath
43. Presence of cough
44. Presence of hemoptysis
45. Feeling of weakness
46. Presence of increased sweating
47. Presence of nausea or vomiting
48. Is pain aggravated by movements?
49. History of previous chest pain
50. Recent injury to chest in falls or while exercising
51. History of tuberculosis
52. History of cigarette smoking

Turn to page 382 for answers

DECISION POINT C-6

The patient appears anxious. Respiratory rate is 28/min. Skin is warm and slightly moist. Heart rate is 92/min and regular tones of good quality. Blood pressure is 160/108 mm Hg. To which of the following items in the physical examination would you wish to give special attention as possibly relevant to the present problem?

53. Examination of lungs
54. Examination of heart
55. Comparison of heart rate at rest and after exercise
56. Examination of color of skin and mucous membranes
57. Examination of veins in neck
58. Temperature
59. Examination of chest wall
60. Examination of legs
61. Homans sign
62. Response to carotid sinus massage

Turn to page 382 for answers

DECISION POINT C-7

With the information you now have, which of the following diagnostic examinations would you order at this time?

63. Complete blood count (CBC)
64. Roentgenogram of chest
65. Electrocardiogram (ECG)
66. Serum levels of "cardiac" enzymes
67. Arterial blood gas studies
68. Roentgenogram of ribs
69. Ventilation-perfusion scan of lung
70. Doppler ultrasound examination of legs
71. Phlebogram of legs (at bedside)
72. Myocardial isotope scan
73. Thallium-201 exercise scan
74. Pulmonary arteriogram
75. Bronchoscopy

Turn to page 382 for answers

DECISION POINT C-8

With the information you now have, which of the following would you choose for the management of this patient?

76. Therapy with nasal oxygen, 3 liters/min
77. Therapy with intravenous heparin sodium by continuous infusion
78. Therapy with warfarin sodium
79. Cardiac monitoring
80. Therapy with heparin sodium, 5,000 units subcutaneously, twice daily
81. Therapy with urokinase
82. Therapy with dipyridamole and aspirin
83. Therapy with mild sedation and analgesics
84. Use of elastic stockings
85. Pulmonary physical therapy
86. Therapy by intermittent positive-pressure breathing
87. Therapy with antibiotics

Turn to page 382 for answers

DECISION POINT C-9

Five and one-half weeks after admission to the hospital, the patient no longer needs the facilities of an acute-care hospital. Which of the following items of information would you regard as important in order to give appropriate advice concerning arrangements for her discharge and continuing care?

88. Patient's ability to walk
89. When will she be able to bear full weight?

90. Patient's ability to transfer unassisted from bed to chair
91. Patient's ability to negotiate steps
92. Current state of bladder function
93. State of bowel function
94. Patient's nutritional status
95. Patient's ability to dress independently
96. Patient's ability to bathe independently
97. Patient's mental status
98. Review of current medications
99. Need for other professional services
100. Patient's monthly income
101. Patient's monthly rent
102. Availability of family members for assistance
103. Where does patient live?
104. Does patient's apartment building offer support services?
105. Accessibility of shelves and the like in patient's kitchen
106. Is patient's apartment carpeted?
107. Type of patient's health insurance
108. Amount of patient's life insurance
109. Accessibility of patient's bathroom and its fixtures
110. Accessibility to apartment from outside

Turn to page 382 for answers

DECISION POINT C-10

With the information you now have, you would recommend:

111. Patient can live in her apartment alone with visiting nurse twice weekly.
112. Patient needs full-time nonprofessional help, visiting nurse once weekly, and physical therapist once weekly.
113. Patient can remain in her apartment but will require full-time nurses.
114. Until patient can walk with full weight bearing, her daughter should move in with her.
115. Until patient can walk with full weight bearing, she should go to a skilled nursing facility.
116. Patient should give up her apartment and move to a home for the aged.
117. Until patient can walk with full weight bearing, she should move in with her daughter.

Turn to page 382 for answers

ANSWERS

DECISION POINT C-1

1. Bladder feels full
2. Not at present
3. None
4. None
5. No
6. No
7. No
8. Two
9. No

DECISION POINT C-2

10. Large suprapubic mass present
11. Lower abdomen moderately tender
12. None
13. Present; within normal limits
14. Within normal limits; good sphincter tone
15. Within normal limits; no bulging on cough
16. Within normal limits
17. Within normal limits
18. Present and equal bilaterally
19. Within normal limits; sphincter contracts on perianal cutaneous stimulation

DECISION POINT C-3

20. Albumin, trace; 5 to 7 leukocytes/HPF
21. Gram-negative rods less than 10,000 colonies/ml
22. 780 ml
23. No elimination of urine on cough
24. 24 mg/dl (normal, 8 to 20)
25. 1.1 mg/dl (normal, 0.7 to 1.3)
26. 3.8 mEq/liter
27. Large distended bladder
28. Renal pelvis and ureter normal
29. Moderate osteoarthritis
30. Normal bladder contours; no vesicoureteral reflux
31. A few internal hemorrhoids
32. Few diverticula in sigmoid colon
33. Bladder fills to 800 ml and then empties by overflow; feeble detrusor activity; no detrusor-sphincter dyssynergia
34. No filling defect of dye column

DECISION POINT C-4

35. Ordered
36. Ordered
37. Ordered
38. Ordered

DECISION POINT C-5

39. Left lateral chest with radiation to the front
40. Increased by deep inspiration
41. Sharp, "like a knife"
42. Moderate
43. Mild, dry cough on deep inspiration
44. No
45. Present
46. Cold sweat of moderate intensity
47. No
48. No
49. No
50. No
51. None
52. None for 10 years; never smoked more than five cigarettes daily

DECISION POINT C-6

53. Depressed breath sounds over left base; remainder of examination within normal limits
54. Tones of good quality; P-2 accentuated and split
55. At rest, 92/min; after exercise, 112/min
56. Pale; no cyanosis
57. Not prominent during sitting
58. 37.2°C (99.0°F)
59. No tenderness; pain not aggravated by movement
60. No swelling; no veins palpable
61. Negative
62. Heart rate slows to 84/min

DECISION POINT C-7

63. Hemoglobin, 12 g/dl; hematocrit, 38%; leukocyte count, 8,200/mm³ with normal differential
64. Lungs clear; heart of normal size; left diaphragm slightly elevated
65. Sinus tachycardia present; no change compared with previous tracing
66. GOT, CPK, LDH within normal limits
67. Po_2, 58 mm Hg; Pco_2, 32 mm Hg; HCO_3, 20 mEq/liter; pH 7.46
68. No fractures present
69. No defect on ventilation scan; defect in left lower lung field on perfusion scan
70. Within normal limits
71. Within normal limits
72. No abnormal uptake of isotope
73. No areas of ischemia
74. Intraluminal filling defect in left pulmonary artery
75. No evidence of bronchial obstruction

DECISION POINT C-8

76. Ordered
77. 40,000 units/24 hr
78. Initial loading dose of 10 mg
79. Ordered
80. Ordered
81. Ordered
82. Ordered
83. Ordered
84. Ordered
85. Ordered
86. Ordered
87. Ordered

DECISION POINT C-9

88. Uses walker without bearing weight on right foot, which she uses for balance only
89. Orthopedist estimates six weeks if roentgenogram shows adequate bone formation

90. Able to transfer; pivots independently on left leg
91. Only with much help
92. Urinates five to six times during day, twice at night; some urgency; occasional incontinence when she cannot get to toilet quickly enough
93. Good control; mild constipation
94. Adequate intake of food; fairly good appetite
95. Needs help with elastic stockings
96. No; needs help to get in and out of tub or shower
97. Within normal limits
98. Coumadin for next four months; stool softeners
99. Determination of prothrombin time once weekly
100. Social Security benefits plus $400.00 from pension, dividends, and interest
101. She pays $180.00
102. One married daughter has three adolescent children and works full-time; limited availability
103. Efficiency apartment in apartment building for senior citizens
104. Manager lives on premises and can be called in emergencies
105. Shelves, gas stove and refrigerator can be reached
106. Yes
107. Medicare plus supplemental insurance
108. $10,000
109. Accessible with walker; elevated toilet seat
110. Five steps with railing from street to entrance; self-service elevator

DECISION POINT C-10

111. Recommendation given
112. Recommendation given
113. Recommendation given
114. Recommendation given
115. Recommendation given
116. Recommendation given
117. Recommendation given

CRITIQUE

CASE SUMMARY

This 79-year-old woman develops bladder distention and overflow incontinence three days after surgical repair of a fractured hip under spinal anesthesia. Differential diagnoses include: uninhibited neurogenic bladder due to cerebral disease; atonic distended bladder caused by trauma and operation; cystitis, which may have been the result of earlier catheterization; cystourethrocele, a preexisting condition that should have caused rather characteristic symptoms; and a cauda equina lesion due to spinal anesthesia, which would present with other neurologic defects.

Following resolution of her urinary problem, on the seventh postoperative day the patient develops severe and persistent chest pain accompanied by tachypnea. She has been partially immobilized during this time, and pulmonary embolus appears to be the most probable diagnosis. Other diagnostic possibilities to be considered include myocardial infarction, pneumonia with pleurisy, and injury to the chest wall, possibly sustained in physical therapy. The diagnosis of pulmonary embolus is made probable by the pleuritic character of the pain, and the normal roentgenogram of the chest. Fever is sometimes found in patients with pulmonary embolism, even in the absence of infection. The diagnosis is confirmed by the positive perfusion scan of the lung.

When the patient no longer needs care in an acute-care hospital, discharge plans must be made; these should consider the character and extent of the patient's remaining disability, her personal family resources, and the physical characteristics of her place of residence. Possibilities include: discharge to her home, with professional or nonprofessional full-time or part-time care; temporary discharge to a skilled nursing home until such time as she becomes fully ambulatory; permanent discharge to a custodial care facility; or discharge to the care of her daughter in her home.

DECISION POINT C-1   Score

Assuming that a thorough history will be taken, to which of the following points in the history would you give particular importance in the evaluation of this complication?

1. Is the patient aware of bladder distention
    It is important to know whether the sensory input from the bladder is intact, and if the patient is alert to her symptoms of need to urinate.
    If you had selected this option your score would be . . . .   +3

2. The patient's sensation of having to have a bowel movement
    In some patients a fecal impaction may contribute to distention

of the bladder; in such instances, it is important to know whether the patient is having difficulties with bowel movements.

If you had selected this option your score would be . . . .   + 1

3. Sensation of "burning" or pain during urination
    Absence of "burning" or pain on urination almost completely rules out the diagnosis of cystitis. Little or no pain will be perceived by patients who have cauda equina lesions, uninhibited neurogenic bladders, or distended atonic bladders.
    If you had selected this option your score would be . . . .   + 3

4. History of previous incontinence
    A positive history of incontinence would suggest an uninhibited neurogenic bladder or cystourethrocele. Absence of incontinence virtually rules out these possibilities.
    If you had selected this option your score would be . . . .   + 3

5. History of kidney stones
    A history of kidney stones is irrelevant to the care of the patient at this time.
    If you had selected this option your score would be . . . .   − 3

6. Family history of bladder problems
    Family history of bladder problems is irrelevant, there being substantially no familial bladder conditions that might account for the patient's difficulty.
    If you had selected this option your score would be . . . .   − 1

7. Presence of bulging into the vagina when bearing down
    A history of bulging tissues into the vaginal area would suggest cystourethrocele. Such bulging is often accentuated with straining or coughing, and is commonly accompanied by incontinence.
    If you had selected this option your score would be . . . .   + 3

8. Number of childbirths
    The likelihood of development of cystourethroceles increases with multiparity.
    If you had selected this option your score would be . . . .   + 1

9. Numbness or weakness of legs
    Absence of weakness or numbness of the legs makes the likelihood of a lesion of the cauda equina very small. It is important that this possibility be excluded.
    If you had selected this option your score would be . . . .   + 3

With the understanding that a thorough physical examination will be done, to which of the following items of the physical examination would you wish to give particular emphasis with regard to the present complication?

10. Palpation of abdomen for masses
    The examination of the abdomen is particularly important in a patient with the problem presented. An enlarged distended bladder should be easily felt; it would suggest an atonic distended bladder or neurogenic bladder secondary to a lesion of the cauda equina. Inability to feel the bladder in a patient voiding small amounts of urine would suggest cystitis. The possibility of oliguria secondary to a renal disturbance would also need to be considered.
    If you had selected this option your score would be . . . .   +5

11. Palpation of abdomen for tenderness
    The tenderness of the abdomen should be assessed; a distended bladder would be tender unless it were the result of a lesion of the cauda equina.
    If you had selected this option your score would be . . . .   +3

12. Palpation of abdomen for rebound tenderness
    The finding of rebound tenderness will not be helpful in this patient. Rebound tenderness indicates peritoneal irritation, which is unlikely to be present for any of the differential diagnostic possibilities being considered.
    If you had selected this option your score would be . . . .   −1

13. Examination for bowel sounds
    The auscultation of bowel sounds is routine, but irrelevant to this patient's problem, which resides in the urinary tract rather than in the gastrointestinal tract.
    If you had selected this option your score would be   0

14. Rectal examination
    A rectal examination should be done to determine whether a massive fecal impaction is in some way contributing to urinary tract obstruction.
    If you had selected this option your score would be . . . .   +3

15. Vaginal examination
    Examination of the vaginal area would be appropriate, even under the difficulties imposed by the immobilization of a patient

with a recent hip fracture. If there is a cystocele, it should become apparent or be felt when the patient strains.

If you had selected this option your score would be ....

+1

16. Sensory examination of lower limbs
    It is important to assess the sensory status of a patient with urinary retention; sensory impairment of the lower limbs will be present in the case of a lesion of the cauda equina. Motor impairment may also be present under such circumstances. Deep tendon reflexes should be impaired.

    If you had selected this option your score would be .... +3

17. Motor examination of lower limbs
    (See critique 16.)

    If you had selected this option your score would be .... +3

18. Examination of reflexes of lower limbs
    (See critique 16.)

    If you had selected this option your score would be .... +3

19. Examination of perianal sensation
    In the case of a lesion of the cauda equina, perianal sensation should be impaired; the anal sphincter should have lost some of its normal tone and may not respond with constriction to stimulation of the perianal skin.

    If you had selected this option your score would be .... +3

DECISION POINT C-3

Score

With the information you now have, which among the following further examinations would you order as important to the diagnosis of the patient's problem?

20. Urinalysis
    Urinalysis is essential in the evaluation of this patient in order to determine if infection is present. The examination should be supplemented by culture of a properly obtained specimen; in elderly women this may involve catheterization or suprapubic aspiration.

    If you had selected this option your score would be .... +3

21. Culture of urine
    (See critique 20.)

    If you had selected this option your score would be .... +3

22. Catheterization for residual urine   **Score**
    The catheterization of the bladder is, of course, essential for
    the patient with urinary retention. The residual volume will be
    high in the presence of an atonic bladder or with retention from
    a cauda equina lesion. Residual volume would be little or none
    if the problem were due to cystitis.
    If you had selected this option your score would be . . . .   +5

23. Catherization; then, fill bladder through catheter with water and
    ask patient to cough
    This is a useful maneuver for detection of cystourethrocele.
    Water will squirt from the catheter or around it if a cystou-
    rethrocele is present.
    If you had selected this option your score would be . . . .   +3

24. Blood urea nitrogen (BUN)
    (See critique 26.)
    If you had selected this option your score would be . . . .   +1

25. Serum creatinine level
    (See critique 26.)
    If you had selected this option your score would be . . . .   +1

26. Serum potassium level
    These screening tests for renal function and fluid and electrolyte
    status will ordinarily be done to set a baseline for further studies.
    Elevation of BUN or serum creatinine levels might indicate
    dehydration or preexisting renal impairment.
    If you had selected this option your score would be . . . .   +1

27. Plain roentgenogram of abdomen
    A roentgenographic examination of the abdomen will probably
    add little new information at this time, other than to show a
    large distended bladder or possibly a high fecal impaction not
    felt on rectal examination. There is no reason as yet in this
    patient to expect evidence of ileus.
    If you had selected this option your score would be . . . .   +1

28. Intravenous pyelogram (IVP)
    An IVP would be a strenuous procedure for this patient at this
    time and would add no useful information.
    If you had selected this option your score would be . . . .   −3

29. Roentgenogram of lumbosacral spine
    A roentgenogram of the lumbosacral spine might show an occult
    spina bifida or other spinal lesion that might have contributed

to the problem of bladder difficulties; in this patient, the possibility is sufficiently small so that the examination is not warranted.

If you had selected this option your score would be ....   −1

30. Cystogram
A cystogram would be contraindicated in the presence of cystitis and is not likely to produce important new information under the circumstances described.
If you had selected this option your score would be ....   −3

31. Proctoscopy
No basis has been laid for this uncomfortable and invasive procedure in this patient.
If you had selected this option your score would be ....·.   −5

32. Roentgenogram of bowel with barium enema
There is no indication of need for a barium enema in this patient at this time. She is not obstructed, and gives no indication of any primary gastrointestinal problem.
If you had selected this option your score would be ....   −5

33. Urodynamic studies
Urodynamic studies should not be done in the presence of an infection. They will yield valuable information about the function of the bladder destrusor and sphincter, but would be better left for a later evaluation in this case.
If you had selected this option your score would be   0

34. Myelogram
Only if there were evidence of a lesion of the spinal cord or cauda equina would a myelogram be indicated. This patient has given no such evidence.
If you had selected this option your score would be ....   −5

DECISION POINT C-4   Score

With the information you now have, which of the following would you choose for the management of this patient?

35. Therapy with nitrofurantoin
In this patient with urinary retention, the use of nitrofurantoin will not be indicated as primary therapy, since urinalysis has not indicated infection. Administration of antibiotics will increase the risk of emergence of resistant organisms.
If you had selected this option your score would be ....   −1

36. Insert indwelling catheter for 72 hr; then remove and observe **Score**
    if patient can now void
    The insertion of an indwelling catheter for a period of 72 hr
    should be the definitive treatment for an atonic distended blad-
    der under the circumstances described here. Keeping the bladder
    empty for this period of time will allow the destrusor tone to
    be reestablished, following which the patient should be able to
    void satisfactorily.
    If you had selected this option your score would be . . . .   +5

37. Have patient void every 2 hr during day and once at night;
    nurse must see that bladder is emptied completely each time
    To ask or to require the patient to void on schedule would be
    inappropriate and unhelpful, since the patient cannot voluntarily
    empty her bladder. Residual urine would likely reaccumulate,
    and the problem would remain unresolved.
    If you had selected this option your score would be . . . .   −3

38. Therapy with bethanecol chloride
    The use of cholinergic drugs will improve the tone of the des-
    trusor: the pharmacologic effect will be inadequate, however,
    to restore normal bladder function in a patient such as this.
    If you had selected this option your score would be . . . .   −3

DECISION POINT C-5   **Score**

On the seventh postoperative day the patient complains of chest pain
located in the left side of the chest. The pain started while she was
eating. She has been sitting in a chair much of the time, and she has
attended physical therapy once daily. Assuming that a complete interval
history will be taken, to which symptoms would you give particular
importance for the evaluation of the present complaint?

39. Location of pain
    The location of pain will be useful in localization of the lesion.
    In this patient, a myocardial infarction is a distinct possibility
    for pain on the left side of the chest.
    If you had selected this option your score would be . . . .   +3

40. Is pain aggravated by breathing?
    To know whether chest pain is affected by breathing will help
    answer the question of whether the pleura is involved.
    If you had selected this option your score would be . . . .   +3

41. Character of pain
    The character of the pain can provide useful information, but
    a clear description may be difficult to obtain from the patient.

Pain from a myocardial infarction is usually described as a feeling of pressure rather than as a sharp pain.

If you had selected this option your score would be . . . .   +1

42. Presence of shortness of breath

Inquiry as to shortness of breath may be less helpful than determining the character of pain. Absence of shortness of breath would strongly contraindicate the diagnosis of pulmonary embolus. Dyspnea may be secondary to pain itself.

If you had selected this option your score would be . . . .   +3

43. Presence of cough

Whether or not cough is present is less helpful than determining the character of the pain. Cough may be due to a variety of causes, such as pleuritic involvement or pulmonary congestion.

If you had selected this option your score would be . . . .   +1

44. Presence of hemoptysis

The presence of hemoptysis might indicate a pulmonary embolus with infarction. Absence of this symptom, on the other hand, does not help with the diagnosis.

If you had selected this option your score would be . . . .   +1

45. Feeling of weakness

A feeling of weakness is not a specific enough symptom to provide much information; it may be due to pain, anxiety, or any of the differential diagnoses under consideration.

If you had selected this option your score would be . . . .   +1

46. Presence of increased sweating

The symptom of sweating is not specific enough to provide useful information. It often occurs in myocardial infarction; it may also be the accompaniment of fever in pneumonitis; and it may occur in any of the differential diagnoses under consideration, especially if the pain is severe.

If you had selected this option your score would be . . . .   +1

47. Presence of nausea or vomiting

Nausea and vomiting in a patient with chest pain would suggest myocardial infarction.

If you had selected this option your score would be . . . .   +1

48. Is pain aggravated by movements?

It is often difficult to get a precise response to a question as to whether pain is aggravated by movement. The occurrence of such pain would suggest musculoskeletal injury to the chest wall.

If you had selected this option your score would be . . . .   +1

391

49. History of previous chest pain
A history of previous chest pain has little relevance to the present condition. A positive answer might indicate angina pectoris and would increase the level of suspicion that coronary heart disease and myocardial infarction might be present.
If you had selected this option your score would be   0

50. Recent injury to chest in falls or while exercising
A question as to recent injury to the chest will be useful only if there is a positive answer. Many elderly people will have fractures of ribs with relatively trivial injury or with exertion. Sometimes the event has seemed rather trivial.
If you had selected this option your score would be . . . .   +1

51. History of tuberculosis
Even if a history of tuberculosis were positive, it would be unlikely to be relevant to the present acute condition.
If you had selected this option your score would be . . . .   −1

52. History of cigarette smoking
A question regarding cigarette smoking is not likely to be relevant in the present situation, though smoking predisposes to coronary artery disease and to myocardial infarction.
If you had selected this option your score would be . . . .   −1

DECISION POINT C-6   Score

The patient appears anxious. Respiratory rate is 28/min. Skin is warm and slightly moist. Heart rate is 92/min and regular with tones of good quality. Blood pressure is 160/108 mm Hg. To which of the following items in the physical examination would you wish to give special attention as possibly relevant to the present problems?

53. Examination of lungs
Examination of the lungs is an important and routine part of the general examination, but may not contribute much at this point to the evaluation of this patient. Decreased breath sounds may be due to splinting, secondary to pain, or may be the first abnormal physical finding in a patient with pneumonitis.
If you had selected this option your score would be . . . .   +3

54. Examination of heart
The intensity of heart sounds may be decreased in a patient with myocardial infarction. Splitting and accentuation of the second pulmonary sound (P2) will indicate increased pressure in the pulmonary arterial system and point toward the possibility of pulmonary embolus.
If you had selected this option your score would be . . . .   +3

55. Comparison of heart rate at rest and after exercise **Score**
This patient should not have an examination of heart rate response to exercise. Tachycardia frequently accompanies pulmonary embolism; in this case, the patient's marginal tachycardia is consistent with her anxiety or pain. Exercise should be avoided at this time; moreover, the test would give no important information.
If you had selected this option your score would be . . . .   −5

56. Examination of color of skin and mucous membranes
The significance of the color of the skin and mucous membranes will be limited. Pallor may be due to pain as well as to anemia. Cyanosis would indicate hypoxemia and may be a sign of pulmonary embolus, myocardial infarction, or extensive pneumonitis.
If you had selected this option your score would be . . . .   +1

57. Examination of veins in neck
Examination for the distention of neck veins would help evaluate the possibility of a right-sided heart failure.
If you had selected this option your score would be . . . .   +1

58. Temperature
Elevation of the patient's temperature must be interpreted conservatively. Elevations may occur in patients who have pulmonary embolism or atelectasis, as well as with pneumonitis. On the other hand, aged patients may have inadequate responses of temperature to infections, and a normal temperature would not rule out the possibility of infection.
If you had selected this option your score would be . . . .   +1

59. Examination of chest wall
Careful examination of the chest wall will assess the possibility of musculoskeletal injury; the absence of tenderness makes such injury unlikely.
If you had selected this option your score would be . . . .   +3

60. Examination of legs
When the possibility of pulmonary embolus must be considered, the legs should be examined for evidence of phlebothrombosis. A negative examination does not rule out the possibility of pulmonary embolus, since the source of emboli may be pelvic rather than in the limb veins.
If you had selected this option your score would be . . . .   +3

61. Homans sign
When Homans sign is present, it is useful in the evaluation of

the possibility of phlebothrombosis; on the other hand, a negative test does not exclude this possibility.

If you had selected this option your score would be .... +3

62. Response to carotid sinus massage
There is no indication for the use of carotid sinus massage in this patient. It would give no useful information and may be dangerous through causing bradycardia.
If you had selected this option your score would be ....   −5

DECISION POINT C-7   Score

With the information you now have, which of the following diagnostic examinations would you order at this time?

63. Complete blood count (CBC)
A CBC would be part of a routine workup. The leukocyte count and differential may be helpful when they give indication of the possibility of infection, in an increase in leukocytes or in a shift to the left.
If you had selected this option your score would be ....   +1

64. Roentgenogram of chest
A roentgenogram of the chest is a very important element in the evaluation of this patient. Pneumonitis or pneumonia may be manifested by an infiltrate. A pulmonary embolus would probably show splinting of the diaphragm.
If you had selected this option your score would be ....   +3

65. Electrocardiogram (ECG)
An ECG will be an important element in the evaluation of the patient, especially since a previous ECG is available for comparison. There may be evidence of myocardial infarction or of right ventricular strain, which might indicate a massive pulmonary embolus.
If you had selected this option your score would be ....   +3

66. Serum levels of "cardiac" enzymes
The measurement of the level of "cardiac" enzymes will give no immediately useful information, but will establish baseline levels against which later changes can be compared. It is particularly expected that lactic dehydrogenase (LDH) activity will rise in the case of pulmonary infarction.
If you had selected this option your score would be ....   +3

67. Arterial blood gas studies　　　　　　　　　　　　**Score**
Measurement of arterial blood gases and pH will be helpful in evaluation of the patient. In pulmonary embolism, P_{O_2} will be reduced, whereas P_{CO_2}, pH, and bicarbonate levels will show evidence of mild respiratory alkalosis.
If you had selected this option your score would be . . . .　　+3

68. Roentgenogram of ribs
It is unlikely that roentgenograms of the ribs will be helpful unless there is a history of high suspicion of skeletal injury. In this patient, examination has shown no tenderness over the rib cage.
If you had selected this option your score would be . . . .　　0

69. Ventilation-perfusion scan of lung
The ventilation-perfusion scan will be most important to the differential diagnosis of pulmonary embolism. One would expect to see a defect on the perfusion scan, with a normal ventilation scan. The examination will be less helpful if the roentgenogram of the chest has shown an infiltrate, in which case there may be expected impairment of ventilation as well as of perfusion.
If you had selected this option your score would be . . . .　　+5

70. Doppler ultrasound examination of legs
The Doppler examination of the legs is a simple, noninvasive, bedside procedure that may detect phlebothrombosis, which has not been apparent on physical examination.
If you had selected this option your score would be . . . .　　+3

71. Phlebogram of legs (at bedside)
The phlebogram of the legs will make definitive the diagnosis of phlebothrombosis. This will be particularly important when there have been repeated episodes of pulmonary embolism and when consideration of surgical ligation of the vena cava or other interventions must be made. This need not be regarded as a routine examination.
If you had selected this option your score would be . . . .　　+1

72. Myocardial isotope scan
A cardiac scan will be important if the diagnosis of myocardial infarction needs to be definitively established in patients for whom the ECG has not been adequately discriminating. In this case, all the evidence accumulated so far points to a pulmonary embolus; accordingly, this examination is not needed.
If you had selected this option your score would be . . . .　　−3

73. Thallium-201 exercise scan
There is no need for this evaluation, in view of other information obtained. Tests involving exercises may be harmful at this stage of the patient's illness.
If you had selected this option your score would be .... −5

74. Pulmonary arteriogram
A pulmonary arteriogram is not indicated for this patient, in whose case the ventilation-perfusion scan has been positive and all other examinations point to pulmonary embolism.
If you had selected this option your score would be .... −5

75. Bronchoscopy
There is no indication for bronchoscopy in the data accumulated so far. There is no substantial evidence of airway obstruction, nor of any other condition for which bronchoscopy would be helpful.
If you had selected this option your score would be .... −5

DECISION POINT C-8 Score

With the information you now have, which of the following would you choose for the management of this patient?

76. Therapy with nasal oxygen, 3 liters/min
The administration of oxygen will be helpful to the patient, in relief of her respiratory and cardiac work load.
If you had selected this option your score would be .... +3

77. Therapy with intravenous heparin sodium by continuous infusion
The intravenous infusion of heparin is the definitive treatment at this time for pulmonary embolism. It is particularly the treatment of first choice for acute embolism. Chronic anticoagulant therapy with warfarin sodium will be indicated after the acute phase, and will be continued for four to six months. It should be initiated 7 to 10 days after the onset of the acute episode, at which time heparin will be phased out.
If you had selected this option your score would be .... +5

78. Therapy with warfarin sodium
(See critique 77.)
If you had selected this option your score would be 0

79. Cardiac monitoring
Cardiac monitoring has as its chief indication myocardial infarction. On the other hand, it may become important in aged

patients who are seriously ill with pulmonary vascular disease, and it may bring essential care to them on short notice.

If you had selected this option your score would be . . . .

+ 1

80. Therapy with heparin sodium, 5,000 units subcutaneously, twice daily

Low-dose heparin therapy is not indicated in the management of acute pulmonary embolism. It is used only prophylactically against the development of such embolism.

If you had selected this option your score would be . . . .

− 3

81. Therapy with urokinase

Urokinase therapy, or therapy with other fibrinolytic enzymes, carries grave risks and is very costly. It would be indicated only if the embolus were massive and the patient's condition critical. These conditions do not pertain to this patient at this time.

If you had selected this option your score would be . . . .

− 5

82. Therapy with dipyridamole and aspirin

Antiplatelet therapy, useful as it may be in the prevention of transient ischemic attacks in males, is useless in pulmonary embolism.

If you had selected this option your score would be . . . .

− 3

83. Therapy with mild sedation and analgesics

The use of sedation and of analgesic medication is appropriate, but care must be taken not to suppress the respiration. The needs of the patient for this supportive therapy ought to be established on an individual basis.

If you had selected this option your score would be . . . .

+ 1

84. Use of elastic stockings

Elastic stockings should be used. Even though the patient has no evidence of thrombosis in the legs, they will have prophylactic value.

If you had selected this option your score would be . . . .

+ 3

85. Pulmonary physical therapy

Pulmonary physical therapy is not indicated in the treatment of pulmonary emboli.

If you had selected this option your score would be . . . .

− 1

86. Therapy by intermittent positive-pressure breathing

There is no indication for intermittent positive-pressure breathing in patients with pulmonary embolism. Bronchospasm is not a substantial element, and no aerosolized medication is indicated.

If you had selected this option your score would be . . . .   **Score**

−3

87. Therapy with antibiotics
The use of antibiotics in patients with pulmonary embolism must be regarded as of prophylactic value only. Whether or not they will be used should probably be decided on an individual basis.

If you had selected this option your score would be   0

DECISION POINT C-9   **Score**

Five and one-half weeks after admission to the hospital, the patient no longer needs the facilities of an acute-care hospital. What information do you need in order to give appropriate advice concerning arrangements for her discharge and continuing care?

88. Patient's ability to walk
The patient's mobility will be an important consideration in the decision as to whether she can get safely about her own home. It is indicated that she is now using a walker, and it is likely that she will be able to improve and sustain her mobility in the next weeks. The walker may permit her to reach areas of her apartment inaccessible by wheelchair. Wheelchairs are often felt by patients to offer easier mobility, but should be prescribed sparingly and for certain functions only, lest the patient become too dependent on the chair and lose the advantages of the walker.

If you had selected this option your score would be . . . .   +3

89. When will she be able to bear full weight?
The patient's ability to bear full weight will be important in establishing a timetable for her discharge, and ultimate mobilization.

If you had selected this option your score would be . . . .   +3

90. Patient's ability to transfer unassisted from bed to chair or vice versa will be an important consideration in the decision as to the patient's further care.

If you had selected this option your score would be . . . .   +3

91. Patient's ability to negotiate steps
In the case of this patient, her ability to negotiate steps is not critical, since she lives in a one-level apartment. On the other hand, this will determine her restrictions of mobility outside her own apartment.

If you had selected this option your score would be . . . .   +1

92. Current state of bladder function   **Score**
The state of bladder function is an important consideration. The patient described has urgency and occasional incontinence, which demand that she be able to reach a toilet reasonably expeditiously. If a toilet is not easily accessible, she will need to have help available at all times.
If you had selected this option your score would be ....   +1

93. State of bowel function
The state of bowel function for the patient is not substantially relevant. Her voluntary bowel control has not been compromised at any time during her illness.
If you had selected this option your score would be ....   −1

94. Patient's nutritional status
The patient's food intake and nutrition will be important considerations for her general health, but have little relevance to the planning of her discharge and convalescent care.
If you had selected this option your score would be   0

95. Patient's ability to dress independently
(See critique 96.)
If you had selected this option your score would be ....   +1

96. Patient's ability to bathe independently
The patient's ability to care for herself will be an important consideration in planning. If she cannot dress or bathe independently, she will need periodic or continuing help during the day.
If you had selected this option your score would be ....   +1

97. Patient's mental status
The patient's mental status is a very important consideration in all aspects of planning current and future care. It may need periodic reassessment.
If you had selected this option your score would be ....   +3

98. Review of current medications
To know the medications the patient will be receiving at home is important, since some medications will require ongoing monitoring, such as periodic prothrombin levels.
If you had selected this option your score would be ....   +1

99. Need for other professional services
The decision has been made that the patient will be on anticoagulant therapy for four to six months. This will require the

measurement of prothrombin time at regular intervals. The blood drawing and adjustment of dosage will be necessary professional services.

If you had selected this option your score would be .... +3

100. Patient's monthly income
The patient's income and expenses will not be the ultimate determinant of her care, but they must be considered if expensive professional help, such as full-time nurses, were to be desired or recommended.
If you had selected this option your score would be .... +1

101. Patient's monthly rent
(See critique 100.)
If you had selected this option your score would be .... +1

102. Availability of family members for assistance. To know the family setting in which the patient lives is very important for planning, and may be crucial to some aspects. One will need to know who is available, how much assistance they will be able to give, and what their emotional, economic, and physical resources are.
If you had selected this option your score would be .... +3

103. Where does patient live?
(See critique 106.)
If you had selected this option your score would be .... +3

104. Does patient's apartment building offer support services?
(See critique 106.)
If you had selected this option your score would be .... +1

105. Accessibility of shelves and the like in patient's kitchen
(See critique 106.)
If you had selected this option your score would be .... +1

106. Is patient's apartment carpeted?
The details of the patient's dwelling will be very important to planning, including the nature of services immediately available. Accessibility of the bathroom has been referred to earlier. The accessibility of kitchen facilities and implements is equally important. The patient has to be able, at the very least, to prepare simple meals or snacks, unless she has full-time attendance. The nature of the floor covering in the apartment is less important, but may have some effect on ambulation.
If you had selected this option your score would be 0

107. Type of patient's health insurance   **Score**
    The evaluation of the patient's health insurance coverage will
    be important in planning skilled nursing home care or home
    health services.
    If you had selected this option your score would be ....   +1

108. Amount of patient's life insurance
    Life insurance is quite irrelevant and should be regarded as an
    intrusive and unnecessary question.
    If you had selected this option your score would be ....   −5

109. Accessibility of patient's bathroom and its fixtures
    (See critique 106.)
    If you had selected this option your score would be ....   +3

110. Accessibility to apartment from outside
    (See critique 106.)
    If you had selected this option your score would be ....   +1

DECISION POINT C-10   Score

With the information you now have, you would recommend:

111. Patient can live in her apartment alone with visiting nurse twice
    weekly.
    This arrangement is possible, but not a safe one, since the
    patient is still handicapped in her ability to get about. Some
    factors other than those already mentioned will be important in
    assessment of the adequacy of the patient's home. Many elderly
    persons find that the elevation of the toilet seat makes the use
    of the commode much easier and more comfortable than if the
    seat is at a lower level. A bathtub is more difficult for many
    elderly persons to negotiate than a shower. Within the shower
    a mat should be supplied for secure footing, and a stool to sit
    on may be found convenient and helpful.
    If you had selected this option your score would be ....   −1

112. Patient needs full-time nonprofessional help, visiting nurse once
    weekly and physical therapist once weekly.
    For the patient to live at home with full-time nonprofessional
    help will be safer than living alone, but appropriate help may
    be hard to find and costly as well.
    If you had selected this option your score would be   0

113. Patient can remain in her apartment but will require full-time
    nurses.
    No need in this instance has been established for full-time nurs-

ing care. Moreover, the patient could not afford it, and it would not be covered by Medicare nor by the usual supplemental health insurance.

If you had selected this option your score would be ....

−3

114. Until patient can walk with full weight bearing, her daughter should move in with her.

It is often unwise in circumstances such as this to thrust on the children the care of their elderly parents. There may be major disruption of the children's work and family responsibilities.

If you had selected this option your score would be ....

−3

115. Until patient can walk with full weight bearing, she should go to a skilled nursing facility.

This arrangement appears to be the best possible. The patient would be in a protected environment and would receive needed professional services, including periodic blood tests. Inasmuch as her medication will need to be monitored, Medicare might well cover the cost of a stay in a skilled nursing facility.

If you had selected this option your score would be ....

+5

116. Patient should give up her apartment and move to a home for the aged.

There is no indication as yet for the patient to give up her apartment and to move into a retirement home. Her disability should be temporary, and once her fracture has healed she will function almost as well as she did before.

If you had selected this option your score would be ....

−5

117. Until patient can walk with full weight bearing, she should move in with her daughter.

It is not advisable to move elderly patients into their children's homes unless it has been well established that such an arrangement will be a completely happy one; otherwise, there will be disruption of the family life in the children's household, and the patient would, in any case, still be alone during a major portion of each day, since all family members have occupations outside the home.

If you had selected this option your score would be ....

−5

SUMMARY

A 79-year-old woman has developed two common complications of surgery and immobilization in elderly patients. These are an atonic distended bladder and pulmonary embolism. Each has been accurately identified by appropriate tests, and the indicated management has been carried out. The final concern will be the extent and character of her remaining disability and her personal and family resources. Ambulation is limited and will remain so for several weeks. For reasons brought out in the evaluation of her home and circumstances, she will not be able to function safely in her own apartment except with full-time help. The most practical solution will be discharge to a skilled nursing facility. Once walking with full weight bearing becomes possible, she may return to her own apartment.

BIBLIOGRAPHY

Brocklehurst, J. C. (1978): *Textbook of Geriatric Medicine and Gerontology*, 2nd ed. New York, Churchill Livingstone, pp. 306–326.

Coe, R. M. (1976): The geriatric patient in the community. In: *Cowdry's The care of the Geriatric Patient*, 5th ed., edited by F. V. Steinberg. St. Louis, C. V. Mosby.

Harrison's Principles of Internal Medicine, 8th ed. pp. 1402–1496. New York, McGraw-Hill, 1977.

Pearson, R. M., and Noe, H. N. (1979): Why urodynamic studies are important in urologic problems of the elderly. *Geriatrics* 34:45.

Rossman, I., Ed. (1979): *Clinical Geriatrics*, 2nd ed. Philadelphia, J. B. Lippincott, Chap. 38.

Viamonte, M. K., Koolpe, H., Janowitz, W., and Hilder, F. (1980): Pulmonary thromboembolism—update. *JAMA*, 243:2229.

PROBLEM D

Congestive Heart Failure in a 74-Year-Old Woman

David E. Johnson

GENERAL INFORMATION

In the emergency room, you are asked to see a 74-year-old woman of Eastern European descent who has had increasing breathlessness, anorexia, and weakness for several weeks. She is now brought in by her son and his wife who can give no details as to her deteriorating condition. The patient herself states, in broken English, that she has "borderline" diabetes mellitus and hypertension, but that neither of these has previously required treatment. It is difficult to elicit any further history from her. She is carrying pill bottles that indicate that digoxin, 0.125 mg daily, and furosemide, 20 mg daily, have been prescribed, presumably for congestive heart failure.

The patient is a fully conscious, oriented, tired-appearing woman who is mildly dyspneic at rest, while she is breathing oxygen, given at a rate of 2 liters/min via nasal prongs.

Her vital signs are as follows: blood pressure, 170/90 mm Hg; pulse rate, 110/min and regular; respiratory rate, 30/min; temperature, 38°C (100.4°F) rectally. Her weight is 72 kg (162 lb). Examination of the chest discloses fine bibasilar inspiratory crackles with dullness and decreased tactile fremitus in the right base of the lung, distant heart sounds, an S4, a II/VI systolic murmur along the left sternal border, and increased jugular venous pulsations. There is 2+ pitting edema of the ankles without tenderness of the calves. Her skin is warm and moist. There is no exophthalmos or lid lag. Her thyroid gland is palpable but not enlarged.

An electrocardiogram (ECG), done before your arrival, demonstrated left ventricular hypertrophy, left-axis deviation, sinus tachycardia with supraventricular ectopics, and no ischemic changes. Roentgenogram of the chest demonstrates left ventricular prominence, pulmonary vascular congestion, and a right-sided pleural effusion.

DECISION POINT D-1

With the information you now have, which of the following studies would you order as appropriate at this time?

1. Complete blood count (CBC)
2. Serum digoxin level
3. Serum electrolyte levels
4. Blood urea nitrogen (BUN) and serum creatinine levels

7. Thoracentesis
8. Arterial blood gas studies and pH
9. Pulmonary function studies
10. Perfusion scan of lung
11. Venograms of legs

Turn to page 407 for answers

DECISION POINT D-2

The patient declines to be admitted to the hospital. Her children indicate that they will take her to their home. She agrees to a follow-up office visit and to immediate admission to the hospital if her condition worsens. Prior to her leaving the emergency room, which of the following do you wish to prescribe or arrange for in the management of this patient?

12. Furosemide, 20 mg intravenously
13. Increase furosemide to 40 mg orally, daily, with potassium supplementation
14. Prothrombin time and partial thromboplastin time
15. Warfarin sodium, 40 mg for three days; then, 5 mg daily
16. Aspirin, 650 mg twice daily
17. Procaine penicillin G, 1.2 million units intramuscularly; then, penicillin V potassium, 500 mg intramuscularly, four times daily for 10 days
18. Cefaclor, 250 mg orally, three times daily
19. Consultation with oncologist
20. Aminophylline, 200 mg orally, four times daily
21. Prednisone, 20 mg orally, twice daily for one week; then, taper to 10 mg orally, daily

Turn to page 407 for answers

DECISION POINT D-3

The patient seemed to improve for a day or two following her visit to the emergency room, but then she slipped into her earlier state. After a week, she finally agrees to be admitted to the hospital. Physical examination, including vital signs, remains essentially unchanged except for less dullness than before at the base of the right lung. For further evaluation, you would order:

22. CBC
23. Serum electrolyte levels
24. Serum thyroxine (T4) level by radioimmunoassay and serum triiodothyronine (T3)-resin uptake
25. Repeat ECG
26. Echocardiogram
27. Cardiac consultation for left heart catheterization
28. Consultation for pulmonary angiogram
29. Gentamicin, 80 mg intravenously, three times daily, and aqueous penicillin G, 2 million units intravenously, every 4 hr after blood cultures drawn
30. Heparin sodium, 6000 units intravenously; then, 1000 units/hr by continuous infusion after coagulation studies drawn

31. Propylthiouracil followed by iodine-131
32. Consultation for bronchoscopy
33. Refer to surgeon for thyroidectomy

Turn to page 407 for answers

DECISION POINT D-4

Following appropriate therapy, the patient makes an uneventful recovery and returns to her former independence. After a year of stable health, she experiences progressive breathlessness of one month's duration and returns to your office. You admit her to the hospital. Physical examination is generally the same as last year except that her blood pressure is 145/85 mm Hg, she has an S3, and she is afebrile. An ECG demonstrates an infarction of undetermined age of the anterior myocardial wall. She denies having had any pain or heaviness in her chest, but she has been feeling tired. All other laboratory tests, including thyroid studies, are within normal limits. You increase the dosage of furosemide to 80 mg orally, daily, and continue all other medications.

After one week of hospitalization, she is less breathless, but she now has postural lightheadedness, constipation, and listlessness. You note that her blood pressure drops from 135/80 to 95/60 mm Hg when she goes from the supine position to standing. For the first time, she has periods of confusion; however, there are no focal neurologic deficits.

At this time, you would order:

34. Serum electrolyte levels
35. BUN and serum creatinine levels
36. Serum glucose level
37. Arterial blood gases on room air
38. Technetium-99m scan of brain
39. Psychiatric consultation
40. Serum digoxin level

Turn to page 407 for answers

DECISION POINT D-5

Given the information you now have, which of the following therapeutic measures would you now order?

41. Increase digoxin to 0.25 mg orally, daily
42. Discontinue furosemide temporarily
43. Increase dose of furosemide
44. Begin hydralazine therapy immediately
45. Begin hydralazine therapy in five days
46. 20 units NPH insulin, subcutaneously, daily
47. Chlorpropamide, 100 mg orally, twice daily
48. Neurologic consultation
49. Social services consultation for planning continuing care

Turn to page 407 for answers

ANSWERS

DECISION POINT D-1

1. Hb, 12.5 g/dl; leukocyte count, 7,500/mm³ with normal differential
2. Results available in 24 hr
3. Na, 135 mEq/liter; K, 3.8 mEq/liter; Cl, 99 mEq/liter; total CO_2, 26 mEq/liter
4. BUN, 18 mg/dl; creatinine, 0.9 mg/dl
5. Few leukocytes; normal oropharyngeal flora
6. None seen; specimen sent to state lab for culture. Negative PPD
7. 1,200 cm³ of clear fluid removed; protein, 1.0 g; pleural/serum LDH ratio, 0.3; no organisms seen on Gram stain; 40 lymphocytes/mm³ and 5 erythrocytes/mm³; no malignant cells seen
8. PO_2, 65 mm Hg; PCO_2, 32 mm Hg; HCO_3, 23 mEq/liter; pH 7.48
9. Ordered
10. Decreased uptake in area of right base; findings not diagnostic of pulmonary embolus
11. Left leg normal; attempts on right leg abandoned after dye extravasation

DECISION POINT D-2

12. Administered
13. Ordered
14. Both normal
15. Ordered
16. Ordered
17. Ordered
18. Ordered
19. Consultation requested
20. Ordered; poorly tolerated; discontinued after three days
21. Ordered

DECISION POINT D-3

22. Hb, 12.5 g/dl; leukocyte count, 8300/mm³ with normal differential
23. Na, 135 mEq/liter; K, 3.8 mEq/liter; Cl, 99 mEq/liter; total CO_2, 26 mEq/liter
24. 17 µg/dl (normal, 5 to 12); and 40% (normal 25 to 35)
25. Unchanged
26. Minimal calcification of aortic cusps and thickening of valve; mobility not impaired; LVH with dilation; no dyskinesia
27. Consultation requested
28. Consultation requested
29. Ordered
30. Ordered
31. Ordered
32. Consultation requested
33. Referred

DECISION POINT D-4

34. Na, 122 mEq/liter; K, 3.4 mEq/liter; Cl, 89 mEq/liter; total CO_2, 32 mEq/liter
35. BUN, 55 mg/dl; creatinine, 1.2 mg/dl
36. 180 mg/dl
37. PO_2, 70 mm Hg; PCO_2, 38 mm Hg; HCO_3, 30 mEq/liter; pH 7.48
38. Ordered
39. Consultation requested
40. 1.8 ng/dl

DECISION POINT D-5

41. Ordered
42. Ordered
43. Ordered
44. Ordered
45. Ordered
46. Ordered
47. Ordered
48. Consultation requested
49. Consultation requested

CRITIQUE

CASE SUMMARY

Congestive heart failure is a condition with high morbidity and mortality that is common in elderly individuals; it requires prompt recognition and thoughtful management by physicians caring for elderly patients.

Determination of the etiology of increasing dyspnea in an elderly patient, who previously had stable congestive heart failure, is a therapeutic and diagnostic challenge. There is nothing in the original presentation of this patient that would provide an unequivocal diagnosis. The nature of the pleural fluid, the unremarkable sputum smear, and the findings from the CBC help to justify the decision to treat the worsening heart failure with a higher dose of diuretics. Only after this measure fails is it really necessary to pursue a more specific cause. The presence of a silent myocardial infarction, new or old valvular lesions, infection, poor compliance in the taking of medication, hypophosphatemia, hypoxemia, pulmonary thromboembolus, constrictive pericarditis, dysrhythmias, significant myocardial dysfunction (ventricular aneurysm), and thyrotoxicosis are examples of treatable causes for refractory failure in elderly patients; although they may not respond to "standard" therapy, they are nonetheless potentially treatable.

There are no clinical, historical, or physical clues that are diagnostic of thyrotoxicosis in elderly patients. This diagnosis should be considered in any elderly person who has experienced unexplained, new, or worsening cardiac failure, atrial fibrillation, confusion, lethargy, personality change, loss of weight, diarrhea, constipation, anorexia, or gluttony. Significant thyromegaly and eye signs are often not present with thyrotoxicosis in people more than 60 years of age. When pretreatment with propylthiouracil is followed by ablation of the thyroid with iodine-131, L-thyroxine is occasionally required for maintenance of thyroid function.

The incidence of silent myocardial infarctions in diabetics, hypertensive patients, and the elderly has not been established; the sensation of heaviness in the chest may not be reported, experienced, or remembered by patients.

Therapy with vasodilators is becoming a proven, useful, long-term alternative to increasing doses of diuretics for patients with refractory heart failure. Although this therapeutic approach clearly can improve the quality of life (if not the functional class of cardiac disability), demonstration of a change in the natural history of life expectancy of those suffering from this devastating condition has not been made.

With the information you now have, which of the following studies would you order as appropriate at this time?

1. Complete blood count (CBC)
   This routine evaluation will help to assess the possibility that anemia or infection may contribute to the worsening of congestive failure in this patient. Here, the findings are reassuring as to both these points.
   If you had selected this option your score would be . . . .   +1

2. Serum digoxin level
   Measurement of the serum digoxin level will provide the best check on the compliance of the patient in following a drug regimen, as well as indicate whether an appropriate dosage of digoxin is being given.
   If you had selected this option your score would be . . . .   +1

3. Serum electrolyte levels
   Measurement of baseline levels of serum electrolytes will be important in management, particularly if modifications in the dosage of digoxin or of diuretics are anticipated or implemented.
   If you had selected this option your score would be . . . .   +1

4. Blood urea nitrogen (BUN) and serum creatinine levels
   Assessment of renal function is important in a patient receiving digoxin, inasmuch as the dosage may have to be modified if renal function is in any way compromised. Here, the results indicate that the patient has satisfactory renal function.
   If you had selected this option your score would be . . . .   +1

5. Gram stain of sputum
   In a patient with respiratory symptoms and congestive failure, the possibility of bacterial pneumonia must be always considered. A Gram stain of sputum may identify an infecting organism, allowing for accurate therapy.
   If you had selected this option your score would be . . . .   +1

6. Sputum smear for acid-fast bacilli and PPD skin test
   Elderly patients are at particularly high risk of reactivation of tuberculosis and may present negative PPD skin tests in the face of active disease, owing to anergy. In this patient, no organisms are seen on smear, and the PPD skin test is negative. It will, nonetheless, be appropriate to culture sputum for acid-fast bacilli.
   If you had selected this option your score would be . . . .   +3

7. Thoracentesis   **Score**

In patients with chronic congestive failure, the appearance or worsening of respiratory distress is commonly due to the accumulation of ascitic or pleural fluid. Generally, it is the pleural fluid that is more likely to be responsible for increasing respiratory distress. In this patient, the physical examination suggests the possibility of an accumulation of fluid on the right side of the chest, and the aspiration of such fluid is likely to be of benefit to the patient. The finding of 40 lymphocytes is consistent with noninfected transudate. A pulmonary thromboembolus is unlikely, but cannot be excluded.

The examination of such fluid should include a measurement of its protein content, of its LDH (which should be compared with the serum level), counts of white and red cells, and a Gram stain of the fluid; culture and examination for malignant cells should be considered. In this patient, the absence of bacteria, the paucity of cells, the low ratio of pleural to serum LDH, and the low level of protein in the fluid indicate a noninflammatory, nonmalignant transudate consistent with cardiac failure. No malignant cells are noted.

If you had selected this option your score would be . . . .   +5

8. Arterial blood gas studies and pH

Studies of arterial blood gases and pH in this patient indicate mild hypoxemia and a mild respiratory alkalosis (low P_{CO_2} and slightly elevated pH), both consistent with congestive heart failure. The respiratory alkalosis reflects the fact that the patient is hyperventilating.

If you had selected this option your score would be . . . .   +3

9. Pulmonary function studies

No need has been established for pulmonary function studies, which would be more appropriate for the evaluation of a primary pulmonary problem. There is no indication that this patient has any mechanical problem in movement of air or in transport of oxygen.

If you had selected this option your score would be . . . .   −3

10. Perfusion scan of lung

The findings in this patient might be consistent with pulmonary embolism, but there has been no acute episode suggesting when an embolus might have reached the lung, and the physical findings are suggestive of pleural fluid.

A perfusion lung scan is not a definitive study for pulmonary thromboembolism when either pleural effusion or pulmonary congestion is present. When indicated, a pulmonary angiogram is the definitive study.

If you had selected this option your score would be . . . .   −3

11. Venograms of legs
In this patient at this time, the evaluation of the possibility of venous thrombosis must be given low priority. It would be indicated only if some indirect evidence of the source of an embolus were required in a case where other tests were equivocal and the possibility of an embolus needed to be assessed.
If you had selected this option your score would be . . . .   −5

DECISION POINT D-2

The patient declines to be admitted to the hospital. Her children indicate that they will take her to their home. She agrees to a follow-up office visit and to immediate admission to the hospital if her condition worsens. Prior to her leaving the emergency room, which of the following do you wish to prescribe or arrange for in the management of this patient?

12. Furosemide, 20 mg intravenously
(See critique 13.)
If you had selected this option your score would be . . . .   +3

13. Increase furosemide to 40 mg orally, daily, with potassium supplementation
In a patient with symptomatic and worsening congestive heart failure, the intravenous administration of a bolus of furosemide can produce a rapid diuresis and relief of distress. In this patient, the maintenance therapy is linked to a general increase in the dose of furosemide, with potassium supplementation to counteract the tendency of this drug to produce hypokalemia.
If you had selected this option your score would be . . . .   +5

14. Prothrombin time and partial thromboplastin time
(See critique 15.)
If you had selected this option your score would be . . . .   −1

15. Warfarin sodium, 40 mg for three days; then, 5 mg daily
The measurement of prothrombin time and partial thromboplastin time would be appropriate if it were planned to use anticoagulant medication for treatment or prophylaxis of thromboembolism. In this patient, however, no substantial basis for the diagnosis of thromboembolism has been uncovered. In any case, the use of coumarin anticoagulant therapy to prevent pul-

monary thromboembolism would be appropriate only after at least one week of adequate heparinization, and its use to prevent systemic embolization is controversial.

If you had selected this option your score would be . . . .   −5

16. Aspirin, 650 mg twice daily
    There is no clear indication that therapy with aspirin would be helpful to this patient.
    If you had selected this option your score would be . . . .   −1

17. Procaine penicillin G, 1.2 million units intramuscularly; then, penicillin V potassium, 500 mg intramuscularly, four times daily for 10 days
    (See critique 18.)
    If you had selected this option your score would be . . . .   −3

18. Cefaclor, 250 mg orally, three times daily
    No adequate basis has as yet been laid for the use of antibiotic medication in this patient. She has a normal white count and no evidence of infection in her sputum. It is particularly inappropriate to use an expensive drug like cefaclor when an inexpensive one such as penicillin will accomplish the same ends.
    If you had selected this option your score would be . . . .   −3

19. Consultation with oncologist
    If it were felt that the pleural fluid in this patient were possibly the result of a malignant growth in or in contact with the pleural space, consultation with an oncologist might be warranted. In this patient, however, there is as yet no such indication. The examination of the chest fluid was reported to show no malignant cells.
    If you had selected this option your score would be . . . .   −3

20. Aminophylline, 200 mg orally, four times daily
    The administration of aminophylline has some theoretical usefulness in the management of acute episodes of cardiac failure, but there is no evidence that it will be helpful here, i.e., no bronchospasm.
    If you had selected this option your score would be . . . .   −3

21. Prednisone, 20 mg orally, twice daily for one week; then, taper to 10 mg orally, daily
    There is no indication for the use of corticosteroid medication in this patient. Its use might lead to retention of salt and water, and to the worsening, in consequence, of her congestive heart failure.
    If you had selected this option your score would be . . . .   −5

The patient seemed to improve for a day or two following her visit to the emergency room, but then she slipped into her earlier state. After a week, she finally agrees to be admitted to the hospital. Physical examination, including vital signs, remains essentially unchanged except for less dullness than before at the base of the right lung. For further evaluation, you would order:

22. CBC
    Repetition of the CBC on this patient would not be harmful, but it is unlikely to provide additional useful information.
    If you had selected this option your score would be   0

23. Serum electrolyte levels
    Measurement of serum electrolyte levels would indicate whether significant electrolyte changes had occurred as a consequence of medication.
    If you had selected this option your score would be . . . .   +3

24. Serum thyroxine (T4) level by radioimmunoassay and serum triiodothyronine (T3)-resin uptake
    Whenever an elderly patient has a worsening of the signs and symptoms of congestive failure, it is important that this not be casually ascribed simply to the worsening of basic underlying structural abnormalities in the heart. Hyperthyroidism not uncommonly is responsible for deterioration of elderly patients with chronic congestive failure, and in such patients it is often not accompanied by the typical clinical features of hyperthyroidism in younger persons. In this patient, who has a low-grade fever, with tachycardia, an assessment of thyroid function is essential. The findings indicate mild hyperthyroidism, and treatment will be appropriate. In patients with heart disease, pretreatment with antithyroid medications is prudent, prior to ablation of the thyroid with the use of iodine-131, which is the treatment of choice. Adjunctive therapy with propranolol should probably not be used routinely in patients such as this, though it may assist in controlling some of the manifestations of hyperthyroidism; in any case, it should not be done without careful monitoring. Following treatment with iodine-131, some patients will require replacement therapy with L-thyroxine.
    If you had selected this option your score would be . . . .   +5

25. Repeat ECG
    Another look at the ECG of this patient would be appropriate, as reassurance that no rapid progression of changes was oc-

curring and that no evidence of myocardial infarction had appeared.

If you had selected this option your score would be . . . .

+1

26. Echocardiogram
Echocardiography is a particularly valuable, noninvasive technique for determining the pathologic anatomy of the heart in elderly patients. In this patient, the findings are consistent with acquired calcific aortic sclerosis, which is a relatively common occurrence in elderly patients, and can be either hemodynamically inconsequential or devastating in its effects on cardiac function. The clinical information available to us in this patient favors the conclusion that the calcific changes in the aortic valve can be regarded as hemodynamically inconsequential. No further evaluation of this patient is indicated at this time.

If you had selected this option your score would be . . . .

+3

27. Cardiac consultation for left heart catheterization
(See critique 28.)

If you had selected this option your score would be . . . .

−5

28. Consultation for pulmonary angiogram
These invasive studies would not be indicated in the evaluation of this patient at this time, since there is no evidence of thromboembolic disease or a surgically correctible heart lesion.

If you had selected this option your score would be . . . .

−5

29. Gentamicin, 80 mg intravenously, three times daily and aqueous penicillin G, 2 million units intravenously, every 4 hr after blood cultures drawn
No basis has been laid for the administration of antibiotics in this patient. If substantial concern were felt with the suggestion that she may have a low-grade fever or if evidence of infection were found in her blood, then it would be appropriate to obtain blood cultures so that a pathogenic organism might be identified. The administration of antibiotic treatment should wait upon such further studies.

If you had selected this option your score would be . . . .

−3

30. Heparin sodium, 6000 units intravenously; then, 1000 units/hr by continuous infusion after coagulation studies drawn
The regimen proposed is appropriate for full heparinization, which would not be indicated in the absence of evidence of pulmonary embolism. Treatment with low doses of heparin might be justified if the patient were required to be kept for a

414

considerable period at complete bed rest, in this case for the prophylaxis of thromboembolism.

If you had selected this option your score would be . . . .   −3

31. Propylthiouracil followed by iodine-131
   (See critique 24.)
   If you had selected this option your score would be . . . .   +5

32. Consultation for bronchoscopy
   This patient appears to have a cardiac rather than a pulmonary problem. There has been no indication brought forward for bronchoscopy.
   If you had selected this option your score would be . . . .   −5

33. Refer to surgeon for thyroidectomy
   (See critique 24.)
   If you had selected this option your score would be . . . .   −5

DECISION POINT D-4   Score

At this time, you would order:

34. Serum electrolyte levels
   (See critique 35.)
   If you had selected this option your score would be . . . .   +5

35. BUN and serum creatinine levels
   The appearance of postural hypotension and periods of confusion in a patient under aggressive treatment for congestive heart failure should always raise the question as to the possibility of electrolyte abnormalities. In this patient, a low serum sodium level is demonstrated, which is consistent with the effects of diuretic medication. BUN and creatinine levels help to assess renal function, and in this instance they seem likely to indicate a prerenal rather than renal azotemia. It is to be expected that with additional salt and water intake, with appropriate attention to potassium economy, her postural hypotension and periods of confusion may be relieved.
   If you had selected this option your score would be . . . .   +5

36. Serum glucose level
   An examination of the blood glucose level will be appropriate in a patient with a history of diabetes mellitus and confusion. The result in this instance does not suggest that she is in the early stages of hyperosmolar state.
   If you had selected this option your score would be . . . .   +3

415

37. Arterial blood gases on room air   **Score**
It is appropriate to examine the possibility that increasing hypoxemia might be a contributing factor in the patient's confusion. In this patient, that is not the case.
If you had selected this option your score would be . . . .   +1

38. Technetium-99m scan of brain
Until other measures for dealing with the confusion in this
patient have been shown to be ineffective, there will be no
indication for a brain scan or for other studies such as computed
tomography or arteriography.
If you had selected this option your score would be . . . .   −3

39. Psychiatric consultation
Until medical and iatrogenic causes of this patient's confusion
have been excluded, there will be no indication to seek psychiatric consultation.
If you had selected this option your score would be . . . .   −3

40. Serum digoxin level
It is not likely that confusion would be associated with the use
of digoxin, although headache, weakness, and apathy are described as effects of overdose. In this patient, the measured
level is at an appropriate therapeutic level.
If you had selected this option your score would be . . . .   +3

DECISION POINT D-5   **Score**

Given the information you now have, which of the following therapeutic measures would you now order?

41. Increase digoxin to 0.25 mg orally, daily
There is no need to increase the digoxin level of this patient,
who is known to have an appropriate therapeutic level.
If you had selected this option your score would be . . . .   −3

42. Discontinue furosemide temporarily
Judicious restoration of this patient's sodium and water balance
will be essential for maximum cardiac output when afterload
therapy is initiated. This form of therapy often results in improved responsiveness to diuretics, presumably owing to improved renal perfusion. The response to drugs affecting afterload
is variable. Increases in the dosage of drugs used should be
made slowly, and central monitoring should be initiated for
patients who have had pretreatment hypotension with a poor

response to therapy, as in those who may have required unusually high dosage of drugs.

The addition of afterload therapy for congestive heart failure management usually requires hospitalization and close observation. The patient's confusion should improve as the serum sodium level returns to normal and her cardiac output improves. If you had selected this option your score would be . . . .   +5

43. Increase dose of furosemide
A further increase in furosemide dosage for this patient is contraindicated, inasmuch as her current symptoms are the probable effect of the heavy dose of furosemide that she is now receiving. If you had selected this option your score would be . . . .   −5

44. Begin hydralazine therapy immediately
(See critique 45.)
If you had selected this option your score would be . . . .   −3

45. Begin hydralazine therapy in five days
The addition of vasodilator therapy must be coordinated with the restoration of fluid and electrolyte balance (here postural hypotension and hyponatremia). Several different combinations of pre- and afterload drugs are possible. Hemodynamic studies and clinical trial-and-error are necessary to achieve the optimal benefits.
At this moment, it must be noted, the patient has both postural hypotension and hyponatremia. Her fluid and electrolyte balance should be restored before hydralazine is added to her regimen. This can be expected to require several days. If you had selected this option your score would be . . . .   +5

46. 20 units NPH insulin, subcutaneously, daily
The blood glucose level of 180 mg/dl does not explain this patient's confusion. Insulin therapy should be initiated only after it has been established that her glucose levels are unacceptably high and uncontrollable by dietary means. If you had selected this option your score would be . . . .   −3

47. Chlorpropamide, 100 mg orally, twice daily
Chlorpropamide is contraindicated for patients who have hyponatremia, and it should probably not be used in patients who are concurrently receiving diuretics. In any case, the dosage suggested here is too high and the frequency of administration excessive. If you had selected this option your score would be . . . .   −5

48. Neurologic consultation **Score**

There is no indication here that a neurologic consultation will be helpful. The neurologic examination is described as normal, and the patient's confusion is adequately explained by the electrolyte abnormality.

If you had selected this option your score would be . . . .   −3

49. Social services consultation for planning continuing care

While it is appropriate that a social service consultation be obtained to plan the continuing care of this patient after her discharge from the hospital, the better time for such a consultation is when the patient is admitted rather than when discharge is imminent. In many communities there are long waiting lists for admission to extended-care facilities. In any case, the decision to explore with a social service consultation the possible needs of the patient at the time of discharge should not be regarded as an anticipation or admission of defeat in an effort to restore her to her premorbid status. It is well to keep all options open as one endeavors to maximize the patient's ultimate independence.

If you had selected this option your score would be   0

SUMMARY

Following the restoration to a relatively normal level of fluid and electrolyte balance, an improved cardiac output was achieved by the use of vasodilators. Within three days her thinking was more clear, and she was again ambulatory. It became clear as time passed, however, that this woman lacked the mental sharpness and physical strength required for her to return to her home. After several frustrating months of delay (in the hospital and at her son's home), she was admitted to a local home for the aged. Unsettled by the move, she became openly hostile toward her family and occasionally disruptive at the home. Despite urging by the staff at the home and pleas from the family, you resisted the temptation to give her "something for her nerves."

Your patient gradually adjusted to the move to the home by making some friends and by having regular family outings and occasional short trips.

The patient died suddenly in her sleep one year after her second hospitalization without any obvious deterioration in her cardiac function.

BIBLIOGRAPHY

Chatterjee, K., and Parmley, W. W. (1977): The role of vasodilator therapy in heart failure. *Prog. Cardiovasc. Dis.*, 19:301–325.
Davis, P. J., and Davis, F. B. (1974): Hyperthyroidism in patients over the age of 60 years. *Medicine*, 83:161–181.

DeGroot, L. J. (1979): The thyroid. In: *Textbook of Medicine*, 15th ed., pp. 2120–2128, 2135–2137. Philadelphia, Saunders.

Ingbar, S. H., and Woeber, K. A. (1980): Diseases of the thyroid. In: *Harrison's Principles of Internal Medicine*, 9th ed., pp. 1703–1709. New York, McGraw-Hill.

Irvine, R. E., and Hodkinson, H. M. (1978): Thyroid disease in old age. In: *Textbook of Geriatric Medicine and Gerontology*, 2nd ed, edited by J. C. Brocklehurst, New York, Churchill Livingstone.

Marjolis, T. R., Kannel, W. B., Feinleib, M., Dawber, T. B., and McNamara, P. M. (1973): Clinical features of unrecognized myocardial infarction—silent and symptomatic. *Am. J. Cardiol.*, 32:1–7.

Mason, D. T., ed. (1978): Symposium on vasodilator and inotropic therapy of heart disease. *Am. J. Med.*, 65.

McKee, P. A., Castelli, W. P., McNamara, P. M., and Kannel, W. B. (1971): The natural history of congestive heart failure: The Framingham study. *N. Engl. J. Med.*, 285:1441–1446.

Moser, K. M. (1977): State of the art: Pulmonary embolism. *Am. Rev. Respir. Dis.*, 115:829–852.

Pacher, M., and Meller, J. (1978): Oral vasodilator therapy for chronic heart failure: A plea for caution. *Am. J. Cardiol.*, 42:686–688.

Pethy, M. S. (1967): Clinical presentation of myocardial infarction in the elderly. *Br. Heart J.*, 29:190–199.

Robin, E. D. (1977): Overdiagnosis and overtreatment of pulmonary embolism: The emperor may have no clothes. *Ann. Intern. Med.*, 87:775–781.

Rodstein, M. (1967): The characteristics of non-fatal myocardial infarctions in the aged. *Arch. Intern. Med.*, 254:577–583.

Thomas, F. B., Mazzafeiri, E. L., and Skillman, T. G. (1970): Apathetic thyrotoxicosis: A distinctive clinical and laboratory entity. *Ann. Intern. Med.*, 72:679–685.

PROBLEM E

Forgetfulness and Withdrawal in a 75-Year-Old Widower

Alvin J. Levenson

GENERAL INFORMATION

A 75-year-old widowed man is brought to your office by his daughter and son-in-law, who indicate their concern that during the past month he has become increasingly forgetful and has tended to withdraw from his usual daily activities and interpersonal relationships. He has been in reasonably good health prior to this time.

On physical examination, you find an elderly man who appears somewhat uncomfortable at the circumstances of this visit, answers questions readily but tersely, and in a monotone, without enthusiasm. He denies any problem, feels it is nonsense that he has been brought to see you. Your routine physical examination discloses no substantial abnormality.

You decide to hospitalize the patient for study.

DECISION POINT E-1

With the understanding that a thorough history will be taken, to which of the following points would you wish to give particular attention in the evaluation of this patient at this time?

1. Recent change in life circumstances
2. Current living arrangements
3. Recent changes in medications
4. History of depression
5. Change in appetite
6. Change in weight
7. History of injury to head
8. History of falls
9. History of alcohol intake
10. Past relationships with family members

Turn to page 423 for answers

DECISION POINT E-2

In your evaluation of this patient, which of the following questions do you regard as appropriate at this time?

11. "How are you feeling?"
12. "What day is it today?"

13. "Can you count backwards from 100 by 7's?"
14. "What sort of hobbies do you have?"
15. "How do you stay busy?"
16. "What kinds of books do you like to read?"
17. "Do you have any friends?"
18. "Are you sleeping well?"
19. "Have you had any thoughts or plans of hurting yourself or others?"

Turn to page 423 for answers

DECISION POINT E-3

Your physical examination has discovered no essential abnormality, except that the patient seemed slow in his movements and his thought processes. With the information you now have, which of the following studies would you order or arrange for?

20. Complete blood count (CBC)
21. Urinalysis
22. Blood urea nitrogen (BUN) and serum creatinine levels
23. Roentgenogram of chest
24. Serum triglyceride levels
25. Serum lactate dehyrogenase (LDH) level
26. Examination of cerebrospinal fluid (CSF)
27. Examination of stool
28. Serum T3 and T4 levels
29. Serum folate level
30. Serum vitamin B_{12} level
31. Venereal Disease Research Laboratory (VDRL)

Turn to page 423 for answers

DECISION POINT E-4

With the information you now have, which of the following further studies would you order or arrange for?

32. Electroencephalogram (EEG)
33. Gastrointestinal roentgenographic series
34. Sigmoidoscopy
35. Barium enema examination
36. Computed tomography (CT scan) of head
37. Pneumoencephalography
38. Carotid arteriography
39. Radionuclide brain scan
40. Evaluation of CSF flow using radioiodinated serum albumin scan

Turn to page 423 for answers

DECISION POINT E-5

With the information you now have, which of the following would you include in your plan of management?

41. Request consultation for carotid arterial surgery

42. Request psychiatric consultation
43. Request neurosurgical consultation
44. Order vasodilator drug
45. Review history for contraindications to drug therapy
46. Order tricyclic antidepressants
47. Order a major tranquilizer
48. Order lithium carbonate
49. Order a combination of major tranquilizer and tricyclic antidepressant
50. Discharge patient now, to have future evaluation at community health center
51. Discharge patient to nursing home
52. Discharge patient for enrollment in day-care center
53. Reassure family that condition is likely temporary and that no intervention is indicated at this time

Turn to page 423 for answers

ANSWERS

DECISION POINT E-1

1. None known
2. Living with son and daughter-in-law in their home since death of wife three years ago
3. None
4. None
5. Appetite has been decreased
6. Loss of 4.5 kg (10 lb) in past six weeks
7. None
8. None
9. Occasional beer
10. Relationships reported to be good

DECISION POINT E-2

11. "No count. I feel tired all the time. I'm not good for anything."
12. "Wednesday. No, I guess it's Thursday. No. I can't remember."
13. "I can try. 100, 93, 86, 81, 74, 64. . . . No. That's not it. Oh, heck, what's the use?"
14. "I cook a little sometimes, and work in the yard."
15. "I don't stay busy anymore."
16. "I don't read much."
17. "Most of them are dead."
18. "I sleep okay."
19. "Yes, I've thought many times of ending it all."

DECISION POINT E-3

20. Within normal limits
21. Within normal limits
22. Within normal limits
23. Within normal limits

24. Mildly elevated
25. Mildly elevated
26. Normal findings
27. No blood demonstrated
28. Within normal limits
29. Within normal limits
30. Within normal limits
31. Nonreactive

DECISION POINT E-4

32. Within normal limits
33. Within normal limits
34. Within normal limits
35. Within normal limits
36. Moderate cortical atrophy and slightly enlarged ventricles
37. Moderate cortical atrophy; slightly enlarged ventricles
38. 30% occlusion of right carotid artery
39. Within normal limits
40. Flow appears within normal limits

DECISION POINT E-5

41. Cardiovascular surgeon will see patient
42. Psychiatrist will see patient
43. Neurosurgeon will see patient
44. Ordered
45. No contraindications discovered
46. Ordered
47. Ordered
48. Ordered
49. Ordered
50. Arrangements made
51. Arrangements made
52. Arrangements made
53. Arrangements made

CRITIQUE

DECISION POINT E-1   **Score**

With the understanding that a thorough history will be taken, to which of the following points would you wish to give particular attention in the evaluation of this patient at this time?

1. Recent change in life circumstances
    Elderly persons are often very sensitive to change in their life circumstances and losses may commonly produce depression. These may range from cancellation of health insurance or of a favorite television show to the loss of a pet or of an old friend. Such losses do not make the diagnosis of depression certain, however, many losses being taken in stride.
    If you had selected this option your score would be . . . .   +3

2. Current living arrangements
    The living circumstances of elderly persons must always be reasonably known if the planning for their care after hospitalization is to be optimal
    If you had selected this option your score would be . . . .   +1

3. Recent changes in medications
    Changes in the mental or emotional states of elderly persons may often accompany the introduction of medications or changes in drugs or in dosage. Drugs used for hypertension, for example, such as propranolol, rauwolfia compounds, or sleep medications, can be responsible for such changes.
    If you had selected this option your score would be . . . .   +5

4. History of depression
    It will always be important to know the past history of mental or emotional illness in the evaluation of changing behavior.
    If you had selected this option your score would be . . . .   +3

5. Change in appetite
    (See critique 6.)
    If you had selected this option your score would be . . . .   +5

6. Change in weight
It is important to know whether change in mental or emotional
status has had an impact on nutrition. Attempts should be made
to quantify loss of weight, since loss of appetite is not necessarily equivalent to loss of weight. Patients may be asked whether
they have found their belts too tight or too loose, their clothes
becoming larger as well as whether they have lost a specific
number of pounds. Loss of weight is not always synonymous
with a psychiatric disturbance, e.g., depression. It may be compatible with cancer, which should always be ruled out first,
while the patient is under close supervision and observation.
Naturally, the two may occur simultaneously.
If you had selected this option your score would be ....   +5

7. History of injury to head
(See critique 8.)
If you had selected this option your score would be ....   +5

8. History of falls
It is important to determine whether elderly patients with changes
in behavior may be suffering the effects of trauma. Some patients who have had falls will be unaware of the fact that they
have suffered injury to the head.
If you had selected this option your score would be ....   +5

9. History of alcohol intake
It is appropriate to ask elderly patients about their intake of
alcohol. Alcoholism occurs among elderly persons, just as among
younger persons.
If you had selected this option your score would be ....   +3

10. Past relationship with family members
It will be useful in evaluating the current condition of the patient, as well as in planning for future care, to know what the
relationships have been with family members.
If you had selected this option your score would be ....   +1

DECISION POINT E-2

In your evaluation of this patient, which of the following questions
do you regard as appropriate at this time?

11. "How are you feeling?"
An open-ended question like "How do you feel?" is likely to
get a reasonably unbiased response from the patient. Such ques-

tions are generally more appropriate than trying to amass details
as to specific daily activities or functions.
If you had selected this option your score would be . . . .   +5

12. "What day is it today?"
    (See critique 13.)
    If you had selected this option your score would be . . . .   +5

13. "Can you count backwards from 100 by 7's?"
    These questions are part of the mental status examination, which
    is absolutely essential to the adequate evaluation of this patient.
    Along with the evidence of his state of feeling, they give evi-
    dence of psychomotor retardation and some disorientation as to
    time. Other questions, which are part of the mental status ex-
    amination, might be expected to show a reduced fund of general
    information and impairment of concrete thinking.
    If you had selected this option your score would be . . . .   +5

14. "What sort of hobbies do you have?"
    (See critique 15.)
    If you had selected this option your score would be . . . .   +1

15. "How do you stay busy?"
    These questions attempt to establish the level of interest and
    activities that the patient displayed prior to this recent deteri-
    oration, and they set the goals of a therapeutic program. In this
    instance, the replies suggest that the patient has generally had
    rather solitary activities and reflect his current feeling of depres-
    sion.
    If you had selected this option your score would be . . . .   +1

16. "What kinds of books do you like to read?"
    This kind of question is less open-ended than "How do you
    feel?" and requires more effort on the part of the patient. It
    assumes that there are kinds of books that he might like to read,
    and if that is not the case, serves no useful purpose.
    If you had selected this option your score would be   0

17. "Do you have any friends?"
    The words with which one makes inquiry of patients should
    always be chosen with great care. A question such as "Do you
    have any friends?" presents to the patient the possibility that
    he has no friends, and in this case, his response seems to reflect
    that this is the feeling that this question engenders. Might it not
    be better to ask "Who are your particular friends?"
    If you had selected this option your score would be . . . .   −1

18. "Are you sleeping well?"
    Questions regarding sleep are helpful in the evaluation of the
    possibility that fatigue or depression may be contributing to the
    patient's current mental or emotional state. Patients with depres-
    sion frequently have sleep disturbances, although the diagnosis
    should not be based on the symptom; it is merely corroborative.
    If you had selected this option your score would be . . . .   +3

19. "Have you had any thoughts or plans of hurting yourself or
    others?"
    With any patient for whom the diagnosis of depression is being
    considered, it is essential to assess the potential for suicide.
    Suicide is relatively common among elderly persons, and par-
    ticularly among elderly men.
    If you had selected this option your score would be . . . .   +5

DECISION POINT E-3   Score

At this point we have the picture of a cognitively impaired and
depressed elderly man, and need to know how much of his recent change
of status may be the result of the intrusion of physical illness on normal
brain function. It will be appropriate to evaluate each major body system, with particular attention to the central nervous system.

We have no clinical evidence of any problem with the pulmonary,
cardiovascular, or gastrointestinal systems. It will be appropriate to
know that the patient does not have any evidence of renal failure, along
with the status of the central nervous system. Your physical examination
has discovered no essential abnormality, except that the patient seemed
slow in his movements and in his thought processes.

With the information you now have, which of the following studies
would you order or arrange for?

20. Complete blood count (CBC)
    (See critique 23.)
    If you had selected this option your score would be . . . .   +5

21. Urinalysis
    (See critique 23.)
    If you had selected this option your score would be . . . .   +5

22. Blood urea nitrogen (BUN) and serum creatinine levels
    (See critique 23.)
    If you had selected this option your score would be . . . .   +5

23. Roentgenogram of chest
    These routine studies are appropriate, although they give no
    evidence of organic difficulty in this man. They indicate that

he is not anemic and has no evidence of diabetes mellitus nor renal failure. **Score**

If you had selected this option your score would be ....   +5

24. Serum triglyceride levels
    (See critique 25.)
    If you had selected this option your score would be ....   −1

25. Serum lactate dehydrogenase (LDH) level
    Metabolic studies such as these give little useful information in a patient such as this. We have no evidence of an organic process with which they can be clearly identified.
    If you had selected this option your score would be ....   −1

26. Examination of cerebrospinal fluid (CSF)
    We have no evidence that examination of the CSF is going to be useful in the evaluation of this patient. He has no signs of meningitis nor of a space-occupying lesion. On the other hand, in elderly persons the signs of tuberculosis or cryptococcal meningitis may be subtle, and these and other conditions may be treacherously indolent, as well as devastating. When the clinical picture leaves any uncertainty whatsoever as to the possibility of an infectious process, examination of the spinal fluid is called for and should include appropriate tests for fungal as well as bacterial or myobacterial infection.
    If you had selected this option your score would be ....   −3

27. Examination of stool
    The examination of the stool is a useful routine study in adults, and particularly in elderly patients in whom the risk of gastrointestinal malignancy may be increased.
    If you had selected this option your score would be   0

28. Serum T3 and T4 levels
    Deterioration in mental function at any age deserves consideration of the possibility of hypothyroidism. In elderly patients, the signs may commonly be obscure, and the recognition of hypothyroidism may rest on a high index of suspicion.
    If you had selected this option your score would be ....   +3

29. Serum folate level
    (See critique 30.)
    If you had selected this option your score would be ....   −1

30. Serum vitamin B_{12} level
    These examinations would be particularly indicated if the patient presented a hyperchromic, macrocytic anemia. Deficien-

cies in these substances are associated with neurologic defects, which are usually associated with anemia. On the other hand, an organic brain syndrome due to vitamin B_{12} deficiency has been reported in patients who have had no evidence of a blood dyscrasia.

If you had selected this option your score would be . . . . -1

31. Venereal Disease Research Laboratory (VDRL)
     It must not be forgotten that syphilis may occur among elderly patients as well as among younger patients. The possibility that a change in mental function might reflect general paresis fully warrants this otherwise routine examination.
     If you had selected this option your score would be . . . . $+3$

DECISION POINT E-4   Score

With the information you now have, which of the following further studies would you order or arrange for?

32. Electroencephalogram (EEG)
     An EEG in an instance such as this is useful in the evaluation of an organic brain syndrome, which, for example, could be mimicked by a seizure disorder or space-occupying lesion that may present as an irritative focus. Any evidence of a focal EEG finding indicates the need for further evaluation.
     If you had selected this option your score would be . . . . $+3$

33. Gastrointestinal roentgenographic series
     (See critique 35.)
     If you had selected this option your score would be . . . . -3

34. Sigmoidoscopy
     (See critique 35.)
     If you had selected this option your score would be . . . . -3

35. Barium enema examination
     No basis has been laid for these examinations. We can imagine that the patient might have a metastatic brain lesion from a malignancy of the lung or gastrointestinal tract, but we would need to have better evidence of that before using these studies to search for a primary tumor.
     If you had selected this option your score would be . . . . -3

36. Computed tomography (CT scan) of head
     In a patient who has had a rapid change in central nervous system function, CT has become the most useful initial measure

in the evaluation of the central nervous system. This exami- **Score**
nation is clearly indicated in this patient, in whom the moderate
cortical atrophy and slightly enlarged ventricles are consistent
with his age, and do not explain his recent change of status.
The absence of evidence of hemorrhage or tumor or significant
hydrocephalus is reassuring.
If you had selected this option your score would be . . . .   +5

37. Pneumoencephalography
    Pneumoencephalography is a generally uncomfortable, and in-
    creasingly obsolete, procedure for evaluation of the central nervous
    system. There is no indication for it in this patient.
    If you had selected this option your score would be . . . .   −5

38. Carotid arteriography
    If this patient's difficulties appear to be the result of transient
    ischemic attacks, carotid arteriography might well be indicated,
    but no basis has been laid for this examination in this patient.
    The finding of 30% stenosis of the right carotid artery can be
    regarded as more or less incidental in a patient of this age, in
    the absence of central nervous system symptoms suggestive of
    transient ischemic disease.
    If you had selected this option your score would be . . . .   −5

39. Radionuclide brain scan
    Radionuclide brain scan might be indicated if there were evi-
    dence of a lesion not detectable on CT scan or evidence of
    hydrocephalus. We have no indication for this examination in
    this patient.
    If you had selected this option your score would be . . . .   −3

40. Evaluation of CSF flow using radioiodinated serum albumin
    scan
    If this patient were felt to have normal-pressure hydrocephalus,
    this examination might be useful. The findings on CT scan,
    however, do not suggest that diagnosis, and no reason for this
    examination has been established in this patient.
    If you had selected this option your score would be . . . .   −5

DECISION POINT E-5

The family, patient, and physician should all approach the needs of a
patient such as this with the goal that, in the absence of irreversible
organic disease setting clear limits, appropriate treatment should restore
him to his previous level of function. This cannot, of course, be made
as a promise, but maintaining a climate of cautious optimism offers the

setting in which this goal has the best chance of achievement.

The appropriate studies carried out above have discovered no organic process that might be responsible for the patient's recent deterioration. Accordingly, treatment of his functional psychiatric state will be appropriate. The goal of treatment should be remission.

With the information you now have, which of the following would you include in your plan of management?

41. Request consultation of carotid arterial surgery
   There is no need for carotid endarterectomy in a patient with moderate unilateral occlusion who has no symptoms indicating transient ischemic attacks.
   If you had selected this option your score would be . . . . -5

42. Request psychiatric consultation
   A psychiatric consultation is just as appropriate for assessment of a depressed elderly patient as it would be for a younger person. Choices of medication or other therapy can often benefit from such consultation. The decision to consult psychiatry should be predicted on the comfort and expertise of the primary physician considering referral and the adequacy of the clinical setting to offer protection to the suicidal patient.
   If you had selected this option your score would be . . . . $+3$

43. Request neurosurgical consultation
   The patient gives no evidence of a neurosurgical condition, and evaluation by this consultant is not indicated.
   If you had selected this option your score would be . . . . -3

44. Order vasodilator drug
   There is no evidence that cerebral vasodilators are effective. In any case, this patient does not have any clear evidence of atherosclerotic cerebral vascular disease.
   If you had selected this option your score would be . . . . -3

45. Review history for contraindications to drug therapy
   The adequate review of the patient's history for contraindications to drug therapy is an essential part of the treatment plan. It is too often overlooked.
   If you had selected this option your score would be . . . . $+5$

46. Order tricyclic antidepressants
   The patient's clinical manifestations clearly indicate a retarded depression for which no reversible organic cause can be found.

He has no evidence of incipient or manifest schizophrenia, no incipient or manifest delusions, nor hallucinations. Under these circumstances, the prescription of tricyclic antidepressant drugs is indicated.

If you had selected this option your score would be . . . .   +5

47. Order a major tranquilizer

Major tranquilizers are not indicated for the condition this patient presents, and might well worsen it.

If you had selected this option your score would be . . . .   −5

48. Order lithium carbonate

Lithium carbonate has no confirmed place in the management of a patient such as this. It is certainly inferior to tricyclic antidepressants.

If you had selected this option your score would be . . . .   −5

49. Order a combination of major tranquilizer and tricyclic antidepressant

Nothing is gained in prescribing a combination of drugs for the management of this patient. It is essential that the effect of each drug be assessed in isolation. It should be pointed out, on the other hand, that minor tranquilizers (such as diazepam) may be indicated for anxious depressions (in contradistinction to retarded depressions) of mild to moderate severity.

If you had selected this option your score would be . . . .   −5

50. Discharge patient now, to have future evaluation at community health center

There is no need at this point to suggest to the patient or to the family that the current problem is going to require a major change in the living arrangements for the patient or for the family. A more optimistic approach to planning is appropriate, with the implicit expectation that the patient will be able to return to former interests and activities. It would be exceedingly imprudent to discharge a suicidal patient.

If you had selected this option your score would be . . . .   −5

51. Discharge patient to nursing home

There is no need at this point to suggest to the patient or to the family that the current problem is going to require a major change in the living arrangements for the patient or for the family. A more cautiously optimistic approach to planning is appropriate, with the implicit expectation that the patient will be able to return to former interests and activities. As with critique 50, it is exceedingly imprudent to discharge a suicidal patient.

If you had selected this option your score would be . . . . −5

52. Discharge patient for enrollment in day-care center
Like placement in a nursing home, the enrollment of this patient in a day-care center would represent in all likelihood a major dislocation in the living arrangements for patient and family. We have no indication as yet that formal involvement in the activities of a day-care center is going to contribute substantially to this patient's sense of well-being. See critique 51 for the inadvisability of discharge of this particular patient.

If you had selected this option your score would be . . . . −5

53. Reassure family that condition is likely temporary and that no intervention is indicated at this time
Shallow reassurance that the condition is temporary and that no intervention is indicated will throw the patient and family upon their own resources, which may be insufficient to restore the balance. The physician has an essential role to play here as therapist, and his or her continuing interest, periodic reevaluation, and treatment to remission, as well as emotional support, will constitute essential intervention.

If you had selected this option your score would be . . . . −5

SUMMARY

In summary, we have considered the problem of an elderly patient with the initial complaint of "forgetfulness." Its recent onset and evidence of cognitive dysfunction indicate a need for immediate medical evaluation and should not be regarded as a normal part of aging. An investigation has been carried out that indicates that the patient has no substantial organic basis for his current clinical presentation, and the prescription of psychotropic medication has become justified, in light of the presence of the retarded depression. In working with the patient and his family, the physician could encourage efforts and expectations that an adequate therapeutic plan has the desired outcome of reapproximating or reattaining the patient's premorbid baseline status, and this can appropriately be made an explicit goal in management, since no indication of irreversibility of the patient's condition has been found.

BIBLIOGRAPHY

Busse, E. W., and Blazer, D., Eds. (1980): *Handbook of Geropsychiatry*. New York, Van Nostrand Reinhold.

Butler, R. N. (1975): *Why Survive? Being Old in America*. New York, Harper & Row.

Dewald, P. A. (1964): *Psychotherapy: A Dynamic Approach*. New York, Basic Books.

Eaton, M. T., and Peterson, M. H. (1969): *Psychiatry, Medical Outline Series*. Flushing, NY, Medical Examination Publishing.

Freedman, A. M., Kaplan, H. I., and Sadock, B. J. (1972): *Modern Synopsis of Comprehensive Textbook of Psychiatry*. Baltimore, Williams & Wilkins.

Hollister, L. E. (1973): *Clinical Use of Psychotherapeutic Drugs*. Springfield, Ill., Charles C Thomas.

Klein, D. F., and Davis, J. M. (1969): *Diagnosis and Drug Treatment of Psychiatric Disorders*. Baltimore, Williams & Wilkins.

Levenson, A. J., Ed. (1979): *The Neuropsychiatric Side Effects of Drugs in the Elderly*. New York, Raven Press.

Levenson, A. J. (1980): *Basic Psychopharmacology for Health Professionals*. New York, Springer.

Levenson, A. J., and Tollett, S. M. (1980): Rapid psychiatric assessment of the geriatric patient for immediate psychiatric referral. *Geriatrics*, 35:113–120.

Levenson, A. J., Ed (1980): *Psychiatric Manifestations of Physical Illness in the Elderly*. New York, Raven Press.

Smith, W. E., and Kinsbourne, M. (1977): *Aging and Dementia*. New York, Spectrum.

Verwoerdt, A. (1976): *Clinical Geropsychiatry*. Baltimore, Williams & Wilkins.

Wells, C. E. (1978): Editorial: Role of stroke in dementia. *Stroke*, 9:1–3.

PROBLEM F

Agitation in an 82-Year-Old Nursing Home Patient

Alvin J. Levenson

GENERAL INFORMATION

You receive a call from a nursing home requesting your assistance in "controlling" an 82-year-old woman who has become "agitated" within the past day. She appears to have no physical illness. Her vital signs are reported to be normal. She has not indicated any tendency towards physical violence against either herself or others. You have no other information about this patient, whom you have not met.

DECISION POINT F-1

You will not be able to see the patient for several hours. With the information you have, which of the following instructions for the nurse would be acceptable?

1. Give head nurse a telephone order for chlorpromazine, to be administered in an intramuscular dose immediately, with further doses every 4 hr as necessary for agitation
2. Give head nurse a telephone order for diazepam, to be given intramuscularly immediately; then every 2 hr as necessary for agitation
3. Give head nurse a telephone order for phenobarbital, to be administered orally immediately; then every 6 hr as necessary for agitation
4. Give head nurse a telephone order to arrange for a relative of the patient to visit, in hope that this will quiet her
5. Give head nurse a telephone order for restraints to be used for patient to control agitation
6. Tell nurse to set firm limits on patient's complaining, confining her to her room or bed if necessary, until she settles down
7. Have nurses tell patient that she will be able to discuss her concerns with you as soon as you get there

Turn to page 437 for answers

DECISION POINT F-2

When you see the patient, she does not appear to be agitated. Except that she is a bit sullen, there are no abnormalities on mental status examination. Physical examination is not remarkable except that you hear soft systolic bruits over both carotid arteries.

In discussing the behavior of this patient at a staff conference, to which of the following points would you wish to give particular attention?

8. Any precipitating event to the patient's "agitation"
9. Patient's usual personality
10. Patient's visitors
11. Patient's religious activities
12. Patient's former occupation
13. Patient's recreational interests
14. History of patient's relationship with her parents
15. History of patient's relationship with her siblings
16. Patient's history of alcohol intake
17. Patient's history of psychiatric illness
18. Patient's use of drugs
19. History of episodes suggesting transient ischemic attacks
20. The nurses' own feelings towards patient and the incident

Turn to page 437 for answers

DECISION POINT F-3

With the information you now have, what further examinations would you regard as appropriate?

21. Computed tomography (CT scan) of head
22. Examination of cerebrospinal fluid (CSF)
23. Carotid arteriography
24. Radionuclide brain scan
25. Study of CSF flow dynamics, using radioiodinated serum albumin

Turn to page 437 for answers

DECISION POINT F-4

With the information you now have, which of the following would you include among your recommendations or orders?

26. Order a major tranquilizer (chlorpromazine)
27. Order a minor tranquilizer (diazepam)
28. Order a tricyclic antidepressant (amitriptyline)
29. Suggest behavior modification techniques for management of patient
30. Suggest that patient's privileges be restricted if an outburst occurs again
31. Request cardiovascular surgical consultation
32. Request psychiatric consultation
33. Request neurosurgical consultation
34. Recommend socialization therapy
35. Recommend greater involvement of patient in religious activities
36. Suggest gardening activity for patient
37. Remind patient that she must conform to daily schedule of the institution in her daily activities

38. Suggest arts and crafts therapy
39. Recommend flexible daily program, within limits of institutional routines and resources

ANSWERS

DECISION POINT F-1

1. Ordered
2. Ordered
3. Ordered
4. Ordered
5. Ordered
6. Ordered
7. Advice given

DECISION POINT F-2

8. Patient became angry when bedtime arbitrarily changed to 1 hr earlier
9. Rigid, independent, introverted
10. Only one or two old friends
11. None
12. Bookkeeper for 45 years
13. Reads a good deal; little else
14. Nothing known
15. No siblings known
16. Has occasional glass of sherry
17. None known
18. Occasional aspirin; no others known
19. None observed or known
20. Discussed

DECISION POINT F-3

21. Mild cortical atrophy
22. Within normal limits
23. Moderate occlusion, bilateral
24. Within normal limits
25. Within normal limits

DECISION POINT F-4

26. Ordered
27. Ordered
28. Ordered
29. Suggestion made
30. Suggestion made
31. Cardiovascular surgeon will see patient
32. Psychiatrist will see patient
33. Neurosurgeon will see patient
34. Recommendation made
35. Recommendation made
36. Suggestion made
37. Recommendation given
38. Suggestion made
39. Recommendation made

CRITIQUE

CASE SUMMARY

The case is presented of an elderly woman in a nursing home who had an emotional outburst upon a change in her expected routine. It is important that such outbursts be evaluated as to whether they represent functional or organic psychopathology or are legitimate reactions to circumstances that can be sympathetically understood when viewed in the patient's frame of reference.

The clinical encounter begins with a telephone call, with some options for intervention presented. It is important that no steps be taken in the absence of adequate evaluation.

DECISION POINT F-1   Score

You will not be able to see the patient for several hours. With the information you have, which of the following instructions for the nurse would be acceptable?

1. Give head nurse a telephone order for chlorpromazine, to be administered in an intramuscular dose immediately, with further doses every 4 hr as necessary for agitation
   No prescription of drugs will be appropriate in a situation such as this until an adequate evaluation of the status of the patient has been made. Psychotropic medications should not be administered over the telephone and especially for a patient whom the physician has never seen. The physician should not ordinarily delegate to the nursing staff the decision as to whether medication is the appropriate treatment for a patient in acute distress. In the absence of a physical examination and personal observation, the physician has no concrete data on which to justify any form of psychotropic medication. If the patient is found to be agitated, the causes of the agitation should be identified and every effort made to produce a remission first without medication.
   If you had selected this option your score would be . . . .   −5

2. Give head nurse a telephone order for diazepam, to be given intramuscularly immediately; then, every 2 hr as necessary for agitation
   (See critique 1.)
   If you had selected this option your score would be . . . .   −5

438

3. Give head nurse a telephone order for phenobarbital, to be **Score**
   administered orally immediately; then, every 6 hr as necessary
   for agitation
   (See critique 1.)
   If you had selected this option your score would be ....   −5

4. Give head nurse a telephone order to arrange for a relative of
   the patient to visit, in hope that this will quiet her
   It is inappropriate to involve the family at this time.
   If you had selected this option your score would be ....   −5

5. Give head nurse a telephone order for restraints to be used for
   patient to control agitation
   (See critique 6.)
   If you had selected this option your score would be ....   −5

6. Tell nurse to set firm limits on patient's complaining, confining
   her to her room or bed if necessary, until she settles down
   On the information that we have, no basis has been laid for
   restriction of the patient's activities, still less for punishment.
   Restraints may worsen a patient's status and should be utilized
   only if the patient's behavior places him or her or others in
   some potential danger. They are not treatment, in any case,
   only interim measures. If restraints are ever to be used, it must
   be only for brief periods, loosely applied, and without interference with such activities as the use of the bathroom; and
   their status must be frequently checked.
   If you had selected this option your score would be ....   −5

7. Have nurses tell patient that she will be able to discuss her
   concerns with you as soon as you can get there
   It is highly appropriate that the patient know that she will have
   a sympathetic ear as soon as possible, and the nurses should
   be encouraged to let the patient know of the physician's interest
   and concern. Personnel should not be permitted to use the calling of the physician as a threat to the patient in the attempt to
   control behavior.
   If you had selected this option your score would be ....   +5

DECISION POINT F-2

The essential feature of evaluation of a patient such as that described
is to identify the patient's status prior to a change in behavior as well
as to try to identify the circumstances under which the change in behavior
took place. It is appropriate to explore the details of a patient's behavior,
to learn whether any seem to represent psychopathology and/or a threat
of violence against herself or others. It is important to know whether

she is displaying purposeful or purposeless hyperactivity. Here we learn **Score** that the patient is responding to an unexpected change in her routine and that she has functioned reasonably well in circumstances where she has had a good deal of reliance on her own independence and resources.

In discussing the behavior of this patient at a staff conference, to which of the following points would you wish to give particular attention?

8.   Any precipitating events to the patient's "agitation"
It is essential to know what circumstances may have precipitated the patient's change in behavior. Here we learn that the patient's change in behavior is most likely a response to a change that she regarded as a major interference with her established lifestyle.
If you had selected this option your score would be . . . .   +5

9.   Patient's usual personality
(See critique 13.)
If you had selected this option your score would be . . . .   +5

10.   Patient's visitors
(See critique 13.)
If you had selected this option your score would be . . . .   +5

11.   Patient's religious activities
(See critique 13.)
If you had selected this option your score would be . . . .   +5

12.   Patient's former occupation
(See critique 13.)
If you had selected this option your score would be . . . .   +5

13.   Patient's recreational interests
These questions are appropriate in exploring the patient's baseline personality and life circumstances, particularly in terms of interpersonal relations, interests, and coping styles. The responses give us a picture of an independent person, for the most part self-reliant in recreation and in life activities.
If you had selected this option your score would be . . . .   +5

14.   History of patient's relationship with her parents
(See critique 15.)
If you had selected this option your score would be   0

15.   History of patient's relationship with her siblings
Little that is useful is likely to be learned from exploring the

history of the patient's relationship with other family members, except as siblings may offer important current contacts with the past. There is usually no need initially to look deeper for the motivation of the patient's behavior than the circumstances in which she lives at the present time.

If you had selected this option your score would be   0

16. Patient's history of alcohol intake
    (See critique 18.)
    If you had selected this option your score would be . . . .   +1

17. Patient's history of psychiatric illness
    It is useful to know whether the patient has manifested any emotional or other psychiatric disturbance in the past. In this case, the response helps us to conclude that the patient's outburst is rooted in her perceptions of her real-life situation.
    If you had selected this option your score would be . . . .   +3

18. Patient's use of drugs
    These questions are appropriate; it is always to be reviewed as a possibility that an acute change in behavior will reflect a response to drugs. This is perhaps more likely when such acute changes are recurrent. In this patient, we are reassured that drugs most likely play no role in the observed behavior.
    If you had selected this option your score would be . . . .   +5

19. History of episodes suggesting transient ischemic attacks
    It is appropriate to know if there is any evidence of chronic or of recurrent central nervous system problems that might account for deterioration in behavior. None have been observed in this patient.
    If you had selected this option your score would be . . . .   +1

20. The nurses' own feelings towards patient and the incident
    It is always essential to review the perceptions of nursing and medical staff with respect to a patient's behavior. These perceptions must be seen in the context of the frustration and fatigue that are commonly generated in institutions that do not always run smoothly. Staff need to be aware that their own emotions may make it difficult for them to make objective judgments about the patient's actual clinical status. Staff should also recognize that they are sometimes the source of a patient's agitation.
    If you had selected this option your score would be . . . .   +5

The patient is fully oriented, but perhaps a little testy. The physical examination disclosed no abnormality except for soft bruits over the carotid arteries, which may be accepted as not unusual in elderly patients and not warranting intervention in the absence of transient ischemic attacks or hypoperfusion of the central nervous system. Neither of those indications for further studies of the carotid arteries is developed in this patient.

With the information you now have, what further examinations would you regard as appropriate?

21. Computed tomography (CT scan) of head
    No basis has been laid for this examination in this patient. Computed tomography has become the preferred first measure for evaluation of the central nervous system in patients in whom some dysfunction is clearly indicated. If it had been done, the finding of mild cortical atrophy would be effectively noncontributory in this 82-year-old patient.
    If you had selected this option your score would be . . . .   −5

22. Examination of cerebrospinal fluid (CSF)
    No basis has been laid for this examination in this patient.
    If you had selected this option your score would be . . . .   −5

23. Carotid arteriography
    No basis has been laid for this examination in this patient. The finding of mild stenosis of the carotid arteries could have been anticipated and would warrant no further intervention in the absence of clinical difficulties.
    If you had selected this option your score would be . . . .   −5

24. Radionuclide brain scan
    No basis has been laid for this examination in this patient. A radionuclide brain scan should ordinarily be done on high suspicion of a lesion not adequately identified on a CT scan.
    If you had selected this option your score would be . . . .   −5

25. Study of CSF dynamics, using radioiodinated serum albumin
    There is no reason to feel that a study of CSF dynamics is indicated in this patient, whose sudden change in behavior is extremely unlikely to represent normal-pressure hydrocephalus.
    If you had selected this option your score would be . . . .   −5

A plan of management for dealing with an acute behavioral disturbance should be as responsive as possible to an understanding of the context in which this disturbance occurred, which includes the realities of the moment as well as the background, lifestyle, and emotional needs of the patient prior to any change in behavior. Some patients will respond to a more structured environment and greater opportunities for controlled activities; others will prefer to be allowed a high degree of flexibility and autonomy in the arrangement of their daily affairs. In this case, what we have learned of the patient suggests that she belongs in the latter category.

With the information you now have, which of the following would you include among your recommendations or orders?

26. Order a major tranquilizer (chlorpromazine)
    (See critique 28.)
    If you had selected this option your score would be ....   −5

27. Order a minor tranquilizer (diazepam)
    (See critique 28.)
    If you had selected this option your score would be ....   −5

28. Order a tricyclic antidepressant
    There is no indication that this patient needs drugs for the modification of behavior. She appears to be in full control of her faculties and probably will need nothing more than a sympathetic understanding and correction of the circumstances precipitating her irritation at what she regarded as an imposition.
    If you had selected this option your score would be ....   −5

29. Suggest behavior modification techniques for management of patient
    (See critique 30.)
    If you had selected this option your score would be ....   −5

30. Suggest that patient's privileges be restricted if an outburst occurs again
    No substantial basis has been laid for any form of psychotherapeutic or behavior modification interventions. Studies of behavior modification techniques suggest that positive reinforcement, in any case, is much to be preferred to punishment.
    If you had selected this option your score would be ....   −5

31. Request cardiovascular surgical consultation
    (See critique 33.)
    If you had selected this option your score would be ....   −3

32. Request psychiatric consultation
(See critique 33.)
If you had selected this option your score would be . . . .   **Score**

                                                                      0

33. Request neurosurgical consultation
Findings at this point do not warrant extensive consultations.
If you had selected this option your score would be . . . .   −3

34. Recommend socialization therapy
There is no indication that this patient will flourish with attempts
to bring her into more active interpersonal relations. She appears
to be a rather self-sufficient woman, preferring her own enter-
tainment and selective associations with others.
If you had selected this option your score would be . . . .   −5

35. Recommend greater involvement of patient in religious activities
The fact that the patient is described as having negligible religious activities does not in any sense indicate that she is not
a religious person; nor does it indicate that she is in need of
any more formal display of her religiosity. This area of her life
is one that can be left entirely to her own discretion except as
she may herself give indications of some need for help.
If you had selected this option your score would be . . . .   −3

36. Suggest gardening activity for patient
There can be no objection to the gentle offering of an opportunity to the patient to become more active in gardening activities, if that should prove of interest to her. Such activities can
be carried out alone or in the company of others, which will
produce results that may be in good accord with the patient's
pace.
If you had selected this option your score would be . . . .   +1

37. Remind patient that she must conform to daily schedule of the
institution in her daily activities
As indicated above, there seems hardly to be a need in the case
of this patient for a more structured daily schedule. The imposition of such a schedule on a patient with the problem described might only be regarded by her as further unwarranted
interference in her life.
If you had selected this option your score would be . . . .   −5

38. Suggest arts and crafts therapy
Opportunities for creative activity should be open to all persons
sharing an institutional environment. Their use can generally

be left to the discretion of the individual. In this case, it is **Score** appropriate to explore the patient's interest in such activities, but there is no need to urge her to become involved in activities that have not been of interest to her earlier in her life.

If you had selected this option your score would be . . . . +1

39. Recommend flexible daily program, within limits of institutional routines and resources

Clearly, a flexible program is likely to be accepted by a patient such as the one described, who will probably be most comfortable with the widest autonomy in choice of activities. On the other hand, the patient's activities ought to be within the same limits of routines and resources of the institution that govern the activities of others.

If you had selected this option your score would be . . . . +5

SUMMARY

A patient has been described in whom an acute change of behavior seemed to occur in response to an imposed change in routine, which angered her. It is pointed out that the evaluation of this kind of episode must integrate what is known about the baseline personality, interests, and resources of the patient prior to such an incident, the setting in which the change in behavior occurred, and the perceptions and feelings of those who are responsible for helping the patient to cope with her life circumstances.

In any case, it was clear that the problem was situational, with no need for diagnostic or psychiatric interventions, though some modest suggestions should be appropriately made to the staff and patient as to how the circumstances might be changed to avoid a recurrence.

BIBLIOGRAPHY

Busse, E. W., and Blazer, D. (Eds.) 1980: *Handbook of Geropsychiatry.* New York: Van Nostrand Reinhold Co.

Butler, R. N. 1975: *Why survive? Being Old in America.* New York: Harper & Row.

Dewald, P. A. 1964: *Psychotherapy: A Dynamic Approach.* New York: Basic Books, Inc.

Eaton, M. T. and Peterson, M. H. 1969: *Psychiatry, Medical Outline Series.* Flushing, New York: Medical Examination Publishing Co.

Freedman, A. M., Kaplan, H. I., and Sadock, B. J. 1972: *Modern Synopsis of Comprehensive Textbook of Psychiatry.* Baltimore; Williams & Wilkins Co.

Hollister, L. E. 1973: *Clinical Use of Psychotherapeutic Drugs.* Springfield: Charles C Thomas.

Klein, D. F., and Davis, J. M. 1969: *Diagnosis and Drug Treatment of Psychiatric Disorders.* Baltimore: Williams & Wilkins Co.

Levenson, A. J. 1980: *Basic Psychopharmacology for Health Professionals.* New York: Springer.

Levenson, A. J., and Tollett, S. M. 1980: Rapid psychiatric assessment of the geriatric patient for immediate psychiatric referral. *Geriatrics*, 35,133–120.

Levenson, A. J. (Ed.). 1979: *The Neuropsychiatric Side Effects of Drugs in the Elderly*. New York: Raven Press.

Levenson, A. J. (Ed). 1980: *Psychiatric Manifestations of Physical Illness in the Elderly*. New York: Raven Press.

Smith, W. L., and Kinsbourne, M. 1977: *Aging and Dementia*. New York: Spectrum Publications, Inc.

Verwoerdt, A. 1976: *Clinical Geropsychiatry*. Baltimore: Williams & Wilkins Co.

Wells, C. E. 1978: Editorial: Role of stroke in dementia. *Stroke: A Journal of Cerebral Circulation*, 9, 1–3.

Subject Index

Abdominal aortic aneurysm,
asymptomatic, 12
Accident liability, 109; *see also* Falls
ACTH, 78
Active incontinence, 120,121,123–
125
and changes in female tract,
124,125
and defective development of
continence, 123
and dementia and confusion, 123
neurogenic, 124–125
and obstruction, 123–124,125
Activities of daily living, in
assessment of cerebral function,
40–41
Activity limitations, 4,26
Acute anxiety, 135
Acute care, and public resources,
26,32
Acute diseases, 5,25
and fluid and electrolyte balance,
70,71
Acute organic brain syndrome, 142–
146,183
cogniactive drugs in, 220,221
and head trauma, 145
and hydrocephalus, 146
iatrogenic factors in, 142–143
and infections, 143
and neoplasia, 146
nutritional and metabolic factors
in, 143–145

and vascular problems, 146
Adaptability, reduction in, 51,56–
59,60
role of endocrine system in, 57–59
role of nervous system in, 56–57
Adipose tissue, increase in,
38,39,296
Adrenocortical diseases, 75–76
Affective disorders, 129–134; *see*
also Depression; Mania
Ageism, 18
Aging
biology of, 37–91
pace of, 9,37
variations in, 52–53
Aging theories, 43–50
genetic, 43,44–48,49
nongenetic, 48–49
Agitation, 435–446
Albumin levels, decrease in, 38
Alcohol
acute organic brain syndrome
caused by, 143
depression caused by, 133
and drug metabolism, 193
Alcoholism, 143
as atypical presentation of
depression, 131,133
Aldosterone antagonists, 210
Aldosterone deficiency, 71
Aldosterone release, 78
Allergic hypersensitivity drug
reactions, 143